Handbook of Cardiac Critical Care and Anaesthesia

This book provides clinical tips on the management of common emergencies that are regularly faced by critical care and acute care cardiologists in resource-limited settings. Based on the current guidelines, it explores the evaluation of the patient, followed by its treatment methodology. It highlights the beneficial effects of the use of cardiac drugs during an emergency. There is also a special section on preoperative evaluation and postoperative management of cardiac patients of different subsets. Medicolegal/documentation points are also discussed where relevant. It is useful as a ready reference for physicians, anaesthetists and cardiologists.

Key Features

- Reinforces practical aspects and recalls certain overlooked clinical points to address emergency situations in a busy, resource-limited setting

- Explains lucidly what the acute cardiac care/anaesthesia registrar or cardiology fellows ought to do in the intensive care and postoperative wards

- Emphasizes the importance of clinical acumen and observation

T0321239

Handbook of Cardiac Critical Care and Anaesthesia

Edited by
Sunandan Sikdar MD, DM, FACC
Department of Cardiology
Narayana Multispeciality Hospital
Kolkata, India

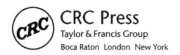

CRC Press
Taylor & Francis Group
Boca Raton London New York

CRC Press is an imprint of the
Taylor & Francis Group, an **informa** business

First edition published 2024
by CRC Press
6000 Broken Sound Parkway NW, Suite 300, Boca Raton, FL 33487-2742

and by CRC Press
4 Park Square, Milton Park, Abingdon, Oxon, OX14 4RN

CRC Press is an imprint of Taylor & Francis Group, LLC

© 2024 Taylor & Francis Group, LLC

ISBN: 9781032455174 (hbk)
ISBN: 9780367462215 (pbk)
ISBN: 9781003027584 (ebk)

DOI: 10.1201/9781003027584

Typeset in Palatino
by KnowledgeWorks Global Ltd.

Access the Support Material: www.routledge.com/9780367462215

Contents

Preface

With the explosive development of interventional cardiology, a change has occurred. We have more critical cases, a larger elderly population and more patients having comorbidities like kidney and lung disease. Intervention in this patient population is riskier, and the post-procedure course requires closer monitoring and deeper interdisciplinary knowledge for better outcomes. In fact, the more difficult or high stakes a procedure is, the more important post-procedure care becomes – as important as the procedure itself – to sail through choppy waters. Knowledge of medical or surgical intensive care strategies may help but may not be enough for cardiac care unit (CCU) needs. Thus, a text is required to bridge the gap between cardiology and intensive care. While I was figuring out an arterial blood gas (ABG) in cardiogenic shock for my resident, I realized that there is a dearth of texts in this field. But a voluminous text will not serve this purpose as the physicians busy in the CCU – residents, trainees, physicians with training in intensive care, cardiologists and anaesthetists – hardly have time. A handbook in the form of dialogue or in question-and-answer format delivers the necessary information to-the-point in a lively way. Just as in the bedside, personal perspectives reinforce education – this aspect has also been incorporated in the text, as are pitfalls, real cases and nightmares. The authors who have been selected for their wide experience in managing cardiac intensive care have been gracious enough to subscribe to this format. We hope this book will provide a much-needed guidance to the "CCU warriors" who toil day in and day out to ensure that critical cardiac patients live to see the light of the day.

Sunandan Sikdar
Kolkata

Acknowledgements

I am indebted to my co-authors, colleagues, editorial staff and family. Special thanks are due for the following close collaborators from Narayana Multispecialty Hospital, Jessore Road, who have helped and stood by me:

- Dr Swarup Paul from the Critical Care Medicine Department who was instrumental in sharing the writing of many chapters with me

- Dr Abhradip Das, Department of Respiratory Medicine

- Dr Apurba Panja, Department of Emergency Medicine

- Dr R.N. Karmakar, Dr A. Kar, Dr Partha Pratim Dey, Dr Sougata Sanyal and Dr G. Agarwal of the Department of Cardiology

- Dr Kowshik Paul and Dr Arunansu Dhole of the Cardiothoracic Department

- Dr Jitendra Ladhania and Dr Subhas Das of the Department of Anaesthesiology

- Dr Gautam Das from Radiology

- Dr Amit Dey, Dr T. Ash, Dr Vikas Maskara and Dr Bodhiswatta Biswas from the Department of Internal Medicine

- Above all, Dr Devi Shetty, Founder-Chairman, Narayana Health, whose care and compassion for the patients and healthcare professionals are exemplary and who has been the greatest source of inspiration to us all. Dr E. Rupert, Managing Director and Group CEO, Narayana Health, has been a source of great support as well.

Dr Jamal Yusuf, Dr Mohit Gupta, Dr Girish M.P., Dr S. Kurien, Dr Vimal Mehta and Dr Saibal Mukhopadhyay have enriched me with their teachings during my days of training in GB Pant Hospital. I have been blessed to have Dr Sanjay Tyagi and Dr Vijay Trehan of G.B. Pant Hospital and Dr J. Naik of RTIICS as my mentors. Dr Anjan Lal Dutta, Dr Debabrata Roy, Dr Mrinal Kanti Das, Dr Biswajit Majumder and Dr Dipankar Ghosh Dastidar from the Cardiological Society of India have provided me with constant encouragement. Special thanks are due to Dr Praloy Chakraborty and Dr Dilip Kumar.

Mr Subhasis Bhattacharya (Facility Director) and Dr Pinaki Banerjee (Medical Superintendent) supported me during preparation of the manuscript. I shall always remember the smiling faces of Shivangi Pramanik and Himani Dwivedi from the Taylor & Francis/CRC Press publishing house while they had to bear my corrections, alterations and overwordiness.

Special thanks are due to my family – my wife Papri, my son Debarghya, my sister Bharati and my parents, Ira and Sudarsan Sikdar and Chandrima and Amarendra Chaudhuri. They cheerfully accepted my absence while I was slogging out hour after hour with the book.

Editor

Dr Sunandan Sikdar MD, DM, FACC, is Attending Physician and Senior Interventional Cardiologist in Narayana Multispecialty Hospital. He graduated from Medical College, Kolkata. He subsequently did his post-graduation and residency in internal medicine in Maulana Azad Medical College, New Delhi. He majored in cardiology from the prestigious Govind Ballabh Hospital, New Delhi (2008). He received further training in the Department of Electrophysiology in Veterans General Hospital, Taipei, Taiwan. He has publications in multiple national and international journals and has been an invited faculty in multiple national and international conferences. He is an active member of the Cardiology Society of India, having been the Interim Secretary of its West Bengal branch. He is actively involved in the social sphere and is the Founder and President of Krishna Science Foundation, a non-profit organization involved in disseminating science and giving cardiopulmonary resuscitation training to the communities living in small villages and towns.

Contributors

Subramanian Anandraja MD, DM Fellowship in Electrophysiology
Heart Care Clinic, Puducherry and
    IGGGH and PGI
Puducherry, India

Dalim Kumar Baidya MD, EDIC
Department of Anesthesiology, Pain
    Medicine and Critical Care
All India Institute of Medical Sciences
New Delhi, India

Soumik Basu MD, DM
Department of Cardiology
Medica Superspecialty Hospital
Kolkata, India

Debabrata Bera MD, DM Fellowship in Electrophysiology
Department of Cardiac Electrophysiology
NH–Rabindranath Tagore International
    Institute of Cardiac Sciences
Kolkata, India

Praloy Chakraborty MD, DM
Department of Cardiac Electrophysiology
Toronto General Hospital and University
    Health Network
Toronto, Canada

Saujatya Chakraborty MD, DM, FSCAI
Department of Cardiology
Ruby General Hospital
Kolkata, India

Debika Chatterjee MD
Department of Non-Invasive Cardiology
NH–Rabindranath Tagore International
    Institute of Cardiac Sciences
Kolkata, India

Sumanta Chatterjee MD, DM
Department of Cardiology
AMRI Hospitals
Kolkata, India

Subhasis Roy Choudhury MD, DM
Department of Cardiology
AMRI Hospitals
Kolkata, India

Abhradip Das MD
Department of Pulmonology
Narayana Multispeciality Hospital
Kolkata, India

Munna Das MD, DM
Department of Cardiology
Narayana Superspecialty Hospital
Howrah, India

Dipankar Ghosh Dastidar MD, DM
Department of Cardiology
Burdwan Medical College
Burdwan, India

Arunansu Dhole MS, MCh
Department of Cardiothoracic
    Surgery
Narayana Multispeciality
    Hospital
Kolkata, India

Indranil Dutta MD
Department of Cardiology
NH–Rabindranath Tagore International
    Institute of Cardiac Sciences
Kolkata, India

Rakesh Garg MD, DNB, FICCM
Department of Anesthesiology,
    Critical Care, Pain and Palliative
    Medicine
All India Institute of Medical
    Sciences
New Delhi, India

Arijit Ghosh MD, DM
Department of Cardiology
AMRI Hospitals
Kolkata, India

Anunay Gupta MD, DM
Department of Cardiology
VMMC and Safdarjang Hospital
New Delhi, India

Arshad Jahangir MD
Aurora Center for Advanced Atrial
    Fibrillation Therapies
Aurora Cardiovascular and Thoracic
    Services
Aurora St. Luke's Medical Center
Advocate Aurora Health
Milwaukee, Wisconsin

Mrinal Kanti Das MD, DM, FACC
Department of Cardiology
B M Birla Heart Research Centre
Kolkata, India

Auriom Kar MD, DM
Department of Cardiology
Narayana Multispeciality
    Hospital
Kolkata, India

Rathindra Nath Karmakar MD, DM
Department of Cardiology
Narayana Multispeciality Hospital
Kolkata, India

Anup Khetan MD, DNB
Department of Cardiology
NH–Rabindranath Tagore International
    Institute of Cardiac Sciences
Kolkata, India

Umesh Kohli MD, DM
Department of Cardiology
Accord Superspeciality
    Hospital
Faridabad, India

Dilip Kumar MD, DM, FHRS
Department of Cardiology
Medica Superspecialty
    Hospital
Kolkata, India

Jitendra Ladhania MD
Department of Anesthesia
Narayana Multispeciality
    Hospital
Kolkata, India

Karan Madan MD, DM
Department of Pulmonary, Critical Care
    and Sleep Medicine
All India Institute of Medical
    Sciences
New Delhi, India

Biswajit Majumder MD, DM, FACC
Department of Cardiology
ICVS and R G Kar Medical College
    and Hospitals
Kolkata, India

Aman Makhija MD, DM, CCDS,
    Fellowship Electrophysiology
Department of Cardiology
Sir Ganga Ram Hospital
New Delhi, India

Amit Mittal MD, DM
Department of Cardiology
Indraprastha Apollo Hospitals
New Delhi, India

Saibal Mukhopadhyay MD, DM
Head of Department of Cardiology
Govind Ballabh Pant Post Graduate
    Institute of Cardiac Sciences
New Delhi, India

Madhav Krishna Kumar Nair MD
Toronto General Hospital and University
    Health Network
Toronto, Canada

Deepak Padmanabhan MD, DM,
    Fellowship in Electrophysiology
Department of Cardiac Electrophysiology
Sri Jaydeva Institute of Cardiac Sciences
Bengaluru, India

Saurabh Pahuja MD
Department of Pulmonary, Critical Care
    and Sleep Medicine
All India Institute of Medical Sciences
New Delhi, India

Arindam Pande MD, DM, FACC
Department of Cardiology
Medica Superspecialty Hospital
Kolkata, India

Neha Pangasa MD, DNB
Department of Anesthesiology, Pain
    Medicine and Critical Care
All India Institute of Medical Sciences
New Delhi, India

Anuradha Patel MD
Yashoda Superspecialty and Cancer Institute
Ghaziabad, India

Kowshik Paul MD, FNB
Department of Cardiac Anesthesia
Narayana Multispeciality Hospital
Kolkata, India

Swarup Paul MD (Anesthesia), FNB
    (Critical Care Medicine)
Department of Intensive Care
Narayana Multispeciality Hospital
Kolkata, India

Debabrata Roy MD, DM
Department of Cardiology
NH–Rabindranath Tagore International
    Institute of Cardiac Sciences
Kolkata, India

Rana Rathore Roy MD, DM
Department of Cardiology
Medica Superspecialty Hospital
Kolkata, India

Simarjot Singh Sarin MD, DM
Department of Cardiology
Patiala Heart Institute
Patiala, India

Biswarup Sarkar MD, DM, FSCAI
Department of Cardiology
ICVS Medical College and Hospital
Kolkata, India

Kaushik Sen MD, DM
Department of Endocrinology
Nil Ratan Sarkar Medical College
Kolkata, India

Devendra Kumar Shrimal MD, DM, FACC
Department of Cardiology
Narayana Multispecialty Hospital
Jaipur, India

Sunandan Sikdar MD, DM, FACC
Department of Cardiology
Narayana Multispeciality Hospital
Kolkata, India

List of Abbreviations

ACEI	Angiotensin Converting Enzyme Inhibitor
ACS	Acute Coronary Syndrome
ADHF	Acute Decompensated Heart Failure
AF	Atrial Fibrillation
AKI	Acute Kidney Injury
AP	Accessory Pathway
AR	Aortic Regurgitation
ARB	Angiotensin Receptor Blocker
ARVC	Arrhythmogenic Right Ventricular Cardiomyopathy
AS	Aortic Stenosis
ASD	Atrial Septal Defect
AVN	Atrio-Ventricular Node
AVNRT	Atrio-Ventricular Nodal Reentrant Tachycardia
AVR	Aortic Valve Replacement
AVRT	Atrio-Ventricular Reentrant Tachycardia
BB	Beta Blocker
BSA	Body Surface Area
CBG	Capillary Blood Glucose
CCP	Chronic Constrictive Pericarditis
CFA	Common Femoral Artery
CHB	Complete Heart Block
CHD	Congenital Heart Disease
CHF	Congestive Heart Failure
CIN	Contrast Induced Nephropathy
CKD	Chronic Kidney Disease
CO	Cardiac Output
COPD	Chronic Obstructive Pulmonary Disease
CPVT	Catecholaminergic Polymorphic Ventricular Tachycardia
CVA	Cerebrovascular Accident
CVP	Central Venous Pressure
DAD	Delayed After Depolarisation
DBP	Diastolic Blood Pressure
D-TGA	D-Transposition of Great Arteries
DORV	Double Outlet Left Ventricle
DT	Deceleration Time
EAD	Early After Depolarisation
EF	Ejection Fraction
EOL	End of Life
EOS	End of Service
ESC	European Society of Cardiology
HCM	Hypertrophic Cardiomyopathy
HCN	Hyperpolarisation Activated Cyclic Nucleotide gated Ion Channel
HF	Heart Failure
HIV	Human Immunodeficiency Virus
HME	Heat and Moisture Exchanger
HMOD	Hypertension Mediated Organ Damage
HOCM	Hypertrophic Obstructive Cardiomyopathy
HR	Heart Rate
HTN	Hypertension
ILD	Intertital Lung Disease
IVRT	Iso Volumetric Relaxation Time
LA	Left Atrium
LAA	Left Atrial Appendage
LAD	Left Anterior Descending Artery
LAFB	Left Anterior Fascicular Block
LAE	Left Atrial Enlargement
LAVI	Left Atrial Volume Index
LBBB	Left Bundle Branch Block
LCX	Left Circumflex Artery
LEAD	Lower Extremity Arterial Disease
LMCA	Left Main Coronary Artery
LPFB	Left Posterior Fascicular Block
LV	Left Ventricle
LVD	Left Ventricle Dysfunction
LVEF	Left Ventricle Ejection Fraction
LVH	Left Ventricular Hypertrophy
LVOT	Left Ventricular Outflow Tract
MAP	Mean Arterial Pressure
MAT	Multifocal Atrial tachycardia
MI	Myocardial Infarction
MINOCA	Myocardial Infarction with Non Obstructive Coronary Arteries
MR	Mitral Regurgitation
MS	Mitral Stenosis
MV	Mitral Valve
MVA	Mitral Valve Area
NASPE	North American Society of Pacing and Electrophysiology
PAEDP	Pulmonary Artery End Diastolic Pressure
PAH	Pulmonary Arterial Hypertension
PAM	Pulmonary Artery Mean Pressure
PAPI	Pulmonary Artery Pulsatility Index
PAPVC	Partial Anomalous Pulmonary Venous Connection
PASP	Pulmonary Artery Systolic Pressure
PCI	Percutaneous Coronary Intervention
PCV	Pressure Controlled Ventilation
PCWP	Pulmonary Capillary Wedge Pressure
PDA	Patent Ductus Arteriosus
PEA	Pulseless Electrical Activity
PJRT	Permanent Junctional Reciprocating Tachycardia
PM VSD	Perimembranous Ventricular Septal Defect
PR	Pulmonary Regurgitation
PS	Pulmonary Stenosis
PTMC	Percutaneous Transluminal Mitral Commisurotomy
PVR	Peripheral Vascular Resistance
RA	Right Atrium
RBBB	Right Bundle Branch Block
RCA	Right Coronary Artery
RCMP	Restrictive Cardiomyopathy
RFA	Radiofrequency Ablation
RRT	Recommended Replacement Time
RV	Right Ventricle
RVEDA	Right Ventricle End Diastolic Area
RVH	Right Ventricular Hypertrophy
RVOT	Right Ventricular Outflow tract
RWMA	Regional Wall Motion Abnormality
SBP	Systolic Blood Pressure
SFA	Superficial Femoral Artery
STEMI	ST elevation Myocardial Infarction
SVR	Systemic Vascular Resistance
SVT	Supraventricular Tachycardia
TAPSE	Tricuspid Annular Plane systolic excursion
TAPVC	Total Anomalous Pulmonary Venous Connection
TDI	Tissue Doppler Interrogation
TEE	Trans-Esophageal Echo
TGA	Transposition of Great Arteries

TIA	Transient Ischemic Attack	**Vp**	Velocity of Propagation (Echo) / Ventricular Pacing (Pacemaker)
TOF	Tetralogy of Fallot		
TR	Tricuspid Regurgitation	**VPC**	Ventricular Premature Contraction
TS	Tricuspid Stenosis	**VSD**	Ventricular Septal Defect
TTE	Transthoracic Echo	**VT**	Ventricular Tachycardia
TV	Tricuspid Valve	**WPW**	Wolf-Parkinson-White Syndrome
UFH	Unfractionated Heparin		

1 Evaluation in Acute Cardiac Care

Sunandan Sikdar and Biswajit Majumder

PERSPECTIVE

In the cardiac care unit (CCU) setting, often the vitals as given by the monitor screen take the place of the general physical exam, and chest X-ray and echocardiography take the place of cardiac palpation and auscultation. The pearls developed over more than a century and given in brief here may appear out of sync with the times. However, the following anecdote makes us painfully aware that even today, the physical examination cannot be discarded.

A 42-year-old female was admitted to the CCU with a troponin-positive acute coronary syndrome with left ventricular (LV) dysfunction. Her echocardiography showed regional hypokinesia, and she was taken for a coronary angiogram. However, the operators, who were radialists, were unable to cross the TIG catheter from the right and left arms (the pulse was palpable in all four limbs). On attempting the femoral route, the guidewire did not cross the aortic bifurcation. A check angiography from the femoral sheath showed an occluded infra-renal aorta. Only then was an auscultation done, revealing a murmur in the bilateral supraclavicular fossa and back. The patient turned out to be suffering from aortoarteritis with coronary involvement as determined by a multi-slice CT aortogram and coronary angiogram.

1. What is the New York Heart Association (NYHA) classification of cardiac disability?

The components of cardiac disability include fatigue, palpitation, dyspnoea and chest pain (**Table 1.1**). Usually dyspnoea and angina are graded. The NYHA classification is the most commonly used and has stood the test of time due to its simplicity.

Table 1.1: NYHA Classification of Cardiac Disability

Class	Description
I	Ordinary physical activity does not cause symptoms
II	Ordinary physical activity causes symptoms
III	Less than ordinary activity causes symptoms
IV	Symptoms even at rest

2. What are the causes of orthopnoea?

Orthopnoea, defined as dyspnoea in the supine posture that is relieved on sitting up, is commonly caused by:

a. Pulmonary edema

b. Chronic obstructive pulmonary disease (COPD) with exacerbation

c. Large ascites (constrictive pericarditis, cardiomyopathies)

d. Diaphragmatic palsy

3. What is platypnoea?

Platypnoea, or dyspnoea in the sitting position that is relieved by lying down, is rare and has been reported in hepatopulmonary syndrome, left atrial (LA) myxoma and ball-valve thrombus.

4. Where do you determine the character of the pulse?

While for the rate, the radial pulse suffices, the brachial and carotid pulses are better suited in terms of character (**Figure 1.1**). Pulse contours are seen in graphical (amplitude vs time) form on the monitor, and this can be used as a surrogate in some cases (**Figure 1.2**).

5. What are components of a normal pulse?

An initial percussion wave and a later tidal wave are its components. While the percussion wave is generated by ejection, the tidal wave is generated by wave reflection at branch points of the aortic vasculature.

DOI: 10.1201/9781003027584-1

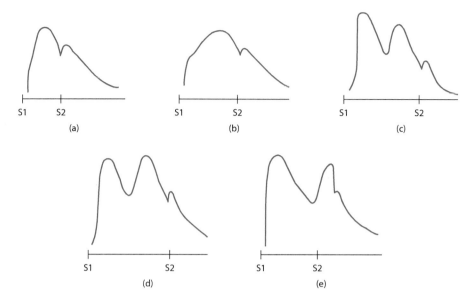

Figure 1.1 Carotid pulse: Characteristics in different conditions. (a) Normal. (b) Pulsus parvus – slow rising, delayed peaking of aortic stenosis. (c) Pulsus bisferiens of AR. (d) Pulsus bisferiens of HCM. (e) Pulse during IABP.

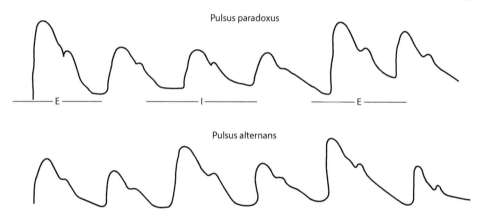

Figure 1.2 Monitors for observation: Pulse contours from plethysmography in the CCU. *Abbreviations:* E: Expiration, I: Inspiration.

6. What are the different types of pulses?

Table 1.2 summarizes the different types of pulses.

Table 1.2: Characteristics of Pulses and Their Clinical Significance

Name	Character	Associated Condition
Pulsus parvus and tardus	• Slow and late rising	Aortic stenosis
Brisk pulse	• Rapid rate of rise	MR, AR,VSD, HOCM
Water hammer pulse	• High volume collapsing	Severe AR, PDA
Pulsus bisferiens	• Double peaking	Severe AR, AS+AR HOCM
Pulsus alternans	• Periodic strong and feeble pulse • Determined by palpation and auscultatory BP • A sudden doubling of pulse occurs as cuff is deflated • Difference in SBP between strong and weak pulse >10 mmHg	LV dysfunction

(Continued)

Table 1.2 (*Continued*): Characteristics of Pulses and Their Clinical Significance

Name	Character	Associated Condition
Pulsus paradoxus	• Decrease in SBP on deep inspiration and increase during expiration. • A fall of 10 mmHg is significant, while in low BP of tamponade, a 5 mmHg drop is sufficient.	Cardiac tamponade Effusive constrictive pericarditis Rarely, constrictive pericarditis
Irregularly irregular	• No periodicity	AF, atrial flutter with variable block, MAT
Regularly irregular	• Periodicity in a pattern	Bigeminy, atrial flutter with 2:1 block

7. What are the causes of cardiac tamponade with absent pulsus paradoxus?

The mechanism of pulsus paradoxus is a stiff pericardium enclosing the cardiac chambers, so that the increased volume in one chamber prevents the inflow of blood to the opposite chamber due to increased intrapericardial pressure. Thus, during inspiration, increased right heart volumes lead to septal shift, decreased pulmonary flow into the left atrium, and left ventricular (LV) underfilling, leading to a reduced inspiratory stroke volume. Thus, in the following cases, paradoxus is not seen even in the presence of tamponade:

a. In aortic regurgitation (AR), as the LV is filled also from the aorta.

b. Atrial septal defect (ASD), as the right side can be decompressed.

c. If left ventricular end-diastolic pressure (LVEDP) is high.

8. What is an auscultatory gap?

The disappearance of Korotkoff sounds after their first appearance while deflating the cuff and their reappearance 10–20 mmHg later.

9. Which is closer to intra-arterial diastolic pressure?

The disappearance of Korotkoff sounds (Phase 5) is closer to intra-arterial pressure rather than muffling (Phase 4).

10. When shall pressure in muffling phase be recorded?

When the difference between Phases 4 and 5 is more than 10 mmHg, muffling should be recorded. In children, in severe AR, in anaemia and post-exercise, muffling is closer to intra-arterial diastolic pressure.

11. What is an adequate cuff?

The width of the cuff must be at least 40% of arm circumference. The cuff is the cloth that houses the bladder. The usual adult cuff bladder size is 12 cm × 16 cm. A smaller cuff may cause overestimation, and a larger cuff may underestimate blood pressure (BP).

12. How high should you inflate the cuff? How rapidly should you deflate the cuff?

It can be inflated 10–30 mmHg above the palpatory BP. It should be deflated at about 5 mmHg/sec.

13. In shock, the Korotkoff sounds are faint. How can they be made more audible?

Elevation of the arm immediately prior to measurement and clenching the fist 5–10 times after cuff inflation will augment the sounds of shock due to vasodilation.

14. What is the cause of the difference in BP between the two arms?

The dominant arm (right) usually has the higher BP, with the acceptable difference being <10 mmHg for systolic and <5 mmHg for diastolic BP. Significant differences may occur in:

a. Aortic dissection

b. Coarctation (usually the left arm has lower BP; however, if the subclavian arises below the lesion, as in arteria lusoria, the right arm may have lower BP)

c. Vascular diseases like atherosclerotic obstruction of the subclavian artery

d. Takayasu arteritis

e. Scalenus anticus syndrome (cervical rib compresses the subclavian)

f. Thoracic outlet obstruction by Pancoast tumour

g. Supravalvular aortic stenosis (AS) (due to the Coanda effect, the right arm has more flow and BP than the left arm)

h. Patent ductus arteriosus (PDA) (a large shunt may reduce left arm BP)

15. When and where do you measure lower limb BP?

In a patient with gangrene, lower limb ischaemic ulcer, discolouration suggestive of ischaemic aetiology and in diabetics, lower limb BP is measured. The measurement is carried out with a large cuff diagonally placed in the popliteal fossa, preferably with the bell of the stethoscope. The systolic BP is usually 20 mmHg or more in the lower limb compared to the upper limb. If it is lower than upper limb pressure, then there may be peripheral arterial disease, coarctation of the aorta, or aortoarteritis. BP can also be measured over the posterior tibia using the bell of the stethoscope. A pressure gradient >20 mmHg suggests a stenosis between the segments. A femoral artery systolic BP (SBP) >20 mmHg more than upper limb suggests presence of AR (Hill's sign).

16. What is radio-femoral delay?

Normally, radial and femoral pulses are simultaneously felt. In coarctation, in the femoral artery, the percussion wave is attenuated, and hence we feel the tidal wave only. The timing of the percussion wave in the radial artery is naturally earlier than the tidal wave in the femoral artery, leading to the sense of delay.

17. Why is the internal jugular preferred over the external jugular for measuring Venous Pressure?

a. The internal jugular is in direct continuation with the right atrium (RA) in systole and the RA and right ventricle (RV) in diastole.

b. In shock, the external jugulars are vasoconstricted.

c. The external jugulars have a smaller diameter.

18. What are the normal waves in a jugular venous pressure (JVP) trace?

The zero or baseline is the sternal angle. If the patient is supine, the upper limit of normal is 2 cm. At an angle of 45 degrees, the upper limit is 4.5 cm from the sternal angle. In order to get a silhouette, shine a torch by bending over from the opposite side to look at the upper level of pulsation.

A wave: Due to atrial contraction

X descent: Due to relaxation of RA

X' descent: Due to descent of the base during ventricular systole

V wave: Due to filling of RA passively

Y descent: Due to emptying of RA and relaxation and filling of RV

Normally in jugular pulsation, only the X descent is visible to the naked eye. The end of the X descent coincides with S2. If the descent does not coincide with S2, then it is probably a Y descent. The pulsation may be made more prominent by elevation of the legs while in the supine position and by breathing deeply.

19. What are the different abnormalities in jugular pulsation and their significance?

Abnormalities of jugular pulsation (**Figure 1.3**) are detailed in **Table 1.3**.

20. How can you make the JVP more visible?

By applying abdominal pressure (by pressing the right upper abdominal quadrant, on the liver), jugular pulsation may be increased. This is called the hepatojugular reflex (HJR).

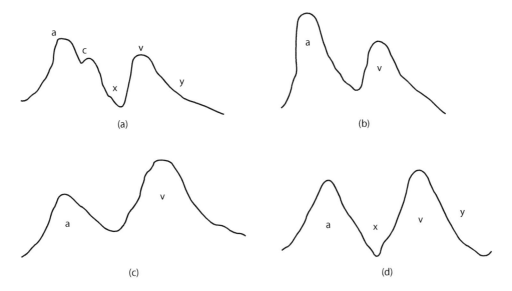

Figure 1.3 Jugular venous pulsation contours. (a) Normal JVP. (b) Tall A wave. (c) Tall V wave. (d) Prominent x and y descents.

Table 1.3: Abnormalities of JVP and Their Significance

Abnormality	Description	Causes
Canon waves	RA empties against closed tricuspid valve	CHB
Giant A wave	RA contraction against obstruction	TS, PAH, PS
Exaggerated X descent	Barely discernible	Cardiac tamponade
Exaggerated Y descent (Friedrich sign)	Perceptible on close observation	CCP, severe TR, RV failure, RCMP
Absent Y descent	Difficult to discern	Cardiac tamponade TS, RA myxoma
Prominent V wave	Due to increased filling of RA or decreased compliance of RV	• Severe TR, ASD, PAPVC • CCP, RV diastolic dysfunction
Kussmaul sign	JVP more prominent on deep inspiration	CCP

In congestive heart failure, due to direct transmission of pressure to the dilated RA, the top of the JVP pulsation rises. If the venous pressure rises by 3 cm and stays elevated for 15 sec, it defines a positive HJR.

In a normal heart, due to the constriction effect of the compression leading to underfilling of the RV, the JVP does not rise – this is called a negative HJR.

A positive HJR suggests an inability of the RV to accommodate any more venous return and is found in RV dysfunction in right ventricular myocardial infarction (RVMI) and also in restrictive cardiomyopathy (RCMP) and chronic constrictive pericarditis (CCP). It is not found in cardiac tamponade.

21. How do you measure JVP when it extends to the cranial vault?

In advanced heart failure (HF), the top of the venous pulsation extends beyond the neck. In the Gaertner technique, the upper limb extended upwards is used as the manometer. The vertical distance from the sternal angle to the height where the superficial veins collapse on the arm is the JVP in centimetres.

22. What is slow and fast oedema?

■ *Slow oedema*: Pitting disappears in 1 min – suggests heart failure.

■ *Fast oedema*: Pitting disappears in <40 sec – suggests hypoalbuminemia.

23. How much fluid accumulation is required before oedema occurs?

Accumulation of 4.5 litres of fluid is required.

24. Where is fluid seen in a bedridden patient?

The presacral area.

25. What are the different respiratory patterns?

A normal respiratory rate is about 12–16/min. However, most sources define tachypnoea as a respiratory rate >20/min. The respiratory rate is easily seen in a CCU multi-channel monitor. **Table 1.4** summarizes the respiratory patterns.

Table 1.4: Respiratory Patterns and Their Significance

Respiratory Pattern Description	Name	Cause
Rapid and shallow	—	Pulmonary oedema Pulmonary embolism Obstructive airway Pneumonia Anxiety
Deep and rapid	Kussmaul	Diabetic ketoacidosis
Snoring with episodic apnoea	—	Obstructive sleep apnoea
Hypopnea alternating with apnoea	Cheyne-Stokes	Advanced heart failure Sedation Uraemia CNS disease
Irregularly irregular (yet equal) breaths alternating with periods of apnoea	Biot	Damage to medulla oblongata
Completely irregular with increasing periods of apnoea	Ataxic	Medulla oblongata, severe damage
Occasional gasps	Agonal	Cardiac arrest/terminal CNS disease

26. What is cyanosis?

Bluish discolouration of the skin and mucous membrane due to increased amounts of reduced haemoglobin (>5 gm%) in capillary blood. Cyanosis manifests when SaO_2 <85%.

27. What is polycythaemia?

Increased red blood cell (RBC) mass above normal (males Hb >17 gm/dL, haematocrit >60%; females Hb >15 gm/dL, haematocrit >55%).

28. What is the difference between central and peripheral cyanosis?

Table 1.5 below sets out the difference.

Table 1.5: Difference between Central and Peripheral Cyanosis

Points	Central	Peripheral
Site	Skin and mucous membrane	Only skin
Mechanism	Low oxygen saturation	Sluggish flow causing increased oxygen extraction
Breathing 100% O_2	Cyanosis improves in lung disease but no effect on right-to-left shunt	No effect
Warming limb	No effect	Cyanosis improves
Clubbing and polycythaemia	Present	None
Periphery	Warm	Cold

29. What is an apex beat?

The apex beat is the heart striking the chest wall, usually the LV apex, but may also be the RV in conditions where the RV is hypertrophied. The apex beat is generated by two forces: Counterclockwise movement of the LV when observed from the apex and recoil force from LV ejection into the aorta during ventricular systole.

30. What position is best for palpation of the apex?

In a majority of children, the apex beat is palpable in a sitting position and leaning forward, but in older adults, the apex beat is palpable in the left lateral decubitus position. The latter position, though commonly used in practice, is inaccurate compared to the sitting position. Astute clinicians may palpate the apex both from the front and back. A palpable apex in an obese patient implies cardiomegaly.

31. What is the definition of normality of apical impulse?

The following aspects must be described:

a. *Location*: The normal apex is commonly described as being in the left fifth intercostal space in the midclavicular line. A more accurate way is to state that in a sitting position, the apical impulse is within 10 cm lateral from midline. A more lateral apex is an enlarged apex. A normal apex is not felt in more than one interspace during the same phase of respiration and not more than 3 cm (one and half fingers) in the side-to-side extent.

b. *Character*: (i) *LV apex vs RV apex*: The LV apex is localized, with medial retraction, while an RV apex is diffuse, with lateral retraction. Both medial and lateral retraction occurs in biventricular enlargement (e.g. large ventricular septal defect [VSD] with pulmonary arterial hypertension [PAH]). (ii) *Ill-sustained vs well-sustained apex*: A normal (and also ill-sustained/hyperdynamic) apex remains outward in systole and goes away before S2. A (well-) sustained apex is defined as an apex that remains outward during systole and goes away only after S2. An ill-sustained apical impulse occurs in LV volume overload (increased preload): VSD, PDA and moderate AR. A well-sustained apical impulse suggests LV pressure overload (increased afterload): Left ventricular hypertrophy (LVH) (hypertension, AS), LV aneurysm and LV dysfunction. As AR severity increases and LV dysfunction sets in, the ill-sustained apex becomes a well-sustained apex.

32. What is an atrial hump or A wave?

The forceful contraction of the LA during the last third of ventricular diastole causes expansion of the LV cavity, leading to the A wave felt at the apex. This is the palpable equivalent of S4 and is found in a hypertrophied and noncompliant ventricle.

33. What are the different areas of the hand that are used for palpation?

■ *Fingertips*: Small pulsation

■ *Distal palm*: Thrill

■ *Base of palm*: Parasternal lift

34. What is a mid-systolic dip?

The mid-systolic dip is an outward impulse just before the apical beat. It occurs in hypertrophic cardiomyopathy where three outward movements are palpable: A wave, mid-systolic dip and apical impulse (triple ripple).

35. When does the left parasternal impulse suggest right ventricular hypertrophy (RVH)?

The normal left parasternal impulse is a subtle inward movement. In RVH the outward impulse (felt with the base of the palm) occurs until the middle of systole. Causes include RV pressure overload states: Pulmonary stenosis and pulmonary hypertension. The parasternal lift caused by *RV volume overload* occurs in *early systole*, while the parasternal lift due to *left atrial enlargement in mitral regurgitation (MR)* occurs at *end systole*. A dilated pulmonary artery can be felt in the left second intercostal space, giving a clue to pulmonary hypertension.

36. What is the grading of parasternal lift?

Dressler's grading of parasternal lift:

I: Visible, not palpable

II: Palpable, obliterable

III: Palpable, not obliterable

37. What are the uses of the diaphragm and bell of the stethoscope?

The bell is designed to catch lower frequencies like S3 and S4 and also the diastolic murmurs of the mitral and tricuspid valves (where the pressure gradient is low). The diaphragm is better suited for higher frequencies.

Low frequency (25–125 Hz, bell): Diastolic murmur of mitral stenosis, S3, S4

Medium frequency (125-300 Hz, diaphragm): Systolic murmur of aortic stenosis, pulmonary stenosis

High frequency (>300 Hz): Regurgitant murmurs of aortic and mitral valves

38. What are the heart sounds and their interpretations?

The four heart sounds and their interpretation in health and disease is detailed in **Table 1.6**.

Table 1.6: Interpretation of Heart Sounds

Heart Sound	Character Observed	Interpretation
S1	Loud	MS, hyperdynamic state, tachycardia
	Soft	Immobile/calcified mitral valve, severe AR, MR, long PR, LV dysfunction
	Variable (caused by AV dissociation in some form)	AF, atrial flutter with variable block, CHB, VT with VA dissociation
Split S1	Wide M1–T1 (usually delayed T1)	RBBB, Ebstein anomaly and, rarely, ASD/TAPVC
	Reverse split S1 (T1–M1)	LBBB
S2	Loud	Pulmonary hypertension, systemic hypertension, dilated aorta
	Soft	AR
Single S2	Absent A2	Severe calcified AS, aortic atresia
	Absent P2	Severe PS, TOF, absent pulmonary valve, pulmonary atresia
	A2 overlaps with P2	Eisenmenger syndrome
A2–P2 split (normal split 30–60 msec and heard during inspiration but not during expiration)	Wide >60 msec (split even during expiration and standing)	*Early A2*: Severe MR, VSD *Late P2*: RBBB, severe PS, pulmonary embolism, RV failure, LV ectopic
	Wide fixed	Large ASD, RV failure
	Paradoxical/reversed P2–A2	*Late A2*: LBBB, severe hypertension, severe AS *Early P2*: Right-sided accessory pathway, TR
S3	Low-frequency thud, 100–200 msec after S2, best heard with a bell at apex in left lateral decubitus position	Heart failure, MR, VSD, PDA and hyperdynamic states like anaemia; S3 occurs at the transition between the first rapid filling phase and diastasis due to sudden tensing of the ventricle
S4	Low frequency, 70 msec after S2, best heard at apex with a bell; prominent after handgrip/squatting; disappears when the pressure on the stethoscope is increased or is moved away from the apex – different from split S1	• LV hypertrophy due to hypertension or AS/HCM; RVS4 in PS. • Presence of S4 implies severe AS. • S4 is the result of vibrations caused by forceful atrial contraction filling a stiff ventricle

39. What is the significance of a paradoxical split in aortic stenosis?

It implies the AS is severe and the valvular gradient is near 100 mmHg.

40. What is the hangout interval?

The point of pressure crossover between the ventricle and corresponding great artery at the end of ventricular systole corresponds to a diastolic notch or incisura. The time interval between the incisura and the actual valve closure is called the hangout time. It is about 30 msec for the aorta and 80 msec for the pulmonary artery.

41. What is the importance of the pulmonary hangout interval?

On deep inspiration, there is split in S2 in normal subjects. This A2–P2 gap is about 30–40 msec and is due to pulmonary hangout time increasing in deep inspiration due to reduced pulmonary resistance. As pulmonary hypertension sets in, pulmonary resistance rises and hangout time decreases, leading to a decreased A2–P2 gap and often a single S2.

42. How is a murmur described?

A murmur is described according to the following aspects:

a. Site of best audibility

b. Grade

c. *Timing*: Systolic, diastolic, continuous

d. *Frequency*: High, medium and low frequency

e. *Character*: Rumbling/blowing

f. Radiation

g. Dynamic auscultation

43. How do you grade a murmur?

Levine graded the murmurs thus:

- *Grade I*: Soft, difficult to hear
- *Grade II*: Soft but easily heard
- *Grade III*: Loud murmur, no thrill
- *Grade IV*: Loud murmur with thrill
- *Grade V*: Very loud murmur, heard with partially applied stethoscope
- *Grade VI*: Very loud murmur heard without stethoscope

A high gradient with relatively low flow produces blowing murmurs (e.g., MR), while a low gradient with varying flow produces rumbling murmurs (e.g., mitral stenosis [MS]). High gradient and high flow produce mixed frequencies (e.g. AS).

44. How do you differentiate between systolic murmur at the apex as that of AS and MR?

The difference is set out in **Table 1.7**.

Table 1.7: Difference between AS and MR Murmurs

Aortic Stenosis Murmur	Mitral Regurgitation Murmur
Mid- and late- systolic (crescendo decrescendo – diamond shape), the more severe the AS, the longer the murmur	Usually holosystolic
Medium frequency Selected high-frequency components may radiate to apex – Gallavardin phenomenon	High frequency
No axillary radiation, may radiate to carotids	Axillary radiation (anterior papillary muscle involvement), base radiation (posterior papillary muscle involvement)
Associated with ejection click if valve bicuspid	No ejection click
Associated with S4	Associated with S3

45. How do you clinically differentiate between the holosystolic murmur of acute MR and that from chronic severe MR?

The sicker acute MR patients need to be immediately differentiated from stable chronic MR (**Table 1.8**).

Table 1.8: Difference between Acute and Chronic Severe MR

Features	Acute MR	Chronic MR
Haemodynamics	Unstable, pulmonary oedema	Stable
S1	Soft	Normal
Diastolic sound	S4	S3

46. How do you a differentiate a holosystolic murmur + mid-diastolic murmur of mixed rheumatic MR + MS from pure MR?

The difference is set out in **Table 1.9**.

Table 1.9: Difference between MS + MR and Pure MR

Features	MR +MS	MR
Diastolic murmur	Presystolic component present	No presystolic component
Opening snap	Present	Absent
S3	Absent	Present

47. How do you determine the loudness of different sounds?

Normally, S1 is louder than S2 at the apex. At the apex only the A2 (but not P2) component of S2 is heard. Normally, A2 is louder than P2 in both left and right second intercostal spaces. A loud P2 is recognized by P2 being present at the apex and P2 louder than A2 at the base.

48. What is the only right-sided event that reduces on inspiration?

Ejection click of the pulmonary valve in pulmonary stenosis. This is because the raised diastolic pressure due to a thick and stiff RV causes the pulmonary valve to be almost half-open even before the systolic ejection starts. So during actual opening at systole onset, the excursion made by the leaflet is progressively smaller as the severity of stenosis increases.

49. What are the different types of additional sounds?

There are five additional sounds (**Table 1.10**).

Table 1.10: Additional Sounds and Their Characteristics

Feature	Ejection Click (EC)	Mid-systolic Click (MSC)	Opening Snap (OS)	Pericardial Knock (PK)	Tumour Plop (TP)
Where found	Bicuspid AS	MVP	MS, TS	CCP	LA myxoma
Timing	Early to mid-systole at start of ejection systolic murmur, 40–60 msec after S1	Mid to late systole at start of late systolic murmur, about >140 msec after S1	Diastole at onset of mid-diastolic murmur, 40–140 msec after S2	Diastole, 60–120 msec after S2	Varies in intensity and timing with posture change, but about 100 msec after S2
Where heard	Aortic area	Left parasternal	Apex, but radiates widely	Left parasternal	Apex
Frequency	High (160–180 Hz)	High	High (130–150 Hz)	Medium	Low

The timing of the sounds can be remembered as:
S1 - EC – MSC - A2 - P2 – OS – PK – TP - S4 - S3

50. How do you differentiate A2–P2 from A2–OS?

The difference is given in **Table 1.11**.

Table 1.11: Difference between A2–P2 and A2–OS

Feature	A2–P2	A2–OS
Best heard	Base	Apex
Inspiration	Increased A2–P2 gap	No effect
Standing	No effect	Increased A2–OS gap

51. What are the different diastolic murmurs?

The characteristics of diastolic murmurs are summarized in **Table 1.12**.

Table 1.12: Diastolic Murmurs and Their Characteristics

Feature	AR	MS	Austin Flint	Carey Coombs
Timing	Early diastolic	Mid-diastolic and presystolic	Mid-diastolic	Mid-diastolic
Location	• Right parasternal (valvular AR) • Left parasternal (root dilation AR)	Apex	Right parasternal	Right parasternal
Frequency	High	Low	High	High
Additional sound	S3	OS	S3	S3
S1	Soft	Loud	Soft	Soft

52. How do you recognize a valvular lesion by examination?

The typical auscultograms in different conditions are given in **Figure 1.4**. A comparison of physical examination findings in stenotic and regurgitant lesions is given in **Tables 1.13** and **1.14**.

Table 1.13: Comparing Stenotic Valvular Lesions

Feature	MS	TS	AS	PS
Pulse	Usually low volume	Usually low volume but raised JVP	Slow rising delayed peak	Low volume in severe PS
Palpation	Tapping apex	NS	Apex forceful, sustained	*LLSB*: Heaving
S1	Loud	NS	NS	NS
S2	Loud S2 indicate PAH	NS	Paradoxical split P2–A2 (late A2) or single S2 (absent A2)	Wide split S2 (A2–P2) due to delayed P2 Single S2 (soft/absent P2)
S3/S4	Absent		S4	S4
Murmur	• Mid-diastolic rumbling murmur with presystolic accentuation • Longer murmur, more severe MS	Crescendo-decrescendo presystolic murmur in sinus rhythm	Late peaking ejection systolic murmur with mixed frequencies	Late peaking ESM, may cross A2 as severity of PS increases
Additional sound	OS A2–OS <80 msec in severe MS	TV–OS	EC in bicuspid AS	• EC of pulmonary valve (softens on inspiration) • S1–EC interval shortens as severity increases and S1 may merge with EC

Table 1.14: Comparison of Physical Examination Findings in Regurgitant Lesions

	MR	TR	AR	PR
Pulse	NS	NS	High-volume collapsing pulse	NS
Palpation	Apex forceful ill-sustained	Parasternal lift	Apex forceful ill-sustained	Parasternal lift
S1	Soft	NS	soft	NS
S2	Wide split (A2–P2) due to early A2	Organic TR: S2 normal Functional TR: S2 loud	Single S2 (soft A2)	Single (Soft P2)
S3/S4	LVS3	RVS3	LVS3	RVS3
Murmur	Holosystolic blowing murmur; apical thrill in severe MR	*Organic TR (fourth ICS):* Early systolic medium pitch murmur *Functional TR (second ICS):* Pansystolic murmur	Early diastolic murmur, length of murmur correlates with severity	*Organic PR:* High-pitch diastolic decrescendo (Graham Steell) murmur starting at S2 *Functional PR:* Low-frequency, early to mid-diastolic murmur
Additional sound	NS	NS	NS	Pulmonary EC

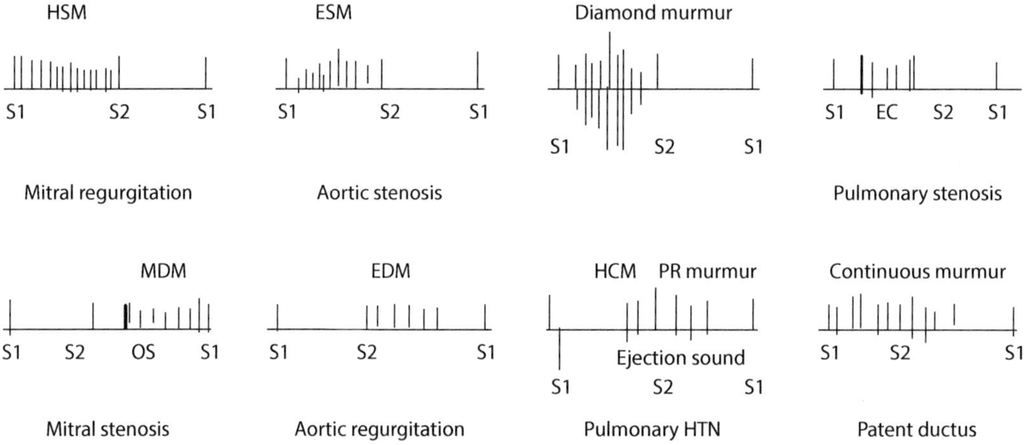

Figure 1.4 Typical auscultograms in common conditions.

53. How do you differentiate hyperkinetic Pulmonary Hypertension (PH) from obstructive PH?

Differentiating hyperkinetic PH, treated by device closure, from obstructive PH (largely untreatable) is important (**Table 1.15**).

Table 1.15: Differentiating Hyperkinetic from Obstructive PAH

Parameters	Hyperkinetic PH (Left-to-Right Shunts)	Obstructive PH (Eisenmenger's)
Cardiomegaly	Present	Absent
Parasternal lift	Early systole	Mid-systole (sustained)
Pulmonary ejection click	Absent	Present
A2–P2 split	*ASD*: A2–P2 wide fixed *VSD*: Wide variable split *PDA*: Paradoxical split	*ASD*: A2–P2 Split remains *VSD*: S2 Single *PDA*: Normal split
Flow murmur (LLSB)	Present	Absent
Shunt murmur (MDM at apex)	Present	Absent

54. How do you determine the significance of a left-to-right shunt on physical exam?

Significant left-to-right shunting is suggested by the following:

a. Cardiomegaly

b. *S2*: In ASD S2 is wide fixed split but is no help in determining the degree of shunt. In VSD a wide variable A2–P2 split implies a large defect, while a loud P2 implies PAH has set in. In PDA, paradoxical P2–A2 suggests a large shunt.

c. LVS3

d. *Shunt murmur*: Continuous murmur of PDA suggests medium size, while the presence of only a systolic component suggests developing PAH.

e. *Flow murmur*: Mid diastolic murmur (MDM) at apex in post-tricuspid (VSD/PDA) suggests large shunt.

55. What are the different causes of continuous murmur?

Meyer's classification:

A. *By rapid blood flow*: Venous hum, mammary soufflé

B. *High to low pressure shunts*:

   a. *Systemic to pulmonary*: PDA, aortopulmonary window, truncus arteriosus, tetralogy of Fallot (TOF) with pulmonary atresia with collaterals, Anomalous origin of Left Coronary Artery from Pulmonary Artery (ALCAPA)

   b. *Systemic to right heart*: Rupture of sinus of Valsalva (RSOV), coronary cameral fistula

   c. *Atrial shunt*: Lutembacher syndrome (ASD+MS), mitral atresia with ASD

   d. *Venovenous*: Anomalous pulmonary vein, portosystemic shunt

   e. Arteriovenous fistula

C. *Localized obstruction*: Coarctation, branch pulmonary artery stenosis

56. What are the different murmurs?

The locational significance of a murmur is given in **Table 1.16**.

Table 1.16: Location of Murmurs

Murmur	Apex	Parasternal	Aortic Area (Right Second ICS)	Pulmonary Area (Left Second ICS)
Holosystolic	MR	TR (High pressure)	—	—
Ejection/Mid-systolic	MVP		AS/HCM	PS
Late systolic	MVP			
Early diastolic		TS	AR	PR (High pressure)
Mid-diastolic	MS	—	—	PR
Late diastolic	MS	—	AR	
Systolodiastolic	MR+MS	TR+TS	AS+AR	PS+PR PDA

57. What are the effects of dynamic auscultation on different murmurs?

General principles of dynamic auscultation listed in **Table 1.17**:

a. Except hypertrophic obstructive cardiomyopathy (HOCM) and mitral valve prolapse (MVP), most murmurs decrease in length and intensity with Valsalva.

b. All murmurs of stenosis and regurgitation (MR and AR) and VSD increase with handgrip except HOCM and AS.

c. Most murmurs diminish on standing and increase on squatting except HOCM and MVP, which respond in the opposite way.

d. Arterial occlusion of the arm by bilateral cuff inflation 20 mmHg above systolic pressure augments the murmur of MR, VSD and AR.

Table 1.17: Response to Dynamic Auscultation of Different Murmurs

Manoeuvre	TR	PS	VSD	MR	AS	HOCM	AR	Remarks
Inspiration	I	I						Right-sided murmur increased
Expiration	D	D		I				Left-sided murmur increased
Leg elevation						D		Increased venous return, increased SVR
Standing	D	D	D	D	D	I	—	HCM and MVP murmur increased, all others decreased
Handgrip	—	—	I	I	D	D	I	Afterload increased

Note: I: Increased, D: Decreased.

58. What is the Sequential Organ Failure Assessment (SOFA) score?

In order to assess critically ill patients, various tools have been validated, among which the SOFA score is widely used (**Table 1.18**).

Table 1.18: SOFA Score

SOFA score	1	2	3	4
Respiration (PaO_2/FiO_2)	<400	<300	<200	<100
Coagulation (Platelet × $10^3/mm^3$)	<150	<100	<50	<20
Liver, bilirubin (mg/dL)	1.2–1.9	2–5.9	6–11.9	>12
Cardiac (MAP, mmHg)	<70	Dopamine <5 mcg/kg/min	Dopamine 5–15 mcg/kg/min or noradrenaline <0.1	Dopamine >15 mcg/kg/min or noradrenaline >0.1 mcg/kg/min
CNS (Glasgow CS)	>13	10–12	6–9	<6
Renal, creatinine (mg/dL)	1.2–1.9	2–3.4	3.5–4.9	>5

CONCLUSION

In a busy CCU, with a patient being monitored by numerous gadgets and being treated by various devices, a comprehensive physical examination is challenging and should be improvised according to the situation. This technique of improvisation comes only with the experience of working in a CCU.

FURTHER READING

1. Constant Jules. Essentials of Bedside Cardiology. 2003. Humana Press.
2. Abrams Jonathan. Essentials of Cardiac Physical Diagnosis. 1987. Lea and Feibger.

2 The ECG in Cardiac Critical Care and Anaesthesia

Sunandan Sikdar

**CLINICAL PEARL: WHY DOES THE ECG AT THE BEDSIDE MONITOR
LOOK DIFFERENT FROM THE 12-LEAD ECG I HAVE AT HAND?**

The answer is filtering. The diagnostic ECG should be recording with filtering at 0.05–100 Hz
(a frequency near the lower ranges gives a better picture of the low-frequency ST segment,
while those on higher side give a better resolution of high-frequency P and QRS segments).
The bedside monitor ECG may be filtering at 0.5–40Hz. Hence, bedside monitor and surface
ECGs may look subtly different from each other, especially with regard to the ST segment.
Filtering may reduce electrical noise that causes a fudgy baseline.

2.1 INTRODUCTION AND DEFINITION

The surface ECG is the summation of the electrical activity of the entire heart over a cardiac cycle
recorded between two electrodes. The three limb leads (I, II, and III) generate bipolar electrograms
(the potential difference between two electrodes), while the augmented limb leads (aVL, aVF, and
aVR) and six chest leads (V1–V6) generate unipolar electrograms (the potential difference between
the exploring electrode and an indifferent electrode, created by connecting the arm and leg electrodes through high-impedance resistors called Wilson's Central Terminal). However, currently all
leads are considered as being effectively bipolar. The ECG is basically a graph generated by the
changing transmembrane potential of the cardiac cells during depolarization and repolarization,
with time in its x-axis and voltage in its y-axis. The recorded voltage is not an absolute value, but the
voltage difference between two electrodes at a given instant. One electrode is designated as positive
and the other as negative (for example, in lead I, the left arm is positive), and the electrical vector
represented travels from negative to positive.

2.2 BASICS OF RECORDING

Before starting to interpret, it is important to ensure that the ECG is recording properly. Asking the
patient to hold their breath may reduce wandering of the baseline. Lead I (left arm and right arm), lead
II (left leg and right arm), and lead III (left arm and left leg) are the standard limb leads. The positive/
negative contribution can be easily recalled by remembering this simple rule – the left leg is always a
positive input while the right arm is always the negative input by convention. The three leads follow
the vectorial law: I + III = II. On the other hand, augmented leads use the exploring electrode (e.g., left
arm for aVL) as the positive input, while the two other limb leads serve as the negative input. There
is an increase in amplitude using this technique. Chest leads V1 and V2 use an exploring electrode
on the fourth intercostal place on the right side (V1) and left side (V2) and the Wilson terminal for the
negative pole. V4, V5, and V6 are placed on the left fifth intercostal space in the midclavicular line,
anterior axillary line, and midaxillary line, respectively. Lead V3 is placed midway between V2 and
V4. The potential of each precordial lead (positive input) is in reference to the Wilson central terminal
(WCT), which is the mean of the potential of the three limb leads (WCT = RA + LA + LL/3).

   The paper speed is usually 25 mm/sec and the amplitude is 1 mV = 10 mm. The graph paper on
which the ECG is recorded has 1-mm small boxes on the side, which represent the smallest unit.
Each smallest division in the horizontal axis represents 40 msec and on the vertical axis 0.1 mV. The
next larger division (five small square boxes) represent 200 msec on the horizontal axis. Usually, a
quick determination of heart rate can be obtained by dividing 300 by the number of larger squares
between two consecutive R waves. The different waves, segments, their normal values and clinical
significance are given next.

P wave (<120 msec): Represents atrial depolarization – right followed by left. Normally, the P wave is
   upright in lead II, inverted in lead aVR and biphasic in V1.

PR interval (onset of P to onset of Q or R: 120–200 msec): Represents the time required for the impulse
   to travel from the sinoatrial (SA) node to Purkinje fibres.

QRS (80–120 msec): The QRS represents ventricular depolarization (endocardium to epicardium).
   There are two vectors – the first vector is the result of *septal activation* from left to right as identified

DOI: 10.1201/9781003027584-2

by rV1/qV6. The second vector, SV1/RV6, represents subsequent simultaneous *free wall activation* of the left and right ventricle and depolarization of the terminal posterobasal segment of the left ventricle (this area is depolarized last).

ST segment: This segment is isoelectric and is the manifestation of the phase 2 ventricular action potential.

T wave: Corresponds to Phase 3 of the ventricular action potential. Repolarization from the epicardium to endocardium (opposite in direction to the depolarization wavefront, where the area depolarized last is repolarized first) creates concordancy with the QRS. The T wave may be negative in III and V1. In vectorial terms, the QRS-T angle is normally within 45 degrees (QRS and T in nearly the same direction). A discordant T wave (QRS and T opposite in polarity) may indicate ischaemia.

U wave: This is a small hump, <1 mm, concordant with the T wave. It is caused by Purkinje depolarization.

QT interval (onset of Q/R to end of T: <440 msec): Represents ventricular systole.

1. How does the heart rate of children compare with that of adults?

The normal heart rate range of children is higher than in adults, as shown in **Table 2.1**.

Table 2.1: Normal Heart Rate Range of Children

Age	Heart Rate Range (beats/min)
New-born to 1 year	100–180
4 years	70–130
12 years	60–120

2. What is the QRS axis?

The vector summation (direction plus magnitude) of the depolarization electric forces of the ventricles in space is the QRS axis. By convention, ECG leads record a positive deflection when a depolarizing wavefront approaches its positive pole. If the limb leads with their positive or negative poles are visualized as being situated on a dial of a clock where instead of time we have plus and minus 180 degrees (180 is a single point written as 180±, opposite to 0 degrees by convention) with four quadrants, then an axis can be determined. There are many pedantic ways to do this, but an approximate method suitable for the critical care setting is discussed in **Table 2.2**. Positive or negative QRS is determined by subtracting the S depth from R height. For example, if S is deeper than the height of R, then in that lead QRS is negative.

Table 2.2: Determining the QRS Axis

Terminology	QRS Axis	Morphology of QRS (Dominant Wave)	Causes
Normal	−30 to +100 degrees	Lead I, aVF both positive	Normal
Left axis	−30 to −90 degrees	Lead I positive, aVF negative	Normal, LAFB, old inferior wall MI, LBBB, LVH
Right axis	+90 to 180 degrees	Lead I negative aVF positive	Normal (children up to 1 month), LPFB, right ventricular pressure overload, lateral wall MI, left pneumothorax, dextrocardia
Extreme/Northwest axis	−90 to 180 degrees	Lead I, aVF all negative	Severe COPD

3. How do you know that the ECG is correctly recorded?

The following are usually seen in a normally recorded ECG:

1. In sinus rhythm, the P wave is positive in lead aVL.

2. There is a QRS progression from V1 to V6, though exceptions are common.

In an ECG with improper leads, though the sequence of P and QRS will remain the same, the morphology of the waves will change.

PRACTICAL TIPS: RECOGNIZING THE WRONGLY RECORDED ECG

A brief shortcut to the myriad mistakes in recording is as follows, compared to ECG with correctly placed leads (**Figure 2.1a**):

1. If P and QRS is negative in aVL and positive in aVR, then possibly the *right and left arm* electrodes are reversed (**Figure 2.1b**). In the presence of atrial fibrillation, a predominantly negative QRS in lead I but positive QRS in lead V6 suggests the same mistake.
2. Interchange of the *left arm* and *left leg* produces right axis deviation (**Figure 2.1c**).
3. If in *lead II*, P and QRS are isoelectric, then check if the *right arm and right leg* electrodes are wrongly interchanged (**Figure 2.1d**); if *lead III* is isoelectric, then the *left arm and right leg* may be wrongly connected. A perfectly isoelectric *single* lead means that rather than disconnection, the right leg and arm electrodes have been wrongly placed.
4. A pseudo-inferior infarct pattern may appear with aVF resembling aVR if the right arm and left leg are reversed.
5. Interchange of right and left legs may not change the ECG substantially.
6. Placing precordial leads one or two intercostal spaces upwards (V1 and V2 in the third or second intercostal spaces) may create an incomplete right bundle branch block (RBBB) pattern with inverted P and T waves.
7. If an individual precordial lead is placed wrongly, in the case of a normal ECG, the smooth progressive increase in the amplitude of the R wave and T wave from V1 to V6 is hampered for that particular lead. This clue may not be valid for disease states.

After the ECG is checked for any recording errors, check for artefacts:

1. Improper gain may create false low voltages.
2. A tremor may mimic atrial or ventricular fibrillation.

The ECG is now analysed for rhythm.

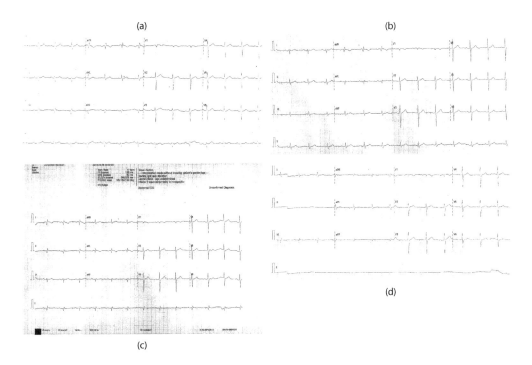

(a)   (b)   (c)   (d)

Figure 2.1 ECG with misplaced leads: (a) An elderly person with COPD, with correctly attached leads. (b) ECG with left and right arm electrodes interchanged – aVR looks like aVL and vice versa. (c) Left arm and left leg interchanged – there is apparent right axis deviation. (d) Right arm and right leg interchanged – lead II is isoelectric.

4. How do you approach bradyarrhythmias in critical care?

For bradycardia (ventricular rate <60/min), differentiating sinus bradycardia from atrioventricular (AV) block is paramount. The relation between P and QRS is the key. First-degree heart block (PR interval more than 200 msec) will cause symptoms if the PR is prolonged to the range of 300 msec.

5. How do you differentiate Mobitz Type 1 from Type 2 second-degree AV block?

Both have a 2:1 AV conduction. Gradual prolongation of the PR interval with sudden block of the P wave is characteristic of Mobitz type 1. If the P wave blocks suddenly without prolongation, it is Type 2 (infranodal block – usually requires pacing). Type 1 Mobitz can be discerned by grouped beating or a Wenckebach pattern of QRS complexes. A chance finding on the monitor showing atropine-induced worsening of the block will favour a diagnosis of a Mobitz Type 2 block. The case is similar with treadmill test–induced worsening of the block.

6. What is the tell-tale sign of "complete heart block" or AV dissociation?

The clue lies in demonstrating that one or more P waves fall in the ST segment of the QRS complexes. Often the sign is subtle, with slight distortion of the T wave hump with a relative periodicity (**Figure 2.2**). A wide QRS escape rhythm is more likely to be slower, unstable and lead to syncopal episodes than a narrow QRS escape rhythm.

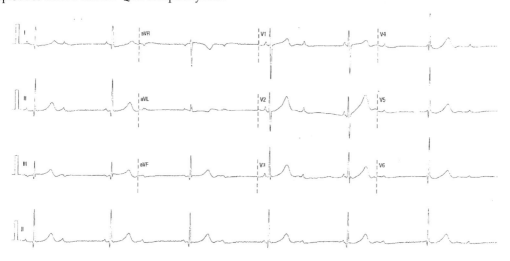

Figure 2.2 A 16-year-old boy with abdominal pain. There is no history of syncope. Although at first glance there are two P waves prior to each narrow QRS complex, a closer look suggests that the PR relation is not constant and there is AV dissociation. So, this bradycardia is due to congenital complete heart block with a narrow QRS escape.

7. How do you diagnose fascicular blocks?

Fascicular blocks can be diagnosed based on the features given in **Table 2.3**.

Table 2.3: Diagnosing Fascicular Blocks

Type	Criteria	Comment
RBBB	rSr' or rSR V1, QRS >120 msec Time to peak R V1 >50 msec	A similar pattern may occur in ASD, Brugada syndrome, WPW, and ARVC
LBBB	rSr' or R in I and V6, QS V1, no septal q in I, V6 QRS >120 msec Time to peak R V6 >60 msec	A similar pattern may occur in RV pacing (small spike), WPW, and anteroseptal MI
LAFB	Left axis, qR I, L	Resembles lateral wall MI
LPFB	Right axis, qR II, II, aVF	Resembles inferior wall MI
RBBB + LAFB	rSr' V1 + left axis	
RBBB + LPFB	rSr' V1 + right axis	

8. What are the criteria for chamber enlargement?

Echocardiogram is a better tool than ECG to determine chamber enlargement. ECG as a surrogate marker of a structural anomaly suffers from a lack of sensitivity but is more specific (**Table 2.4 a,b**). This is particularly true in the case of the atrium, as the structure is smaller, and the right ventricle, which is overwhelmed by the left.

Table 2.4a: ECG Criteria for Chamber Enlargement in Adults

Chamber	Criteria	Sensitivity	Specificity
Right atrium	P wave height in II >2.5 mm (P pulmonale) ++	< 20%	>90%
Left atrium	• P wave wide (>120 msec)	85%	35%
	• P notched with interhump interval >40 msec	–	–
	• *Morris index*: Biphasic P with terminal negative component >40 msec and V in depth duration	60%	90%
	• *Macrucz Index*: P duration/PR segment duration (end of P to onset of QRS) > 1.6 denotes enlargement	58%	–
Right ventricle	V1 R >7 mm	6%	98%
	V1 qR	5%	99%
Left ventricle	S V1 + R V5 >35 mm*	22%	100%
	R I + S III >25 mm	10%	100%
	R aVL >11 mm	11%	100%

++ Pseudo–P pulmonale: ECG change is present but echocardiogram shows normal-sized right atrium.

* This criteria from *Sokolow and Lyon* is best used in patients over 50 years of age. Another simple criteria (*Cornell*) for left ventricular hypertrophy is R aVL + S V3 >28 mm for men and 20 mm for women. The presence of secondary ST depression, often called "strain" in the literature gives, strong support of the presence of left ventricular hypertrophy (LVH).

9. How does the chamber enlargement criteria of children differ from adults?

The basic principle is same but the values are different (**Table 2.4b**).

Table 2.4b: ECG Criteria for Chamber Enlargement in Children

Chamber	Criteria for Hypertrophy	Causes/Comments
Right atrium	P height >3 mm	Ebstein anomaly
Left atrium	P duration >100 msec	Mitral stenosis/atresia, VSD, PDA
Right ventricle	• Tall R, qR in V1, V2 • Deep S in V5, V6 • T wave upright in V1 after 3 days to 6 years of age • Right axis	Pulmonary stenosis
Left ventricle	• Deep Q (>5 mm) V5, V6 • Tall T in V5, V6 • Left axis • Wide QRS-T angle (T wave and QRS of opposite direction)	• Aortic stenosis • Hypertrophic cardiomyopathy
Biventricular hypertrophy	Large equiphasic R and S wave in V2–V5 (Katz-Wachtel phenomenon)	Ventricular septal defect

---

PRACTICAL TIPS: WHAT ARE THE EXCEPTIONS TO THE ECG CRITERIA FOR LVH?

a. *In presence of a left anterior fascicular block (LAFB), limb lead criteria should not be used*, especially in I and aVL.
b. In cases of left bundle branch block (LBBB), the presence of left atrial enlargement, QRS duration >155 msec and precordial leads fulfilling LVH criteria may be acceptable but may not be accurate.
c. In RBBB, the S wave in the right precordial leads is diminished and so is the sensitivity of LVH criteria. The presence of left atrial enlargement, left axis deviation and R in V5–V6 >15 mm may be clues to LVH in this condition.

PRACTICAL TIPS: WHAT ARE THE PITFALLS IN DIAGNOSING RIGHT VENTRICULAR HYPERTROPHY (RVH)?

RVH cannot be attributed in:

a. *Posterior wall MI*: Tall R in V1. If R wave duration >40 msec and T wave is upright in V1, myocardial infarction (MI) is more likely rather than RVH
b. RBBB
c. RVH criteria becomes very insensitive in the presence of chronic obstructive pulmonary disease (COPD)

10. What are the changes in ischaemic heart disease?

Ischaemia affects repolarization, which is an energy-dependent process, and hence the ST segment and T waves are altered. During a significant part of the cardiac cycle, all the cells are in approximately the same potential and are electrically homogenous, and hence the ventricular TQ segment (representing diastole) is isoelectric. When depolarization occurs in a normal heart, different areas of the heart are activated at different times, causing inscription of a non-isoelectric QRS due to the heterogeneity of the electrical field (which causes a net electrical vector to develop). During depolarization in the presence of low perfusion, ischaemia causes abbreviation of the action potential duration in a specific arterial territory. Ischaemic areas have partially repolarized cells in systole, while in normal areas all cells have depolarized. Hence, a systolic voltage gradient develops between the extracellular positivity of repolarized ischaemic cells and extracellular negativity of normally depolarized myocardium. This creates an electric dipole pointing toward ischaemic cells leading to the well-known "ST elevation" phenomenon in the leads facing the vector (systolic current of injury theory). Subendocardial ischaemia occurs in acute coronary syndrome as these areas have high wall stress and oxygen requirements. Thus, V5 and V6, which "look" at the apex and lateral wall, show ST depression as the vector points away from these leads toward the ischaemic ventricular subendocardium. Occluded arteries during an ST segment elevated myocardial infarction (STEMI) cause transmural ischaemia. In these cases, the vector points towards the epicardium and thus towards V5 and V6 (in the case of left anterior descending artery [LAD] occlusion), causing at first a hyperacute T wave and then ST elevation in those leads. As necrosis progresses, the infarcted area acts as an electrical window, causing the leads facing them to record the activity of the opposite wall as a negative deflection (Q wave).

Classically it is described that ECG changes of ischaemia pass through three stages: *ischaemia* represented by T-wave inversion/tall T wave (repolarization abnormality), *injury* manifested as ST elevation or depression (repolarization abnormality) and *infarct* denoted by the Q wave (depolarization abnormality).

Subtotal occlusion – Deep T wave inversion in the leads facing the ischemic area (*Wellens* T wave)

Total occlusion – Early stage (minutes): Tall T wave

Hours: ST elevation

Late hours to days: Q wave

Normalization of ST

Days: T wave inversion

Reperfusion may cause the Q wave or ST or T wave to change prematurely. ST resolution by 50% or more is often taken as marker of successful reperfusion. Resolution of <30% of ST segment elevation is considered to be a sign of failure to perfuse the occluded artery. Early T wave inversion in leads with ST elevation is a good sign of reperfusion. Five to twenty-five percent Q wave post-infarction disappears over time.

The J point depression of 0.5 mm in V2 and V3 and 1 mm in all other leads is significant. ST segment elevation in inferior leads may be occasionally found in normal hearts, but ST depression in precordial leads is considered abnormal **Table 2.5a**.

Table 2.5a: ECG Thresholds for Labelling J Point Elevation as Abnormal

Lead	Age	Sex	Amplitude (mm)
V2, V3	<40 yr	Male	2.5
V2, V3	>40 yr	Male	2.0
V2, V3	All ages	Female	1. 5
All except V2, V3	All ages	Any	1
V3R, V4R	<30 yr	Male	1
V3R, V4R	>30 yr	Any	0.5

11. How can you localize the culprit artery in a STEMI situation?

Ischaemia usually occurs in coronary arterial segments, especially in STEMI. The ECG is handy in locating the site of arterial occlusion and thus predicting prognosis. For single-vessel disease, the localization is far more accurate than in triple-vessel disease. For example, in a case of a chronically occluded proximal LAD being well supplied with collaterals from the right coronary artery (RCA), acute RCA occlusion may give an ECG pattern of anteroseptal ischaemia. Difficulty in localization may also occur if there is natural variations like a very large diagonal branch. Here an occlusion at the diagonal ostium may create an anteroseptal infarct pattern, even though the LAD is free of disease. An anomalous artery like a single coronary artery, previous bypass surgery and rotations of the heart may alter the standard ECG features of localization. Keeping all these limitations in mind, one must approach the STEMI ECG looking at ST elevations and depressions, as shown in **Table 2.5b**, to locate the site of occlusion (**Figures 2.3** and **2.4**).

CLINICAL PEARLS: HOW DO YOU DIAGNOSE STEMI IN THE PRESENCE OF LBBB?

Diagnosing an acute anterior wall MI in the presence of LBBB may be difficult. *Sgarbossa* criteria can be used to judge the possibility that this diagnosis is true:

1. ST segment elevation >1 mm and concordant with QRS (highest predictive value) – 5 points
2. ST segment depression >1 mm in V1, V2, and V3 – 3 points
3. ST segment elevation >5 mm and discordant with QRS – 2 points

The algorithm diagnoses acute MI in the presence of LBBB if the score is 3 or more with a sensitivity of 78% and specificity of 90%.

For old MI in presence of LBBB, the following may be helpful:

a. *Cabrera's sign*: Notching of 0.05 sec duration in the ascending limb of the S wave in V3–V4, provided the patient is in sinus rhythm with a normal PR interval. There should be a clear shelf or visible downslope of the notch in Cabrera; otherwise, it may be a false Cabrera.
b. Q in I, aVL, V6 (normally LBBB should not have Q in these leads) and sharp R in V1.

PRACTICAL TIPS: HOW DO YOU DIAGNOSE MI IN THE PRESENCE OF PERMANENT PACING?

Permanent pacing from the right ventricular (RV) apex causes an LBBB-like pattern. The caveat is that a non-apical RV lead may cause the appearance of a Q wave in I or aVL even without ischaemia or its sequelae.

For acute MI, the Sgarbossa criteria is valid, especially >5 mm elevation of precordial leads, which should be of new onset.

For an old MI diagnosis in the presence of RV pacing, it may be challenging but *Kochiadakis* has given a number of features which may be useful: (a) The Cabrera sign described earlier; (b) *Chapman sign*: Notch on the upstroke of the R wave on leads I, aVL and V6; (c) Q waves >0.03 sec in leads I, aVL and V6; (d) Q wave in leads II, III and aVF; and (e) Notch in the first 0.04 sec of the QRS in inferior leads.

Table 2.5b: ECG Criteria for Culprit Artery Localization in STEMI

Territory	ST Elevation	Special Features
Proximal LAD	V1–V5	ST elevation in aVR, RBBB ST depression in inferior leads
Mid-LAD before diagonal	V1–V5, I, aVL	ST depression III, F
Mid-LAD after diagonal	V1–V5, III, aVF	ST depression I, L
Distal LAD	V1–V5, II, III, aVF ST elevation V1 < V3	ST depression I, L
LCX	II, III, F, I, aVL	Elevation II > III, T inversion V4R
RCA proximal before RV branch	II, III, aVF, V4R V1–V3 with ST elevation V1 > V3	• Elevation III > II, ST depression aVL, I • T wave is positive in V4R • Usually, AV blocks
RCA distal to RV branch	II, III, aVF	T wave is isoelectric in V4R AV block may occur
LMCA/triple vessel disease	aVR	ST depression >1 mm in eight or more leads

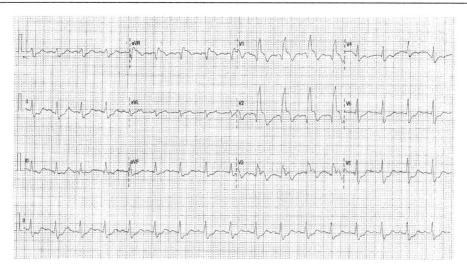

Figure 2.3 Anterior wall STEMI ST elevation in V1–V3 with a Q wave in the same leads. There is an RBBB pattern, ST elevation in aVR and reciprocal ST depression in the inferior and lateral leads. The culprit coronary lesion is localized to the proximal LAD.

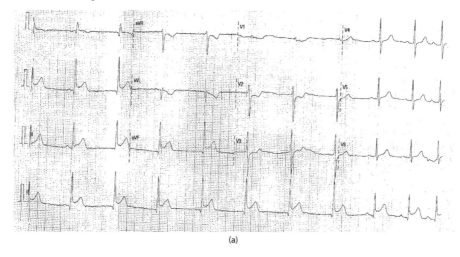

(a)

Figure 2.4   (a) Inferior wall STEMI. ST elevation in II, II and aVF with reciprocal ST depression in I, aVL, V1 and V2.

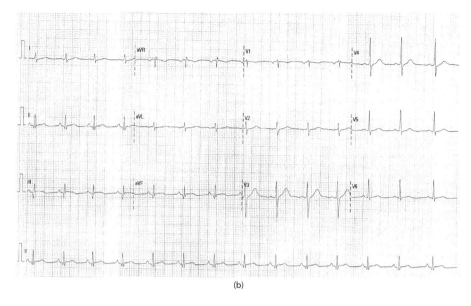

(b)

Figure 2.4 (Continued) (b) Same patient post-primary PCI to RCA. Note the resolution of ST segment >50%, which is a marker of successful reperfusion.

12. What is a pathologic Q wave?

A Q wave with duration >40 msec (one small square) or depth >25% of the height of the corresponding R wave. However, all "pathologic" Q waves may not be pathologic, and all Q waves do not represent an infarct. *Septal or positional Q waves may disappear on deep inspiration.* Q waves are present in inferior leads in more than 50% of normal hearts.

13. What is the non-ischaemic differential diagnosis of different ischaemic patterns?

Each ischaemic pattern has its non-ischaemic differential, which needs to be remembered in every clinical setting (**Table 2.5c**).

Table 2.5c: Non-Ischaemic Causes of Ischaemic Patterns

Pattern	Common Differential	Uncommon Differential
ST elevation	• Athletes • Early repolarization • Pericarditis • Hyperkalaemia • Hypothermia • LBBB/LVH • Myocarditis	• Brugada syndrome • ARVC • Left pneumothorax • Pulmonary embolism • Class IC antiarrhythmic drug • Post-DC cardioversion
ST depression	• Sympathetic overactivity/ tachycardia • Secondary to LVH • WPW • Hypokalaemia • Digitalis	• Mitral valve prolapse • Takotsubo cardiomyopathy
T wave inversion (**Figure 2.5**)	• LVH • CVA • Apical HCM • Memory T waves after pacing	• Global T-wave inversion • Athletes
Q wave	• Normal variant septal Q • WPW (Septal APs) • Left Pneumothorax • Hypertrophy Cardiomyopathy • LVH	• aVL in vertical heart • III in dextrorotated heart • LBBB • Infiltrative disease like amyloidosis, sarcoidosis

Table 2.5c (*Continued*): Non-Ischaemic Causes of Ischaemic Patterns

Pattern	Common Differential	Uncommon Differential
Tall R, V1, V2 (Posterior wall MI)*	• Misplacement of leads • Dextroversion of heart • RVH • HCM • WPW (Left free wall AP)	Duchenne dystrophy

* The pattern referred to as posterior wall MI has been demonstrated to be caused by lateral wall ischemic changes (**Figure 2.6**).

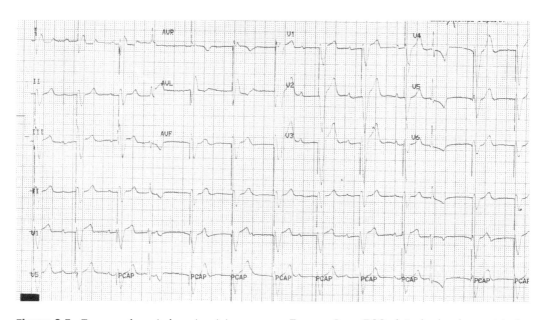

Figure 2.5 T waves of non-ischaemic origin – memory T waves. In an ECG of single-chamber ventricular pacing, the fourth and eleventh beats are native complexes. They have an inverted T wave caused by preceding paced complexes.

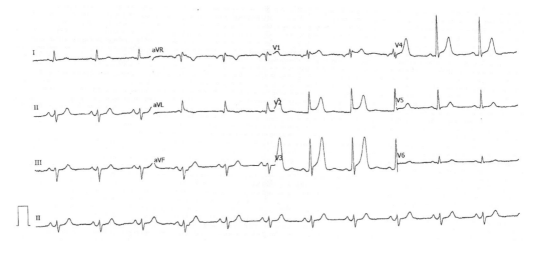

Figure 2.6 Evolved posterior wall MI. Lack of R wave in aVF. There is also an R in V2 and V3 along with a tall T wave. Reversing the ECG paper (upside down) and holding against the light will show a deep Q with T-wave inversion in the mentioned leads.

14. What is the classic ECG of early repolarization?

There is ST elevation with J point elevation in anterior leads V2–V6 (or sometimes in inferior leads II, III and F) with upright T waves. It is found in 50% of athletes (and may be related to increased vagal tone). A common mistake in critical care is to thrombolyse these cases. Previously thought to be innocuous, early repolarization syndrome (ERS), especially the inferolateral variety, may be related to sudden cardiac death due to idiopathic ventricular fibrillation (VF), though the actual risk is very low.

15. How do you define T-wave inversion?

The criteria for T-wave inversion are given in **Table 2.5d**.

Table 2.5d: T-Wave Descriptors: Electrodes I, II, aVL and V2–V6

Terminology	Threshold
Inverted	–1 to 5 mm
Deep negative	–5 to 10 mm
Giant negative T wave	–10 or more negative
Low-amplitude T wave	<10% R-wave amplitude
Flat T wave	–1 to +1 mm

16. What are the ECG changes with respect to right-sided heart pathophysiology?

Often right-sided pathophysiology is the cause of a patient's symptoms. Because the lead V1 overlies the RV, the changes are often more evident in these leads. The RV forces are usually overwhelmed by the left ventricle in a normal heart, but in cases of RV strain, the reverse may be true and may be the cause of poor R-wave progression. Similarly, in a diseased RV, there is increased scar tissue, which causes conduction disturbances leading to RBBB.

Table 2.6: ECG Patterns in Right Ventricular Pathophysiology

Condition	ECG Pattern	Comment
Pulmonary embolism/acute cor pulmonale (**Figure 2.7**)	• Sinus tachycardia • T-wave inversion in precordial leads • Right axis deviation • S in lead I, Q in lead III, T in lead III	S1Q3T3 is uncommon (10%) but a specific sign
Chronic cor pulmonale (lung disease)	• Poor R-wave progression (small r in precordial leads) • Low voltage in limb leads • Right axis deviation	Downward displacement of diaphragm and heart
Right ventricular pressure overload/pulmonary hypertension	• qR in V1 • Right axis deviation • R > S V1 • ST depression/T inversion V1–V4 • Deep S wave V5 and V6	Often seen in pulmonary stenosis or hypertension when right ventricle is working at near systemic pressure
Arrhythmogenic right ventricular cardiomyopathy	• RBBB • Epsilon wave • T-wave inversion in V1–V4	Epsilon wave is an extra hump in the terminal segment of RBBB

17. What are the ECG features of electrolyte abnormalities?

Electrolyte abnormalities are common in critical care setup and often are important in rapidly deciding the course and management of a particular patient. Serum potassium and calcium are the electrolytes most affecting the ECG (**Table 2.7**).

CLINICAL PEARLS: HOW DO YOU DIAGNOSE A TALL T WAVE AND ITS CAUSE?

T waves taller than the corresponding QRS complex can be considered tall. There are two common differentials – hyperkalaemia and ischaemia (earliest phase of STEMI). Hyperkalaemia-related T waves are peaked, pointed and symmetrically limbed with a narrow base (**Figure 2.8**). Ischemic T waves are asymmetric and have a gradually sloped ascending limb and rapid downslope. Picking up a tall T wave is important in critical care, as treating it at this early stage leads to excellent results in both hyperkalaemia and ischaemia.

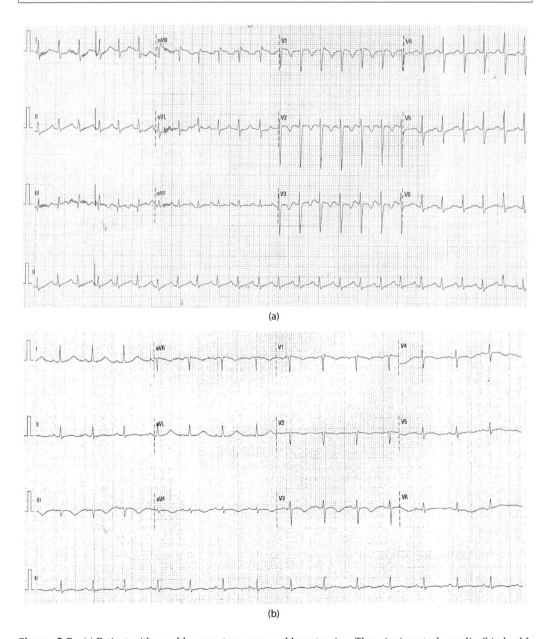

(a)

(b)

Figure 2.7 (a) Patient with a sudden-onset syncope and hypotension. There is sinus tachycardia, S in lead I, Q in lead III and a T wave in lead III and T-wave inversion in the anterior precordial leads. There was right ventricular dilation and dysfunction on echocardiogram, and contrast CT pulmonary angiogram showed occlusive thrombus in the left main pulmonary artery. (b) The same patient as in Figure 2.5a. Note the resolution of the S wave in lead I and aVL after thrombolysis with rtPA (unpublished observation).

Table 2.7: ECG Abnormalities in Dyselectrolytaemias

Electrolyte	Serum Level	ECG Feature
Hyperkalaemia	K 5–6 mEqv/L	Tall T wave, short QT (**Figure 2.8**)
	K 6–7 mEqv/L	Sinus bradycardia, diminution of P wave, AV block, QRS wide
	K >7 mEqv/L	ST elevation V1–V2, sinoventricular rhythm, asystole
Hypokalaemia	K <3.5 mEqv/L	• ST depression • QT prolongation, U wave >1 mm • Atrial and ventricular ectopics/arrythmia • AV dissociation
Hypercalcaemia	Serum calcium >13 mg/L	Short QT, ST elevation, prolongation of PR leading to AV conduction block (>15 mg/dL), Widening of QRS
Hypocalcaemia	Serum calcium <8 mg/L	Long QT due to prolongation of ST segment with normal T-wave duration (specific for hypocalcaemia)

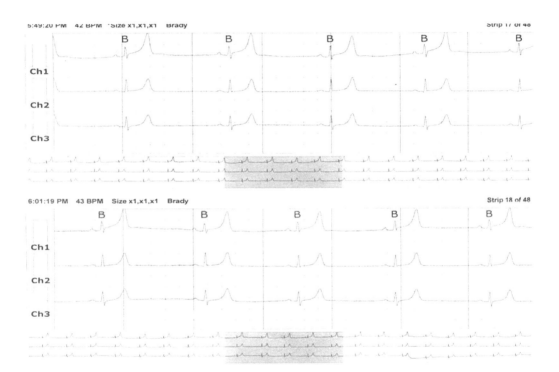

Figure 2.8 This Holter tracing from a chronic kidney disease patient showed sinus bradycardia with tall T waves and T waves taller than the preceding QRS complex, which is classic for hyperkalaemia.

18. What is a normal U wave?

The U wave is a hump that follows the T wave and is 25% or less of its height. The height of a pathologic U wave is often equal to or more than the T wave. U waves are characterized by their presence in hypokalaemia frequently larger than the preceding T wave so that the T (U) wave looks bifid.

19. Can an ECG help in diagnosing drug use/poisoning?

Interesting ECG patterns can often guide an astute clinician to narrow the differential (**Table 2.8**), though they are rarely specific (e.g. bidirectional ventricular tachycardia [VT] in aconite or digoxin toxicity).

Drugs acting on the fast sodium channel cause phase 0 of the upstroke of the ventricular muscle and the conduction system action potential to become delayed. This membrane event is translated to widening of the QRS complex on the surface ECG. Apart from class IA and C antiarrhythmic drugs, carbamazepine and chloroquine can create this toxicity. Sodium channel blockers frequently have anticholinergic effects and thus cause sinus tachycardia in the early stages. Thus, bradycardia in this situation means the toxicity is very advanced. On the other hand, drugs acting on the potassium channel delay Phases 2 and 3 of the action potential, and this manifests on the ECG as prolongation of the QT interval. Digoxin, which inhibits sodium potassium ATPase, acts on Phase 4 of the action potential and causes sodium overload. This cellular overload of sodium leads to Na-Ca exchanger hyperactivity, leading to calcium overload. Oleander causes the same class of effects.

Table 2.8. ECG in Drug Overdose and Poisoning

Substance/Drug	Feature	Comments
Tricyclic antidepressant	• QRS prolongation • QT prolongation • Rightward shift of terminal 40 msec of frontal plane QRS axis – manifests as prominent terminal R (>3 mm) wave in aVR, S in I, aVL	• Class IA antiarrhythmic drug effect • Right-sided conduction system preferentially affected
Aconite (**Figure 2.9**)	Bidirectional VT	Starts with VPC, may be found with homeopathic medicine
Digoxin/oleander	• ST depression • AV block • Shortened QT • VPC • Paroxysmal atrial tachycardia with variable block is specific sign • Bidirectional VT	• Scooped appearance of ST segment is characteristic • Hypokalaemia exacerbates toxicity • Digoxin-specific Fab treatment of choice • Pacing may cause arrhythmia
Theophylline	Multifocal atrial tachycardia	Often in COPD substrate
Cocaine	Ischemia, ST elevation QRS widening, sinus tachycardia, VPC	Coronary spasm may occur, is also a sodium channel blocker and sympathomimetic
Beta-blocker	• Bradycardia, PR prolongation • Propranolol causes QRS prolongation (Na channel effect)	• Always check drug history in sinus bradycardia • Atropine and glucagon are the antidote • Propranolol overdose has a higher mortality
Calcium channel blocker	Sinus bradycardia, AV block, asystole	• Hyperglycaemia may occur • Calcium gluconate injection is the antidote.
Flecainide	• QRS widening, prolonged QT (use dependence – more widening at faster heart rates mimicking wide QRS tachycardia)	• Often given in rhythm control of AF • May convert fibrillation to flutter, causing high ventricular rates
Sotalol	Bradycardia, prolonged QT, U wave – Reverse use dependence	Torsades may occur
Amiodarone	Prolonged QT, U wave (Reverse use dependence – more prolongation of QT at slower rate)	Torsades usually does not occur. QT prolongation may take 2 months or more (oral route)
Lithium	T-wave flattening/inversion Sinus node dysfunction	May take 2 weeks to recover.
Adrenaline	Transient ST elevation	Mimics ischemia
Noradrenaline	T-wave inversion	Change usually subsides

PRACTICAL TIPS: HOW DO YOU MEASURE THE QT INTERVAL?

This is best measured in leads with a visible Q wave or depolarization onset and T-wave termination (crossing the isoelectric line) in leads II, V5 and V6. The T wave may be indistinct, and the U wave may be superposed and inseparable – in such cases the interval begins at the onset of Q or R and is terminated by the point representing the intersection of a tangent to the maximum descending slope of the T wave and the baseline (x-axis or TP segment). By convention, the longest value is used, and usually three to five cardiac cycles must be used to derive these values. Leads V2–V3 often have the longest QT. However, if they differ from other leads by >40 msec, other leads should be used. Leads aVR and aVL do not have U waves, and these leads can be used in special cases. The QT interval should be measured in heart rates near 60 beats/min. Hence, for high and low heart rates, a correction must be applied. Among the many formulae for correction, Bazett's is the oldest (1920) and most widely used. However, it overcorrects at slow heart rates and undercorrects at fast heart rates. For drug-induced QT prolongation, the Hodges formula has been found to be generally acceptable. Ventricular pacing (as seen in bundle branch blocks) prolong the QT by prolonging the QRS duration, and in this situation the Framingham formula may be more useful.

- QT (Bazett) = $QT/\sqrt{R-R}$ (all intervals in seconds)
- QT (Hodges) = QT + 1.75 (heart rate – 60)
- QT (Framingham) = QT + 154 (1 – 60/heart rate)

The normal QT interval is <440 msec (children 1–15 years), <430 msec (adult men) and <450 msec (adult women). Recommendations to consider a QT >460 msec in females and 450 msec in men were made by the American Heart Association (AHA) in 2009.

Drugs prolonging the QT interval often precipitate torsades. This aspect is dealt with in a later chapter on channelopathies. The specific ST-T characteristic of long QT syndrome 1, 2 and 3 – the three most common types – are detailed in **Table 2.9**.

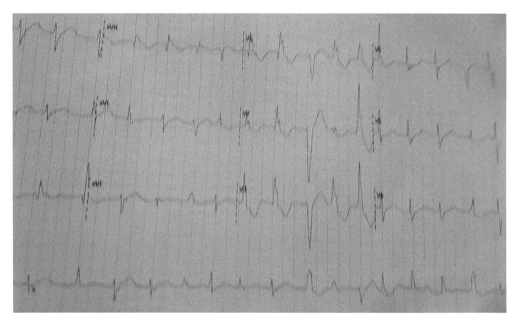

Figure 2.9 A young woman presented with recurrent syncope and had a cardiac arrest in the emergency room. The ECG shows an absence of P waves and VPCs of varying morphology. The third and fourth ventricular complexes have opposite polarity in V1; similarly in long lead II given at the lowermost trace, there is opposite polarity between the second and third and between the eleventh and twelfth complexes. These bidirectional ventricular complexes have few documented causes. An overdose of homeopathic medicine containing aconitine was the cause in this case.

Table 2.9: ECGs in Long QT Syndrome

Long QT Type	T-Wave Morphology	Trigger of Syncope
1	Precordial broad-based T wave	Swimming
2	Low-amplitude bifid T wave	Alarm clock
3	Long isoelectric ST segment followed by a narrow-based "late-onset" T wave	Sleep

---

PRACTICAL TIPS: WHAT IS A LOW-VOLTAGE QRS COMPLEX?

A peak-to-trough QRS amplitude <5 mm in the limb leads and <10 mm in the chest leads is defined as low voltage (**Figure 2.10**).

Causes: Pericardial effusion, left pleural effusion, left pneumothorax and restrictive cardiomyopathy especially amyloidosis.

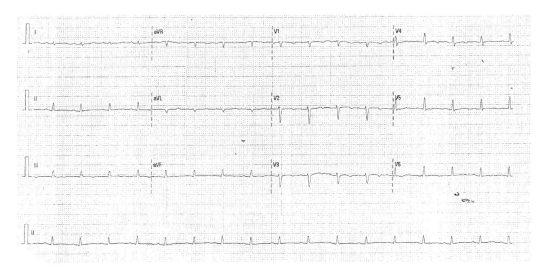

Figure 2.10 Low-voltage complexes in limb and chest leads in a patient with severe dyspnoea. The echocardiography confirmed a large pericardial effusion.

20. What is electrical alternans?

Alternans in the ECG is caused by a periodicity such as an ABABA pattern or AABAAB (2:1 periodicity) and so on. A common cause is a large pericardial effusion where a swinging motion of the heart brings it near to and away from the precordium, alternately creating small and large complexes. This sign is therefore an important and specific feature of large pericardial effusion and tamponade.

Alternans can occur in conditions other than pericardial effusion when the conditions are just right for a periodic response (**Table 2.10**).

Table 2.10: Alternans in Different Situations

Alternans Type	Cause	Comment
QRS amplitude: Small and large QRS in alternate beats	Large pericardial effusion/ tamponade	May require pericardiocentesis
QRS morphology: QRS morphology similar in alternate beats	WPW syndrome	Intermittent preexcitation
ST: Small and large ST elevation in alternate beats often with QT-segment alteration	Coronary spasm	Severe ischaemia may cause this ST-QT alternans
Repolarization alternans: Alteration of T-wave morphology in alternate beats, often with QT alternans	Congenital long QT syndrome Dyselectrolyaemia	Rare

WPW, Wolff-Parkinson-White syndrome.

Making sense of congenital heart disease ECG

Often a physician who treats adults is faced with a dilemma in certain situations where he or she may be required to read a paediatric ECG or an ECG of a suspected congenital heart disease patient not by choice, but by compulsion. The typical ECG features of some congenital heart defects are given next.

Situs Inversus: Right axis P (−ve I, +ve III), P upright in aVR. Atrial ectopic is a differential. Check the chest X-ray for a gastric bubble under the right diaphragm.

Dextrocardia: Absence of QRS progression over precordial leads. QRS and T are inverted in lead I, aVL looks like aVR and vice versa. Check the chest X-ray. Left pneumothorax or COPD is a differential.

Atrial Septal Defect (ASD): RBBB in the ostium secundum, left axis in the ostium primum. Holt-Oram syndrome with ASD has a left axis. Inferior leads show a notch at the top of the R wave (Crotchet sign). qR V1 if pulmonary hypertension. Atrial fibrillation in 20%.

Ventricular Septal Defect (VSD): Biventricular hypertrophy, Katz-Wachtel phenomenon (biphasic RS pattern in mid-precordial leads). Inlet VSD may have left axis. Left atrial enlargement may occur. Chamber enlargement suggests significant shunt flow.

Patent Ductus Arteriosus: LVH, left atrial enlargement. Chamber enlargement suggests significant shunt flow.

Ebstein Disease: Tall (Himalayan) P wave, RBBB, Q II, III, F (RV free wall fibrosis), low voltage in right precordial leads, preexcitation due to right-sided accessory pathway (including atriofascicular path) is common. Manifestation of Ebstein disease can vary according to severity.

Tetralogy of Fallot: Right axis deviation, RVH, RS complexes in mid-precordial lead. Differential of similar pattern: D-TGA (D-Transposition of Great Arteries) PS (Pulmonary Stenosis), DORV-PS (Double Outlet Left Ventricle-Pulmonary Stenosis), single ventricle-PS (Pulmonary Stenosis), TAPVC (Total Anomalous Pulmonary Venous Connection)

Tricuspid Atresia: Left axis of QRS, right atrial enlargement, LVH. This is a very characteristic ECG signature of this condition.

AV Canal Defect: Left axis QRS. S wave II, III, aVF with notched upstroke. Biventricular hypertrophy. Prolonged PR in nearly 50%. Left axis due to inferior displacement of bundle of His and hypoplasia of left anterior fascicle.

D-TGA: Q V1, Q absent in V5 and V6, right axis. RVH. Reversed septal depolarization.

L-TGA: Q in V1–V4 but absent in I, L, V5 and V6. Left axis. T wave upright in all precordial leads (side-by-side ventricles). Reversed septal depolarization. AV dissociation common (yearly incidence 2%).

Pulmonary Stenosis: Right axis deviation. RVH. Right atrial enlargement. Northwest axis of QRS in Noonan syndrome.

Coarctation: LVH in grown-up children. RVH in neonates.

21. What are the characteristics of an ECG in an athlete's heart?

For endurance athletes, the following may be normal:

1. Sinus bradycardia with heart rates 30–40 beats/min

2. First-/second-degree AV block (Mobitz type 1)

3. Increased QRS voltage

4. Normal variant ST elevation

5. Tall T wave, T-wave inversion

MEDICOLEGAL BOOBYTRAPS AND LIMITATIONS

A. Check the name on the ECG before interpreting.
B. The ECG may not show significant changes in acute coronary syndrome or heart failure.

WHAT IS THE IMPORTANCE OF THE aVR LEAD?

The aVR is a unique lead, as it looks at the heart from the base.

a. ST elevation in lead aVR in a STEMI scenario suggests left main coronary or proximal LAD involvement, especially if ST elevation in aVR is more than ST elevation in V1.
b. In this lead PR-segment elevation and ST depression, along with diffuse ST elevation in other leads, suggest pericarditis.
c. In supraventricular tachycardia, a negative P in this lead suggests atrial tachycardia, as it implies a high to low activation of the chamber. This effectively rules out AV-nodal re-entrant tachycardia (AVNRT) and atrioventricular re-entrant tachycardia (AVRT), as in these cases the atrial activation wavefront is retrograde (travelling from the atrioventricular node [AVN] to the roof of the atria).
d. The aVR is the single most important lead in wide QRS tachycardia. A positive QRS in this lead mostly implies VT ("Verickei algorithm" – see the section on wide QRS tachycardia).

FURTHER READING

1. Khairy P and Marelli A J. Clinical Use of Electrocardiography in Adults with Congenital Heart Disease. Circulation 2007;116:2734–2746.
2. Issa Z F, Miller J M, Zipes D P. Electrophysiological Tools and Techniques, in Clinical Arrhythmology and Electrophysiology. 3rd Edition (2019). Elsevier, pp. 81–125.
3. Hancock E W, Deal B. J, Mirvis D M, Okin P, Kligfield P, Gettes L S. ACC/ACCF/HRS Recommendations for the Standardization and Interpretation of the Electrocardiogram: Chamber Enlargement. JACC 2009;53:992–1002.
4. Rautaharju P M, Surawicz B, Gettes LS. ACC/ACCF/HRS Recommendations for the Standardization and Interpretation of the Electrocardiogram: ST, T, U and QT Interval. Circulation 2009;119:e241–e250.
5. Wagner G S, Wellens H J J. AHA/ACCF/HRS Recommendations for the Standardization and Interpretation of the Electrocardiogram Part VI: Acute Ischemia/Infarction. Circulation 2009;119:e262–e270.
6. Mirvis D L, Goldberger A L. Electrocardiography, in Zipes D P, Libby P, Bonnow R O, Mann D L, Tomaselli G F (Eds). Braunwald's Textbook of Cardiovascular Medicine. 11th Edition (2019). Elsevier, pp. 117–150.
7. Goldberger A L. Electrocardiography, in Jameson J L, Fauci A S, Kasper D L, Hauser S L, Longo D L, Loscalzo J (Eds). Harrison's Principle of Internal Medicine. 20th Edition (2018). McGraw Hill, pp. 1675–1682.
8. Surawicz B and Knilans T K (Ed). Chou's Electrocardiography in Clinical Practice. 6th Edition. Elsevier.
9. Baltazar R F. Basic and Bedside Electrocardiography. Wolters Kluwer, Lippincott 2009.
10. Barold S S, Crawford M H (Eds). Advanced 12 Lead Electrocardiography in Cardiology Clinics. 24, (2006). Elsevier, pp 305–504.
11. Luna A B, Batchvarov V N, Malik M. The Morphology of the Electrocardiogram in Camm A J, Luscher T F, Serruys P W (Eds). The ESC Textbook of Cardiovascular Medicine. (2006). Oxford, pp 1–37.
12. Park M K. Electrocardiography, in Paediatric Cardiology for Practitioners. 5th Edition (2008). Mosby (Elsevier).

3 Echocardiography in Critical Care

Sunandan Sikdar and Debika Chatterjee

1. What is the importance of echocardiography in critical care?

Echocardiography plays an important part in rapidly reaching a diagnosis in the critical care setting:

1. Diagnosis of chest pain, dyspnoea, syncope, oedema/anasarca

2. Diagnosis of unexplained hypotension

3. Underlying cause of arrhythmia

4. Assessing volume status

5. Investigating the cause of systemic embolism or stroke

6. Investigating unexplained fever

7. Investigating unexplained hypoxemia

For assessing volume status, refer to the Chapter 4.

2. What is the principle behind an echocardiographic image?

The ultrasound waves emitted by the transducer are reflected at the interface of structures of different densities and at different depths. These returning reflected waves are coded by the transducer as *location* (based on the return time) and *amplitude* (based on the intensity of the reflection). This information is processed by software and represented as grey-scale image on the monitor. The higher the frequency (or shorter the wavelength) of the beam, the better the spatial resolution (ability to distinguish two closely located points) but the poorer the depth of tissue penetration.

3. What are the different echocardiographic modalities available?

The echocardiographic modalities available are summarized in **Table 3.1**.

Table 3.1: Different Modalities Available in Echocardiography

Modality	Features	Principal Use

M-mode	• Motion mode
	• Single-line scan (raster line)
	• High temporal resolution
		a. Chamber measurements (**Figure 3.1**)
		b. Timing of events
		   • RVOT collapse in tamponade
		   • Mitral valve motion in mitral stenosis
		   • Systolic anterior motion in HCM

2D TTE	Linear (phase) array 2D sector scan transducer (64–512) piezoelectric elements) *Adult*: 2.5 MHz–5 MHz *Paediatric*: 5–7.5 MHz	Default modality
3D TTE	Rectangular/matrix (volumetric) scan (2000–3000 elements) which can be: a. Multiplane imaging b. Multibeat imaging c. Real-time 3D	a. Structural heart intervention, especially mitral valve and ASD b. Paravalvular leak evaluation
2D TEE	*Modified endoscopy probe* *Transducer*: 3–7 MHz	a. LAA clot evaluation b. Prosthetic valve evaluation c. Vegetation mitral valve/prosthesis d. ASD rims and device closure e. Intraoperative during cardiac surgery f. Poor window on TTE g. Aortic arch in dissection

(Continued)

DOI: 10.1201/9781003027584-3

Table 3.1 (*Continued*): Different Modalities Available in Echocardiography

Modality	Features	Principal Use
ICE	64-element phased array transducer (5.5–10 MHz) on 8F catheter	a. Septal puncture during AF ablation b. Localization of papillary muscle VT during ablation c. Device and paravalvular leak closure
Doppler	• Pulsed wave (PWD) • Continuous wave (CWD) • Tissue Doppler imaging (TDI)	• *PWD*: Diastolic function • *CWD*: Gradients across valves • TDI: E'
Speckle tracking/ Strain imaging	• Measurement of myocardial deformation • Requires high frame rate (200 fps) • Reflection, scattering and interference of beam produces speckle patterns in myocardium, which are constant and are tracked frame by frame	• Global longitudinal strain • Early detection of cardiomyopathy • LV function before chemotherapy
Contrast echocardiography	Contrast microbubbles like Optison reflect ultrasound, both with linear and non-linear systems depending on the mechanical index, low (<0.2) and high (>0.5), respectively	• Shunt by saline contrast • Detection of LSVC (in case of dilated CS) by saline contrast • Apical LV thrombus • Endocardial border • Stress echocardiography

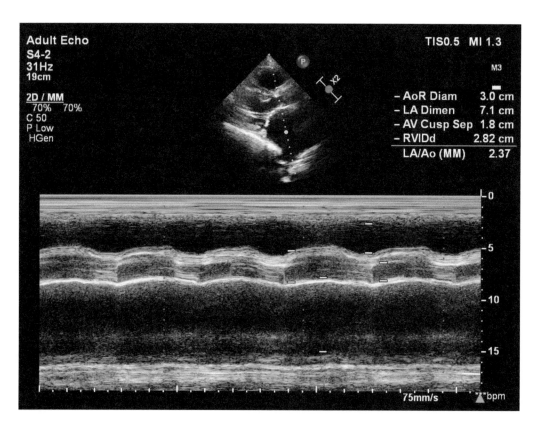

Figure 3.1   Dilated left atrium by M-mode.

4. What are the commonly used views in transthoracic echocardiography?

Though many modified views may be improvised by an experienced operator, the basic views and the structures interrogated are summarized in **Table 3.2.**

Table 3.2: Key Views in Transthoracic Echocardiography

Key View	Main Structure	Common Use
Parasternal long axis (PLAX) (**Figure 3.2**)	LV, LA, aorta, RVOT	RWMA, aortic, mitral valve pathology, PM-VSD
Parasternal short axis at base	LV, RV	RWMA, mitral valve
Parasternal short axis (SAX) at aortic valve level	RVOT, aortic valve	Pulmonary valve, PDA, PM-VSD, outflow VSD, ASD aortic rim
Apical four chamber (A4C)	LV, LA, RV, RA	LV RWMA, MV, TV
Apical two chamber (A2C)	LV, LA	RWMA
Apical five chamber (A5C)	LV, LA, RV, RA, aorta	Aortic valve, LVOT in HCM
Subcostal	LV, LA, RV, RA	Confirming ASD, IVC rim
Suprasternal	Aortic arch, pulmonary artery	Aortic dissection

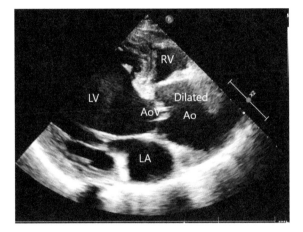

Figure 3.2   Dilated aorta in a case with a bicuspid aortic valve.

5. What is the Doppler principle?

When an ultrasound beam reflects off a moving object (blood or tissue), the frequency of the returning beam is more than the incident beam if the object is moving toward the transducer and less if it is moving away – this is the Doppler principle. This is colour coded as red and blue, respectively, and is the principle of *colour flow mapping* (*CFM*). When the flow is laminar (uniform velocity of RBCs), a pure red or blue colour is seen. But when turbulence takes place, as in a stenotic valve, the mixed velocities (variance) dominate and are displayed as yellow-green.

Pulsed wave Doppler (PWD): In PWD, the transducer element emits an ultrasound pulse and waits for the returning wave to be reflected from a particular depth. This imposes a restriction on the sampling rate (called pulse repetition frequency, PRF). Though it can localize and measure blood velocity at a particular point at a relatively shallower depth, it can only track a velocity <1.5 m/sec.

Continuous wave Doppler (CWD): In CWD, a dedicated element continuously emits, and another element continuously receives the reflected signal. Though it cannot determine the velocity at a given point, it is useful to record velocities >1.5 m/sec. The highest velocity on the line of interrogation is represented on the monitor.

6. What is resolution?

Resolution is simply the ability to see and differentiate closely spaced objects or events. There are four types of resolution: axial, lateral, contrast and temporal (**Table 3.3**).

Table 3.3: Types of Resolution and How to Modify Them

Type of Resolution	Definition (Ability to See)	How to Increase
Axial	In the direction of the beam	Increase pulse frequency
Lateral	Perpendicular to the direction of the beam	Increase gain
Contrast	Differentiating two grey-scale objects	Increase contrast
Temporal	Ability to detect events closely spaced in time	Increase frame rate and reduce depth

7. What is an artefact?

Since echocardiography is an image of real structures that is generated by software processing of reflected ultrasound beams reaching the transducer, errors of representation may arise. These are called artefacts. Commonly they are:

1. *Side lobe artefact*: The transducer interprets the returning ultrasound waves reflected by a peripheral object as coming from the central beam. When a strong reflector is nearby, it may cause the image of a mass to appear in a place/cavity when there is actually none.

2. *Reverberation*: Multiple secondary echoes of a strong reflector, like the posterior left ventricular (LV) wall, may create an impression of pericardial effusion.

3. *Shadowing*: Lack of echoes (dark shadow) behind a strong reflector, like a prosthetic valve.

8. What are the normal range of values in transthoracic echocardiography (TTE)?

The normative values of different dimensions are given in **Table 3.4**.

Table 3.4: Normative Values of Echocardiography Dimensions

Parameter	Male (mm)	Female (mm)	Comments
Septal/posterior wall thickness	6–10	6–9	Mean ± 2D
LV diastolic dimension (LVIDD)	42–58 34–52 (India)	37–52 32–49 (India)	Mean ± 2D
LV systolic dimension (LVIDS)	25–39 22–34 (India)	28–33 20–32 (India)	Mean ± 2D
LVEF	52–72 58–69 (India)	54–74 58–68 (India)	Mean ± 2D
Mild LV dysfunction	41–51	41–53	As per ASE guidelines 2015
Moderate LVD	30–40	30–40	
Severe LVD	<30	<30	
Aorta (at sinus of Valsalva)	31–37	27–33	
LA volume/BSA	<34	<34	
TAPSE	24 ± 3.5	24 ± 3.5	<17 abnormal
RVOT (PLAX)	20–30	20–30	Mean ± D
RV (mid)	19–35	19–35	Mean ± D
RV fractional area change	100× (RV end-diastolic area – RV end systolic area/ RVEDA)		<35% abnormal
RA minor axis	19 ± 3	19 ± 3	Mean ± D
RA major axis	25 ± 3	24 ± 3	Mean ± D

9. How is LV systolic function assessed?

Left ventricular ejection fraction (LVEF): Probably the most commonly used metric is LVEF – a global measure of systolic function. It can be measured by M-mode, 2D and 3D echocardiography.

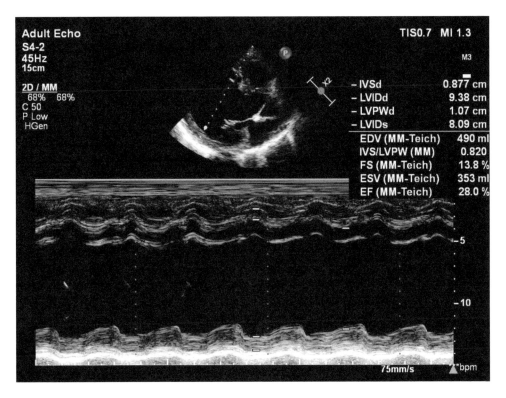

Adult Echo		TIS0.7 MI 1.3
S4-2		
45Hz		M3
15cm		

– IVSd	0.877 cm
– LVIDd	9.38 cm
– LVPWd	1.07 cm
– LVIDs	8.09 cm
EDV (MM-Teich)	490 ml
IVS/LVPW (MM)	0.820
FS (MM-Teich)	13.8 %
ESV (MM-Teich)	353 ml
EF (MM-Teich)	28.0 %

Figure 3.3 Dilated LV and severe LV dysfunction from M-mode.

M-mode: The LV measurements are to done at the mid-ventricular papillary muscle level (**Figure 3.3**). The LVEF is calculated by the Quinones method, although the Teichholz method is still popular, as it is easy, and the automated calculations are available in the machine itself. It is based on the inaccurate assumption that the LV is a prolate ellipsoid.

$$LVEF(Quinones) = (\% \text{ delta } D^2) + (1 - \text{delta } D^2)(\% \text{ delta } L)$$

where the first component is uncorrected ejection fraction (EF):

$$\text{delta } D^2 = LVIDD^2 - LVIDS^2 / LVIDD^2 \times 100$$

And the second component is the apical correction factor, given the following arbitrary values: % delta L = 15% in a normal subject, 5% in apical hypokinesia, 0% for apical akinesia, –5% for apical dyskinesia and –10% for apical aneurysm.

2D: Simpson's method of calculating LV volume as the summing of discs after tracing the endocardial border in diastole and systole is the method of choice in calculating LVEF. Trabeculae and papillary muscles should be included during endocardial tracing. Diastole and systole must have no apical foreshortening and nearly equal long axis lengths.

$$LVEF (\%) = (LVEDV - LVESV / LVEDV) \times 100$$

$$\text{Fractional shortening (FS): FS} = LVIDD - LVIDS / LVIDD \times 100$$

Global longitudinal strain (GLS): Relative length change of LV myocardium between end diastole and end systole compared to end diastole is the GLS derived from strain imaging. Normal peak GLS is less than –20%.

10. How do you grade LV diastolic dysfunction?

Evaluation of diastolic function (**Figure 3.4**) gives us an idea whether the cause of dyspnoea is cardiac (Grade III dysfunction or a restrictive pattern may cause pulmonary congestion).

Diastolic dysfunction grades are classically defined as in **Table 3.5**.

Table 3.5: Diastolic Dysfunction Grades

Parameter	Normal	Grade I: Impaired Relaxation	Grade II: Pseudo-Normal	Grade III: Restrictive
IVRT (ms)	70–90	>90	60–90	<70
E/A	0.8–1.5	<0.8	0.8–2	>2
DT (ms)	140–240	>240	140–200	<140
e′ (septum)(cm/s)	>10	<7	<7	<5
E/e′	<8	<8	8–14	>14
Pulmonary S/D	>1	>1	=1	<1
Pulmonary Ar-A (ms)	<0	Variable	>30	>30
Vp (cm/sec)	>50	<50	<50	<50
LAVI (mL/m²)	16–28	>28	>34	>34

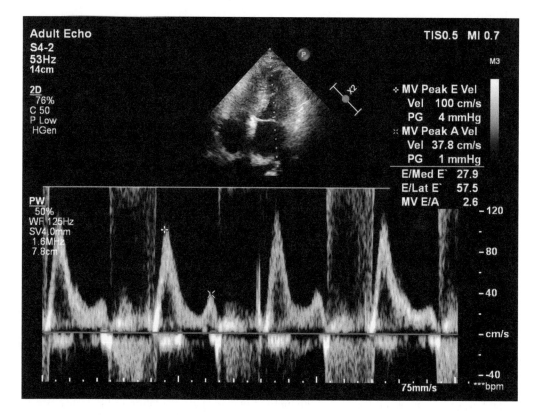

Figure 3.4 Grade III diastolic dysfunction: E/A >2.

The recommended algorithm for diagnosis: The 2016 American Society of Echocardiography (ASE) guidelines altered the way in which we approach diastolic dysfunction. Only four parameters were to be utilized apart from E/A:

a. Average E/e′ >14

b. Tricuspid regurgitation (TR) velocity >2.8 m/sec

c. Left atrial (LA) volume index >34 mL/m²

d. Septal e′ <7 cm/sec, lateral e′ <10 cm/sec

In patients with normal LVEF if three or more criteria are present, diastolic dysfunction is diagnosed.

On the other hand, if the patient has LV systolic dysfunction, the key parameter changes to the E/A ratio, and diastolic dysfunction is diagnosed as per the following protocol:

a. If E/A <0.8 and E <50 cm/sec, then it is normal left atrial pressure/grade I diastolic dysfunction.

b. If E/A is >2, it is grade III diastolic dysfunction (**Figure 3.4**).

c. If E/A is between 0.8 and 2 (or if E/A <0.8 and E >50 cm/sec), then criteria (a), (b) and (c) should be considered. Grade II diastolic dysfunction is diagnosed if two or more criteria are present.[1]

11. What are the common formulae for haemodynamic calculation?

Objective haemodynamics often supplement visual impression by echocardiography, especially valve area, valve/shunt gradients and regurgitant severity. **Table 3.6** summarizes the haemodynamic formulae frequently used.

Table 3.6: Haemodynamic Formulae and Their Underlying Principles

Parameter	Formula	Comment/Assumption
Cardiac output = Stroke volume × HR	(CSA LVOT × VTI LVOT) × HR	• Based on continuity equation • Assumes circular LVOT
RV stroke volume	CSA RVOT × VTI RVOT	• Assumes circular RVOT
Qp/Qs	$\dfrac{\text{CSA RVOT} \times \text{VTI RVOT}}{\text{CSA LVOT} \times \text{VTI LVOT}}$	• Useful for VSD/ASD/PDA for haemodynamic importance of shunt
Aortic valve area	CSA LVOT × VTI LVOT/VTI AoV	• Assumes circular LVOT, based on continuity equation
Mitral valve area	$2\pi r^2 \times (\alpha/180) \times$ (Aliasing velocity/Peak velocity MR)	• Assumes spherical inflow • PISA principle, see later
MVA in mitral stenosis	220/Pressure half time or 759/Deceleration time	• Assumes LA pressure remains constant during diastole and LV compliance is normal • Empiric constant (220) used
LVEDP in AR	SBP – 4 (AR V^2 at end diastole)	• Assumes normal mitral valve • Uses Bernoulli equation
LAP in MR	SBP – 4 (MR peak V^2)	• Assumes normal aortic outflow • Uses Bernoulli equation
RVSP in VSD/PDA	SBP – 4 (Shunt jet peak V^2)	• Assumes normal aortic outflow • Uses Bernoulli equation

12. How do you measure pulmonary artery pressure (PAP?

Measuring PAP is often crucial in critical care, as it gives an idea about the cause of dyspnoea and hypoxia and the intensity of treatment required. PAP gives an idea of *"pulmonary congestion."* Measurement of TR peak velocity may be the most recommended way in determining PAP (**Figure 3.5**), but it may be very faint and other formulae may be necessary (**Table 3.7**).

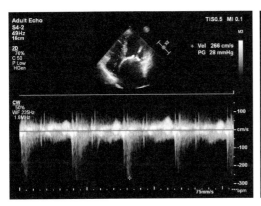
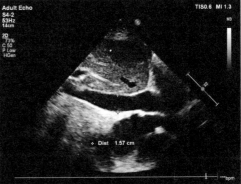

Figure 3.5 Measuring pulmonary artery systolic pressure from TR jet and IVC diameter.

Table 3.7: Assessment of Pulmonary Pressure and Resistances

Parameter	Formula	Cut-Off for Normality	Comment
Pulmonary artery systolic pressure (PASP)	4 (TR peak velocity)^2 + RAP	• TRV <2.8 m/sec • PASP <36 mmHg	RV dysfunction causes underestimation, assumes non-stenotic tricuspid valve
Mean pulmonary artery pressure	4 PRV^2 (peak PR jet velocity) + RAP	mPAP <25 mmHg	Used if TR jet is inadequate
Pulmonary artery end diastolic pressure	4 PRV^2 (end PR jet velocity) + RAP		Use D in calculating PDA gradient
Acceleration time (AT): Use pulse wave Doppler in RVOT	Time to peak of RVOT flow envelope shortens as pulmonary artery pressure increases	>100 msec (<100 msec abnormal)	• Mean PAP (mmHg) = 79 – (0.45 × AT) • Mahan's equation: HR must be between 60 and 100 beats/min
Mid-systolic notch	Seen in pulmonary flow velocity envelope		Predicts increased pulmonary resistance
Pulmonary vascular resistance (PVR)	(TRV/RVOT VTI) × 10 + 0.16 (based on regression equation)	• <0.15 normal • >0.2 implies PVR • >2 Wood U	Differentiates high flow from pulmonary vascular disease
Pulmonary capillary wedge pressure (PCWP)	1.9 + 1.2 × E/E' (based on regression equation)	<15 mmHg	Inflow MV angle dependence. Dilated LA supports raised PCWP

13. How is RA pressure determined?

RA pressure gives an idea of *"systemic congestion."*

Inferior vena cava (IVC) size is the marker used in determining right atrium (RA) pressure, as it is the chamber proximal to the RA (**Table 3.8**). The diameter of the IVC should be measured in the subcostal view with the patient in the supine position at 1–2 cm from the junction with the RA, using the long axis view (**Figure 3.5**).

Table 3.8: Determination of Estimated RA Pressure

IVC Size	Collapse with Sniffing	Estimated RA Pressure (mmHg)
<2.1	>50%	3 (0–5)
<2.1	<50%	8 (5–10)
>2.1	<50%	15 (10–20)

14. What is the Myocardial Performance Index (MPI)?

This index incorporates three distinct time intervals – ejection time (ET), isovolumetric contraction time (IVCT) and isovolumetric relaxation time (IVRT). Systolic dysfunction leads to prolongation of IVCT and shortening of ET, while diastolic dysfunction leads to prolongation of IVRT. Any or both of these abnormalities lead to increase in MPI.

$$MPI = (IVCT + IVRT)/ET$$

LV-MPI >0.5 and RV-MPI >0.43 suggest LV and right ventricle (RV) dysfunction, respectively. Unlike EF, MPI has an advantage in that it is less dependent on preload.

15. What are the echocardiographic findings in ischaemic heart disease?

Ischaemic heart disease may present in an intensive care unit or to an anaesthetist as (1) a cardiac emergency directly or perioperatively or (2) as an associated condition along with a primary surgical/medical problem. Echocardiography frequently determines the severity of the disease, nature of therapy, prognosis and, most importantly, whether the event is a new one that is acute coronary syndrome versus chronic ischaemic heart disease (**Table 3.9**).

Table 3.9: Echocardiography Findings in Ischaemic Heart Disease

Acute Coronary Syndrome	Chronic IHD
RWMA	RWMA
Pericardial effusion (due to post-MI)	Pericardial effusion (due to heart failure)
RV akinesia	LV aneurysm
Ventricular septal defect	LV pseudoaneurysm
Mitral regurgitation	Apical thrombus
Free wall rupture	

16. How is the LV segmented with respect to coronary artery disease?

Segmentation of the LV allows inter-operator communication of the extent of involvement by isch-aemia in a more accurate way.

LV segmentation can be easily remembered in a bull's eye view of the short axis representation as given in **Figure 3.6**. A quick idea of regional wall motion abnormalities (RWMA) requires three views: Parasternal long axis (PLAX), short axis (SAX) and apical four chamber (A4C). The more LV segments involved, the lower the LVEF. As a rough approximation, involvement of the entire antero-septal and anterolateral wall (left anterior descending artery [LAD] territory) by hypokinesia will reduce the LVEF to 40% or below.

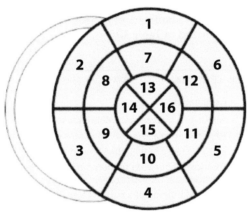

All models

1. Basal anterior	7. Mid anterior
2. Basal anteroseptal	8. Mid anteroseptal
3. Basal inferoseptal	9. Mid inferoseptal
4. Basal inferior	10. Mid inferior
5. Basal inferolateral	11. Mid inferolateral
6. Basal anterolateral	12. Mid anterolateral

Figure 3.6 Standard LV segmentation: Bull's eye short axis, A4C, A2C and long axis (A5C). (Adapted with permission from Lang RM, Badani LP. Recommendations for cardiac chamber quantification by echocardiography in adults. J Am Soc Echocardiogr 2015;28:1–39.)

17. How do you determine the territorial supply of coronary artery disease?

The LAD commonly supplies the largest area of the anteroseptal and anterolateral wall. Whether the inferolateral area is supplied by the right coronary artery (RCA) or circumflex artery (LCx) depends on the dominance of right or left, respectively, and anatomic peculiarities. This is sum-marized in **Figure 3.7**.

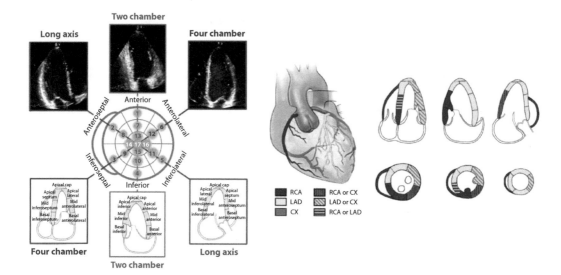

Figure 3.7 Coronary artery territories. (Adapted with permission from Lang RM, Badani LP. Recommendations for cardiac chamber quantification by echocardiography in adults. J Am Soc Echocardiogr 2015;28:1–39.)

18. What are the different types of wall motion abnormalities?

Regional wall motion abnormalities are a hallmark of ischaemic heart disease (IHD). A brief definition of well-known terms is summarized in **Table 3.10**.

Table 3.10. Classification of RWMA

Term	Explanation	Score
Normal/hyperkinetic	About 40% increase in wall thickness in systole	1
Hypokinetic	10%–40% increase in wall thickness (less than normal)	2
Akinetic	<10% increase in wall thickness in systole	3
Dyskinetic	Paradoxical outward motion during systole, often associated with scarring	4
Aneurysm	Outward bulging of a part of LV wall in both systole and diastole, often associated with scarring	5

The wall motion score (WMS) is calculated by adding the score of all 17 segments. The wall motion score index (WMSI) is calculated by:

$$WMSI = Sum\ of\ wall\ motion\ score\ /\ Segments\ visualized$$

Normal WMSI is 1. The larger the infarct, the larger the WMSI. If WMSI >1.7, the perfusion defect is >20%.

19. How do you identify an aneurysm, pseudoaneurysm and diverticula, and why are they important?

Though aneurysm and pseudoaneurysm are sequelae of IHD, the second one is far more dangerous, though rarer (**Table 3.11**). In a patient whose history is not available, they need to be separated from LV diverticula, which is an incidental finding without much significance.

20. What is the role of echocardiography in valvular heart disease?

Echocardiography is the most versatile investigation in relation to valvular heart disease with regard to diagnosis, grading/severity, timing of intervention and also intraoperative and postoperative care.

Table 3.11: Comparison between LV Aneurysm, Pseudoaneurysm and Diverticula

LV Aneurysm	LV Pseudoaneurysm	LV Diverticula
Seen >6 weeks after MI	Earlier after MI	Congenital (not related to IHD)
Outward bulge of scar tissue in both systole and diastole	Contained rupture of LV wall	Outpouching of LV endocardium
Thin wall of fibrous scar tissue, less likely to rupture	Wall of thrombi and parietal pericardium, more likely to rupture	Preserved LV wall thickness
Neck of sac wide	Neck of sac narrower than the maximum transverse diameter	<1 cm in maximum diameter
Measurement of neck accurate	Measurement of neck inaccurate due to presence of thrombus	Seen in inferior wall and apex
Cause of LV thrombus, heart failure, arrhythmia	Sudden fatal rupture	Incidental finding

21. What are the principles of assessment in valvular heart disease?

Assessment of valves is divided into components dependent on each other.

2D Anatomy

a. *Valve*: The leaflets (commissural fusion, calcification, mobility –restricted or prolapsed), annulus (normal, calcified or dilated) and subvalvular apparatus (especially for the mitral valve) should be evaluated and reported. Diastolic doming of the anterior mitral leaflet and restricted mobility of the posterior mitral leaflet are characteristic of rheumatic mitral stenosis. In the mitral valve, measurement of the valve area by planimetry by 2D echocardiography (**Figure 3.8**) is the gold standard (severe <1.5 cm^2). The systolic displacement >2 mm of one or both mitral leaflets into the LA below the plane of mitral annulus in PLAX is the accepted criteria for mitral valve prolapse (**Figure 3.9**), especially if the leaflets are thickened (>5 mm).

b. *Chamber upstream and downstream to the valve*: Dilated or normal. Dilated chambers suggest severe regurgitation.

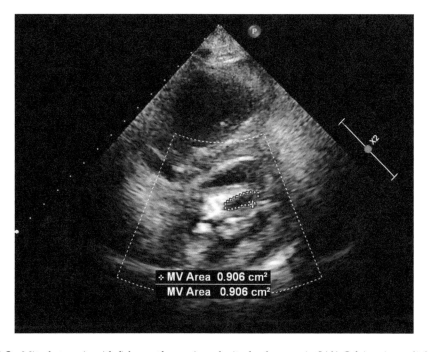

Figure 3.8 Mitral stenosis with fish mouth opening of mitral valve seen in SAX. Calcium in medial commissure is well appreciated.

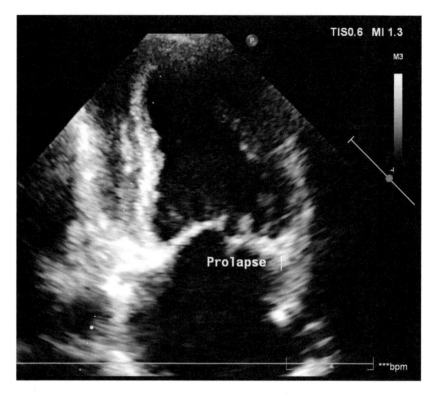

Figure 3.9 Mitral valve prolapse in A2C view.

Haemodynamics

a. *Gradient across the valve for stenotic valves*: Mean and peak. The mean gradient is used to define severity in the aortic (severe stenosis >40 mmHg), mitral (severe stenosis >10 mmHg) and tricuspid (severe stenosis >5 mmHg) valves. The peak gradient is used in the pulmonary valve (severe >64 mmHg). The gradient determination is based on the Bernoulli principle: delta P = 4 (velocity of jet)^2.

b. *Shape of the flow envelope*: The flow of the aortic valve is a half-parabola. The later the peak from the onset, the more severe the stenosis. This is quantified by the parameter, acceleration time (AT), which is useful in assessing prosthetic valve stenosis (AT >100 ms). On CWD, the inflow of the mitral valve shows a double hump in form of fused E and A waves in mitral stenosis. The gentler the downward slope of E or the slower the pressure decay, the tighter the stenosis. This is quantified by pressure half time (PHT) (the time taken by the pressure to reach half its original value – the longer the time, the more severe the stenosis; in severe mitral stenosis, PHT >150 ms). In the case of the mitral valve, an empiric relation exists between mitral valve area (MVA) and PHT: MVA = 220/PHT.

c. *Continuity equation*: This versatile equation, derived from the principle of conservation of flow at any two given orifices connected in series, can be summed up thus:

$$CSA(inflow) \times VTI(inflow) = CSA(valve) \times VTI(valve)$$

where CSA = Cross-section area and VTI = Velocity time integral (available by tracing the flow envelope). The most important application of this is in the calculation of aortic valve area (AVA <1 cm^2, severe stenosis) and effective regurgitation orifice (ERO). In calculating AVA, the left ventricular outflow tract (LVOT) is considered as the inflow, and its diameter (CSA = πD^2) and VTI are measured. The continuity equation can be utilized to calculate the regurgitant volume (RV):

In atrial regurgitation (AR): RV(AR) = Stroke volume (Aortic valve) – Stroke volume (Mitral valve)

In mitral regurgitation (MR): RV(MR) = Stroke volume (Mitral valve) – Stroke volume (Aortic valve)

Stroke volume across a valve = π(Diameter of valve)^2/4 × VTI across the valve

Diameter of the aortic valve = Hinge point to hinge point in PLAX

Diameter of mitral valve = Distance between two ends of the MVA in A4C (inaccuracy of mitral diameter measurement is a limitation)

d. *Jet area and jet width*: For quantification of regurgitation, jet area as a percentage of LA area is used in MR (>50% is severe), while the absolute value of the jet area is used in TR (>10 cm^2 is severe). For the aortic valve, on the other hand, conventionally, jet height/LVOT height is used in AR (>65% is severe AR) and should be calculated in the PLAX view (the axial resolution is better).

e. *Proximal Isovelocity Area (PISA) and ERO*: Regurgitation takes place from the high pressure to the low- pressure side when the valve is closed (ventricular diastole in AR and systole in MR). As flow converges and accelerates toward the orifice of the partially closed valve, a number of concentric shells (with equal velocity at each point on the shell surface) of smaller and smaller diameter is formed. They are called isovelocity surfaces. At the boundary of the shell, there is velocity aliasing and a red-blue interface is formed. This velocity is the Nyquist limit. The Nyquist limit is defined as the upper limit of Doppler frequency that can be accurately characterized by pulsed wave beam – beyond this limit, the PWD will not characterize the direction or velocity of the jet correctly. This can be read from the velocity colour scale shown on the monitor. By adjusting the Nyquist limit (the scale is moved downward in the case of MR as seen from the A4C view), the size of shell can be maximized. In doing so, the outer surface of the shell moves upstream so that its radius increases and can be measured more accurately. Three pieces of data are now required so that ERO is automatically determined by the machine: *The radius of the aliasing surface, aliasing velocity and peak velocity of MR*. Since flow rate is equal across the shell and orifice, using the continuity equation:

$$\text{Surface area of shell} \times \text{Aliasing velocity} = \text{Effective valve orifice} \times \text{MR velocity}$$

$$2\pi r^2 \times \text{Aliasing velocity} = \text{ERO} \times \text{MR velocity}$$

Thus ERO = 2πr^2 × Aliasing velocity/MR velocity

ERO >0.4 cm^2 for severe primary MR

>0.3 cm^2 for severe AR

>0.2 cm^2 for severe secondary MR

ERO leads us to the regurgitant volume (RV): RV = ERO × VTI of MR jet

RV >60 mL/beat implies severe primary MR or AR

>30 mL/beat implies severe secondary MR (ischaemic)

Regurgitant fraction (RF) = RV/Stroke volume (>50% implies severe regurgitation in both aortic and mitral valves)

Limitations of the PISA concept include the fact that (1) shells may not be hemispheric in reality and (2) the flow rate is not constant throughout systole in many cases.

f. *Vena contracta (VC)*: It is the narrowest neck of flow region at the level of the valve immediately below the flow convergence zone. Measured in the PLAX view in AR, it is smaller than the width of the jet in LVOT. *VC > 6 mm is specific for severe AR*. While measuring VC in MR, A4C and another orthogonal view are used and the value averaged. *VC > 7 mm is specific for severe MR*.

g. *Nature of the jet*: An eccentric or wall-hugging jet does not lend itself to quantification (often underestimated by >40% in comparison to the central jet) and are generally severe. One of the reasons for this is that they recruit RBCs only on one side, while central jets recruit RBCs on all sides.

The utilization of 2D and haemodynamics helps us in grading the severity of valvular heart disease, and *the reader is referred to the chapter on valvular heart disease and infective endocarditis* for discussion on the same.

22. How do you evaluate a prosthetic valve by echocardiography?

Echocardiographic evaluation is paramount to determine whether the symptoms are due to a dysfunctional prosthesis. The cardinal signs are reduced movement of the leaflet on 2D and an increased gradient across the valve on Doppler.

2D Echocardiographic Evaluation of a Prosthetic Valve

Normal: The sewing ring has higher echogenicity and can be recognized. The motion of individual leaflets (e.g., in St Jude prosthesis) or the ball (in ball and cage prosthesis) can also be visualized

Degeneration: Thickening of leaflets >3 mm mean calcification

Pannus: A small, firmly fixed structure often on the aortic valve (less mobile) and highly echogenic. Commonly associated with paravalvular leak

Thrombus: Large and mobile, less echogenically dense than pannus

Dehiscence: Rocking motion of prosthesis is characteristic

Doppler Echocardiographic Evaluation of Prosthetic Heart Valves

Jets on colour flow map: Monoleaflet valve – two jets, bileaflet valve – three jets

Peak velocity: Usually <3 m/sec for aortic and <2 m/sec for mitral (if >4 m/sec, likely stenosis for aortic, >2.5m/sec for mitral)

Peak and mean gradient: As per the manufacturer. Generally, the acceptable mean gradient <20 mmHg for aortic and <5 mmHg for mitral prosthesis (>35 mmHg means possible stenosis in the case of aortic prosthesis and >10 mmHg means possible stenosis in the case of mitral prosthesis)

Velocity profile: Maximum velocity in early systole; the later the peak velocity, the more likely the possibility of stenosis

Acceleration time for aortic valve prosthesis: AT <80 ms is normal; if >100 ms, valve is likely stenotic

PHT for mitral valve prosthesis: PHT <130 ms is normal; if >200 ms, valve is likely stenotic

Dimensionless Index:

- For aortic valve: VTI LVOT/VTI aortic valve prosthesis < 0.25 suggests stenosis
  - For mitral valve: VTI mitral valve prosthesis/VTI LVOT. A reading of <2.2 is normal; a reading >2.5 suggests the possibility of stenosis

Doppler Velocity Index (DVI): Velocity LVOT/Velocity aortic valve: Normally >0.3. If < 0.25, it is likely to be stenotic

Effective orifice area (EOA) by continuity equation: CSA inflow × VTI inflow/VTI of valve itself. Values:

>1.2 cm^2 normal, <0.8 cm^2 aortic valve stenosis likely

>2 cm^2 normal, <1 cm^2 mitral valve stenosis likely

Regurgitation: Valvular and paravalvular.

- Physiologic regurgitation (closure backflow during closure, leakage backflow post-closure) is transient, narrow and symmetrical.
  - Pathologic regurgitation is central in bioprostheses and eccentric/paravalvular in mechanical prostheses. They are of high velocity, dense and broad in profile.

Dobutamine Stress Echocardiography may unmask occult prosthetic valve stenosis if there is an increase in the gradient (>15 mmHg for the aortic valve and >18 mmHg for the mitral).

Clinical Scenarios

1. *High gradient with DVI <0.25 and AT >100 ms suggests prosthetic stenosis*

2. *High gradient with normal DVI and normal AT*: High flow (anaemia/regurgitation)

3. *High gradient with borderline DVI and normal AT*: Check EOA to rule out patient-prosthesis mismatch

For possibly stenotic tricuspid valve prosthesis, cut-off values of velocity, gradient and PHT are >1.7 m/sec, >6 mmHg and >230 ms, respectively.

23. What are the characteristics of vegetations?

1. Attached to the native/prosthetic valve on the low-pressure side (atrial side of mitral or tricuspid valve, ventricular side of aortic or pulmonary valve)

2. Oscillating mass

3. Irregular surface

Note: *Echocardiographic mimics of vegetations* – Fibrosis/calcification of leaflet, papillary fibroelastoma, valve/leaflet prolapse with myxomatous appearance, ruptured chordate, thrombus, Lambl excrescences, sutures.

Complications of Vegetations

Abscess: Non-homogenous perivalvular thickening that is echodense or echolucent

Pseudoaneurysm: Perivalvular echocardiographic free space with flow demonstrated on colour Doppler

24. What are the sources of an embolus in the cardiac care unit/intensive care unit (CCU/ ICU)?

When a patient presents with a stroke, peripheral embolism or acute coronary syndrome, a search of an embolic source is justified (**Table 3.12**).

Table 3.12: Sources of Embolus in Intensive Care

Source	Location	Characteristic
LV thrombi	Mostly in the apex, which is akinetic	• Echolucent centre implies fresh thrombus and calcification implies an old one • *DD*: Trabeculae, endocardial fibroelastosis, LV non-compaction
LA thrombi (**Figure 3.10**)	Mostly LA appendage, but may occur in roof or septum	
LA myxoma (**Figure 3.11**)	LA (75%) – fossa ovalis, RA (15%), RV (5%)	Non-homogenous cluster of grapes appearance with or without calcification
Papillary fibroelastoma	Aortic/mitral valve in elderly	Common tumour, embolic episodes occur
Lipoma	Atrial septum	Hyperechogenic septum with dumbbell appearance
Rhabdomyoma	LV, RV in children	Cause obstruction
Fibroma	LV in children	Obstruction, arrhythmia, embolus
Renal cell carcinoma (**Figure 3.12**)	IVC, RA, RV	Inflow obstruction of tricuspid valve, pulmonary embolism, syncope
Lung carcinoma	Pulmonary vein, pericardial effusion	
Melanoma	LV or RV, often in apex	Looks like thrombi
Carcinoid	Tricuspid, pulmonary valve	Obstruction common, embolus rare

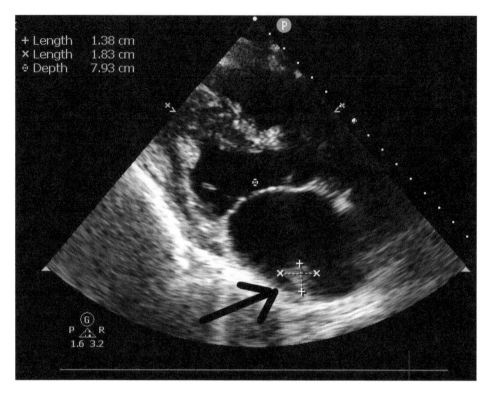

Figure 3.10   Cause of Middle Cerebral Artery infarct: Clot in LA roof.

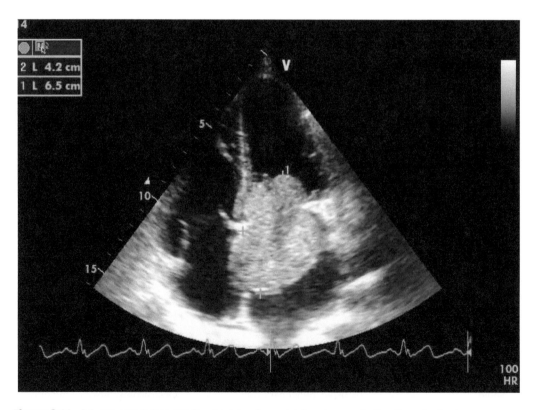

Figure 3.11   LA myxoma (4.2 cm × 6.5 cm) arising from atrial septum occluding the mitral valve.

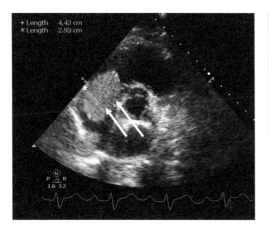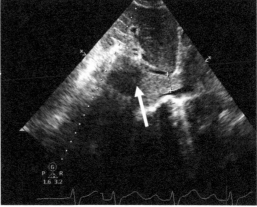

Figure 3.12 A middle-aged man presented with syncope with the ECG showing RBBB. Echocardiography revealed metastasis via the IVC to the right atrium (*single arrow*). An obstructive mass sits across the tricuspid valve impeding RV filling (*double arrow*). An Abdominal CT scan showed renal cell carcinoma.

25. What are the common causes of shock and their respective findings on echocardiography in a CCU/ICU patient?

During stabilization of a hypotensive patient, causes of shock need to be actively investigated. Echocardiography is the first line of investigation in finding its cause (**Table 3.13**).

Table 3.13: Causes of Shock in Intensive Care

Cause	Key Findings	Comment
Pump failure	Dilated LV with reduced contraction	Check ECG/troponin to rule out acute event
Cardiac tamponade	Large pericardial effusion with RV collapse	Urgent pericardial tap
Sepsis/hypovolemia	Non-dilated hypercontractile LV with kissing papillary muscles	IV fluids
Aortic dissection	Dilated aorta with dissection flap	Surgery
Pulmonary embolism	RV dysfunction/dilation, raised PASP, thrombus in pulmonary artery/RA/IVC	Thrombolysis
Severe AS/MS	Deformed valve	Initial stabilization then surgery
Acute AR	IE or aortic dissection related to prolapsed aortic leaflet or perforation with turbulent jet in LVOT filling >65% of normal chamber size	Emergent surgery
Acute MR	• Post PTMC or IE related • Flail valve leaflet • Eccentric turbulent jet/jets in LA • Pulmonary hypertension • Normal chamber dimension	Tall V wave on catheter if during PTMC, emergent surgery

26. What are the echocardiographic signs of cardiac tamponade and pericardial constriction?

Echocardiography can rapidly determine the cause of apparent cardiomegaly on chest X-ray (though most of the time they are due to expiratory films in the supine position in a CCU). Once in a while, sudden diagnosis of an impending tamponade may save lives (**Figure 3.13**). Sometimes a patient with anasarca may turn out to be a case of constrictive pericarditis. Both of these conditions have some similarities and differences on echocardiogram and may be studied together as they are both pericardial pathologies (**Table 3.14**).

Table 3.14. Cardiac Tamponade and Pericardial Constriction

Parameter	Tamponade	Constriction
Pericardium	Effusion predominant, often large if chronic	Thickening predominant
2D/M-mode	• Late diastolic RA collapse-sensitive sign • Early diastolic RV collapse-specific sign	• Exaggerated leftward septal shift with inspiration • Septal bounce • Flattened posterior wall on diastole
IVC dilated	Yes	Yes
PW Doppler	Reciprocal relation of RVOT flow (VTI) vs LVOT flow (VTI), e.g., during inspiration RVOT flow increases but LVOT decreases	Exaggerated respiratory variation of tricuspid and mitral inflow velocity, e.g., during expiration there is >25% increase in mitral inflow velocity
Diastolic pattern	–	Restrictive (E/A >>2)
Tissue Doppler	–	Annulus paradoxus (Medial E' > lateral E')
Hepatic vein	–	Expiratory flow reversal

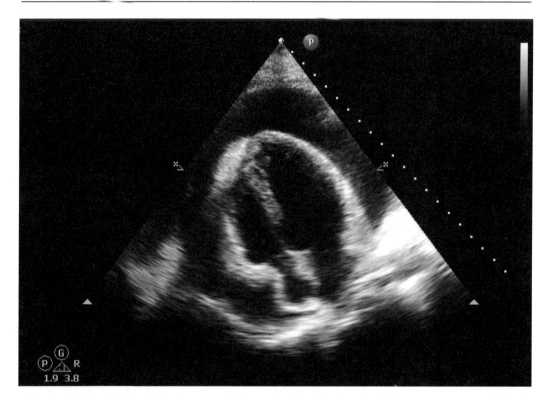

Figure 3.13 Large pericardial effusion causing cardiac tamponade. Notice the Right atrial collapse (Reverse S shape of RA free wall).

27. What are the echocardiographic features of cardiac trauma?

Cardiac trauma (accident/injury) is an emergency where immediate assessment for surgery may be required. Always look for:

1. Pericardial effusion

2. Rupture of valve apparatus

3. Free wall rupture

4. Aortic dissection/intramural haematoma

5. Wall motion abnormalities

28. What segments of the aorta are recognized by echocardiography?

A. *Aortic root*:

    a. Annulus (junction of LVOT and aorta, part of fibrous skeleton, plane of attachment of leaflets)

    b. Sinus of Valsalva (onion-like dilated part above annulus)

    c. Sinotubular junction (STJ, junction of sinus and tubular ascending aorta, the plane of leaflet coaptation)

B. Ascending aorta (tubular structure from STJ to the right brachiocephalic artery

C. Arch of aorta (from right brachiocephalic to the left subclavian)

D. Descending thoracic aorta (left subclavian to the diaphragm)

The aortic arch is not properly visualized by TTE and requires transoesophageal echocardiography (TEE). Aortic measurements should be taken from leading edge to leading edge and at end diastole, except for the aortic annulus, which is taken in end systole.

29. What are acute aortic syndromes?

Acute tearing chest pain radiating to the back requires an urgent echocardiogram to decide whether it is acute coronary syndrome or aortic dissection (**Figure 3.14**). Taking an aortic dissection to the catheter lab or thrombolysing is a potential disaster.

Class I: Classic dissection

Class II: Intramural haematoma

Class III: Localized tear, no haematoma

Class IV: Ulcerated plaque (descending/abdominal aorta)

Class V: Iatrogenic dissection

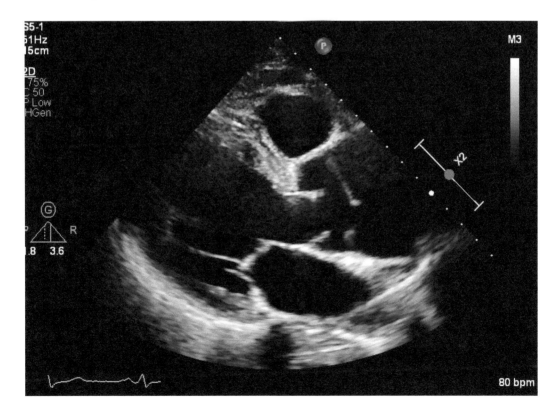

Figure 3.14 Aortic dissection: Note the flap in ascending aorta.

If in doubt after doing the TTE, it is useful to get a contrast-enhanced (CE) CT of the thorax rapidly, as a patient in severe pain rarely tolerates TEE and is frequently in hypotension.

30. What are the echocardiographic features of aortic dissection and its variants?

Variants of aortic dissection must be rapidly differentiated from classic dissection and their extent and location ascertained, as the treatment strategy may differ (**Table 3.15**).

Table 3.15. Aortic Dissection and Its Variants

Aortic Dissection	Intramural Haematoma	Atheromatous Ulcer
Thin undulating flap separating true from false lumen, dilated aorta (often >55 mm)	Thick aortic wall >7 mm, haemorrhage in medial layer but without a luminal exit	Two types: a. *Crescentic*: Smooth crescentic protrusion in the lumen from the wall b. *Complex*: >4 mm pedunculated protrusion
Entry and re-entry sites	Echolucent area in aortic wall with intact intimal surface, with longitudinal and circumferential propagation of haematoma	• Located in descending aorta and arch • Intima intact
Large bulging false lumen and smaller true lumen, identified by colour flow	Displacement of superficial calcification toward lumen	• Intimal thickening, calcification present • Associated with aneurysm
Dissection of proximal ascending aorta associated with AR	Intramural haematoma may find a luminal exit and convert to typical aortic dissection	May develop: a. Penetrating ulcer b. Embolism

FURTHER READING

1. Lang R M, Badani L P, Mor Avi V, et al. Recommendations for Cardiac Chamber Quantification by Echocardiography in Adults: An Update from the American Society of Echocardiography and the European Association of Cardiovascular Imaging. J Am Soc Echocardiogr 2015;28:1–39.
2. Nishimura R A, Otto C M, Bonow R O, et al. 2014 AHA/ACC Guideline for the Management of Patients with Valvular Heart Disease: Executive Summary: A Report of the American College of Cardiology/American Heart Association Task Force on Practice Guidelines. J Am Coll Cardiol 2014;63:2438–2488.
3. Nagueh S F, Smiseth O M, Appleton C P, et al. Recommendations for the Evaluation of Left Ventricular Diastolic Function by Echocardiography: An Update from the American Society of Echocardiography and the European Association of Cardiovascular Imaging. J Am Soc Echocardiogr April 2016;29:277–314.
4. Asch F M, Miyoshi T, Addetia K, et al. Similarities and Differences in Left Ventricular Size and Function among Races and Nationalities: Results of the World Alliance Societies of Echocardiography Normal Values Study. J Am Soc Echocardiogr 2019;32:1396–1406.

4 Assessment of Volume Status in CCU

Swarup Paul and Sunandan Sikdar

Chapter 4 may be accessed online at: www.routledge.com/9780367462215

DOI: 10.1201/9781003027584-4

5 Thoracic Ultrasound

Abhradip Das and Sunandan Sikdar

1. What is the role of thoracic ultrasound sonography (USG) in the cardiac care unit (CCU)?

Air in the lung was once considered the worst enemy of ultrasound, as it creates false images (artefacts). However, typical artefacts and some real images produced by the interaction of the ultrasound beam with the air-fluid interface may help to make an early diagnosis in certain cases. Many bedside real-time protocols (the bedside lung ultrasound in emergency [BLUE] protocol for the immediate diagnosis of acute respiratory failure and the fluid administration limited by lung sonography [FALLS] protocol) are in clinical use now. Recent studies have also demonstrated its high sensitivity and specificity in the diagnosis of heart failure, pneumonia, pneumothorax, pulmonary embolism and pleural effusion. Published performance of lung ultrasounds in critically ill patients compared with CT scanning are given in **Table 5.1**.

Table 5.1: Sensitivity and Specificity for Different Conditions

Ultrasound	Sensitivity %	Specificity %
Pleural effusion	94	97
Alveolar consolidation	90	98
Interstitial syndrome	100	100
Complete pneumothorax	100	96
Occult pneumothorax	79	100

2. What are the types of tools used for thoracic USG?

A linear probe (higher frequency) is used for superficial lung structures. Convex probes (lower frequency) are used for deeper structures. A micro-convex probe is used for various protocols.

There are various methods of examination. Usually, each lung is divided into three spaces on each side. Total six BLUE points are used for protocols (three on each side) (**Figure 5.1**).

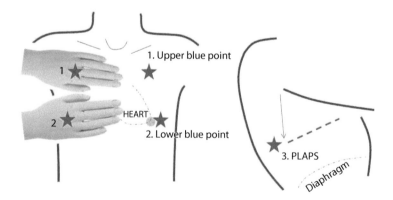

Figure 5.1 Lung ultrasound: Areas of imaging. Note: (1) Upper BLUE point and (2) Lower BLUE point. (3) Posterolateral alveolar and/or pleural syndromes (PAPS) point where horizontal line from lower BLUE point and post-axillary line meet.

3. What is the pleural sliding sign?

The pleura, made of parietal and visceral layers, is seen on-screen as a thick white line, which moves with each respiration. This is called the *pleural sliding sign* (**Figure 5.2a**). *The bat sign*: The ribs on both sides and the pleural line in between outline a silhouette which is reminiscent of a bat. This allows confident recognition of the pleural line in all circumstances, even in patients with acute dyspnoea, patients who are agitated and even in bariatric patients.

DOI: 10.1201/9781003027584-5

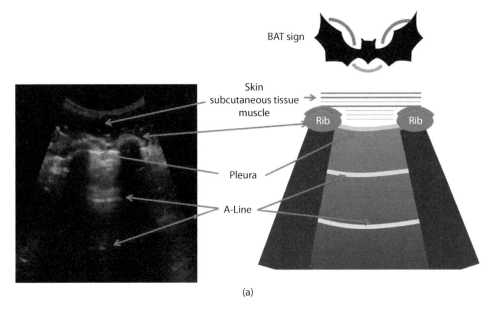

Figure 5.2 (a) Bat sign: Normal lung and A line.

4. What is the seashore sign?

This is a dynamic sign seen in M-mode. The "sea" is described as straight horizontal lines produced by motionless skin, tissue and muscles (real image); and the "shore" is displayed as a granular appearance produced by moving lung (false image). This signifies a normal lung segment in sonological studies.

5. What is the A line?

The A line is a "reverberation" artefact. It is a repetition of the pleural line (white horizontal line), indicating air in the lung. When the ultrasound beam traverses through skin, intercostal muscles, neurovascular bundles and pleura, it produces real images. When it reaches the pleura, it bounces back to the probe and appears as horizontal lines (A line), which are equidistant from the pleural line (**Figure 5.2a**). An A line with pleural sliding signifies a normal lung.

6. What are B lines?

B lines are vertical white thick lines which start from the pleura, traverse throughout and abolish the A line. It is also known as the "lung comet" or "lung rocket" (**Figure 5.2b**). When interlobular septa are enlarged by oedema, the ultrasound waves, while penetrating the lung, suddenly change

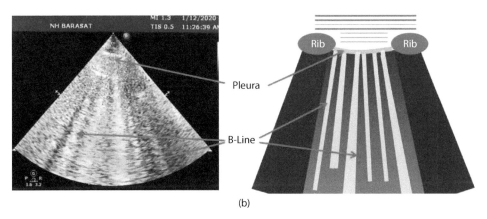

Figure 5.2 (b) Pulmonary oedema and recognition of the B line.

in impedance between gas and fluids, which trap the beam, generating the B line. Fluid in the alveolar space produces multiple B lines in ultrasound (interstitial syndrome). A pattern of three B lines in an intercostal space, called lung rockets, corresponds to the anatomic number of subpleural interlobular septa (oedematous) and are taken as B line positive. Four thoracic ultrasound windows: Right midaxillary, right midclavicular, left midaxillary and left midclavicular, are utilized. If bilateral B lines are found in a symmetric distribution, pulmonary oedema is confirmed. Lung ultrasound plays a crucial role in the bedside diagnosis of pulmonary oedema, especially in patients with preserved ejection fraction and in cases where the chest X-ray is suboptimal, or brain natriuretic peptide (BNP) is not available. It may also differentiate pulmonary oedema from pneumonia in an acutely ill patient.

7. What are Z lines?

Z lines are vertical lines. Unlike B lines, Z lines don't traverse through the screen and don't abolish A lines. They are of normal variant (**Figure 5.2c**).

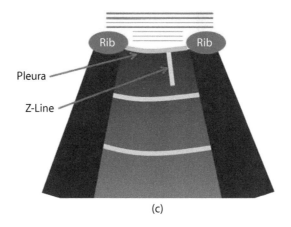

(c)

Figure 5.2   (c) Z line.

8. What are E lines?

These are vertical lines. They originate from above (superficial to) the pleural line (B lines originate from the pleura), i.e., tissue, muscle and skin. These lines are seen in subcutaneous emphysema. As air is a bad conductor of sound, air in the subcutaneous spaces erases all other architectural images with E lines (emphysema lines) (**Figure 5.2d**).

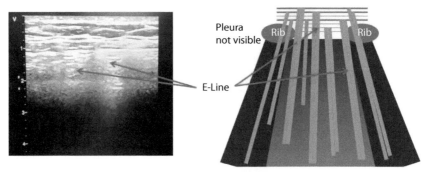

All other images (anterior cortex of rib, pleural line) – erased by E-Line

(d)

Figure 5.2   (d) E line.

9. What are the sonological findings in the case of consolidation (pneumonia)?

Bedside thoracic ultrasound is useful in diagnosing consolidation. The following signs are usually seen:

a. *Shred sign*: At the initial phase of lung consolidation, it appears as patchy B lines. Usually, it is associated with an irregular pleural line, and the B lines originate from various levels of the pleura, unlike the typical wet lung profile, where B lines originate from the smooth pleural line (**Figure 5.3a**).

b. *Tissue-like sign*: As the infective process progresses, more and more lung parenchyma get involved. It looks like a solid tissue (commonly as echogenic as the liver). It is pathologically denoted as "hepatization" of parenchyma of the lung (**Figure 5.3b**).

c. *Air bronchogram*: Movement of air through terminal bronchioles in a consolidated lung parenchyma is well displayed by ultrasound on-screen as moving (in and out) white dots along with respiration. This is called a dynamic air bronchogram (**Figure 5.3b**). It signifies true consolidation (pneumonia). A static air bronchogram may be seen in three conditions: atelectasis, the initial phase of collapse due to blocking of the airway and air trapping.

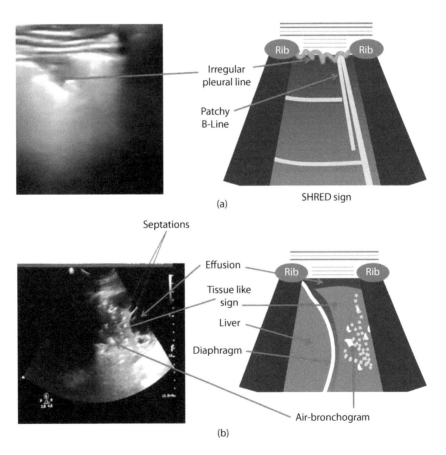

Figure 5.3 (a) Shred sign. (b) Air bronchogram and effusion.

10. What are the sonological findings in pleural effusion?

Bedside ultrasound is a very good tool to pick up a pleural effusion in no time with very high sensitivity and specificity. It appears as an anechoic (black) area between the parietal and visceral pleura. It is picked up earliest at the most dependent part of the pleural cavity as per the patient's position and posture. The size of the effusion changes as the position changes.

The following radiological signs are seen in pleural effusion:

a. *Jellyfish sign*: It is the freely moving collapsed lung with the rhythm of respiration within free fluid (**Figure 5.4a**). Usually, it is seen in large effusions.

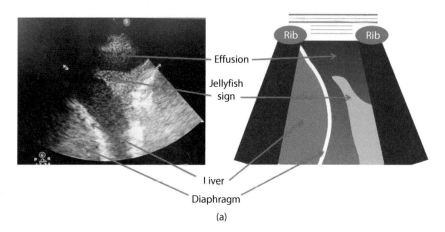

(a)

Figure 5.4 (a) Jellyfish sign for pleural effusion.

b. *Quad sign*: An area of effusion is bounded by the shadow of the adjacent ribs on both sides, by the parietal pleura above and the visceral pleura + lung at the bottom. This is a static sign.

c. *Sinusoid sign*: It is a dynamic sign seen on M-mode. With inspiration, the visceral pleura moves towards the parietal pleura. It is seen in small effusions (**Figure 5.4b**).

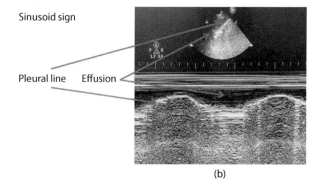

(b)

Figure 5.4 (b) Sinusoid sign for pleural effusion.

d. *Plankton sign*: Floating cellular debris in fluid appears as an internal echo. The debris gets agitated with respiration or cardiac pulsation. It is a real-time dynamic shadow. It signifies the exudative nature of the pleural fluid or a haemothorax.

11. How does ultrasound help to determine the aetiology of a pleural effusion?

An anechoic appearance usually suggests transudative effusion. Transudative effusion is usually seen on both sides.

Fibrotic septa, loculations and echogenic fluid are commonly seen in exudative effusions. An inflammatory process causes the high protein and cellular content of pleural fluid, producing septa and echogenic fluid. A haemothorax may also show the same features.

12. What is the role of USG in thoracentesis or placing an intercostal chest drain (ICD)?

Use of ultrasound in thoracentesis has significantly reduced iatrogenic pneumothorax, bleeding or injury to nearby solid organs.

A. *Marking a safe puncture point*: With a fixed position of the patient, an area of fluid with three or more intercostals placed within an in-plane distance of 1.5 cm or more and in the absence of interposition of any organ can give a good and safe puncture point.

B. With a real-time guide, the needle can be safely placed in the pleural space, avoiding puncture to the visceral pleura.

An ICD can safely be placed under ultrasound guidance by these processes.

13. What are the signs elicited in a pneumothorax?

Rapid diagnosis of a pneumothorax is possible by the following features:

A. In a pneumothorax, there is an absence of lung sliding and the A line.

B. The presence of an A line, B line, lung sliding, lung pulse, consolidation and effusion eventually rules out pneumothorax on that segment.

C. *Barcode sign* or *stratosphere sign*: Horizontal straight motionless lines on M-mode are known as the barcode sign or stratosphere sign. This sign may be seen in a patient with pneumothorax.

D. *Lung point*: This is the point where the lung touches the chest wall during inspiration. This is displayed on-screen on M-mode an as alternate presence of the typical seashore sign on inspiration and the barcode sign on expiration. It is one of the sure signs of pneumothorax. It is seen in a small pneumothorax.

14. What does the diaphragm look like?

The diaphragm is seen on ultrasound as a whiter structure dividing the thoracic and abdominal cavity. It has two echogenic layers – on both sides there is a more whitish pleural and peritoneal line, with a lesser white muscle layer in between. Usually, the thickness of the diaphragm is 22–28 mm in healthy individuals and 13–19 mm in a paralysed diaphragm. Thickness less than 20 mm at the height of expiration indicates diaphragmatic atrophy.

15. What is the BLUE protocol (Figure 5.5)?

At the anterior chest wall, normal lung sliding with predominant A lines defines the **A-profile**. An A-profile indicates a normal lung surface.

Lung sliding with lung rockets defines the **B-profile** and usually indicates **acute haemodynamic pulmonary oedema (AHPE)**. Haemodynamic pulmonary oedema creates a transudative,

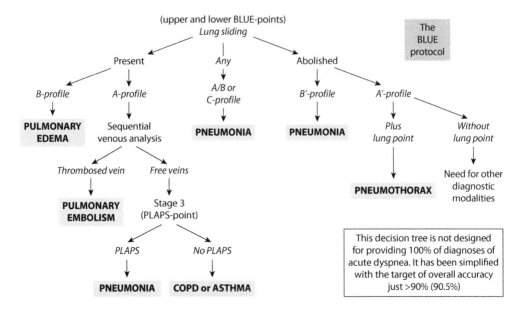

Figure 5.5 The BLUE protocol. (Redrawn with permission from Lichtenstein D, Mezière G A. Relevance of lung ultrasound in the diagnosis of acute respiratory failure: The BLUE protocol. Chest. 2008;134:117–125.)

The FALLS-protocol (Schematic decision tree)

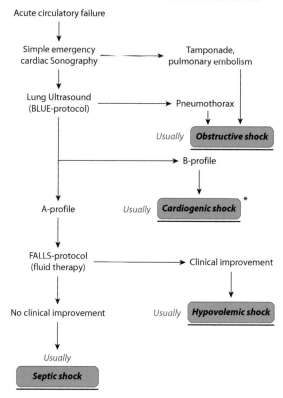

Figure 5.6 The FALLS protocol. *Use SVC or IVC analysis, etc., if non-cardiogenic pulmonary edema suspected. (From Lichtenstein D. Expert Review of Respiratory Medicine. 6(2):155–162.)

pressurized pulmonary oedema, therefore associating lung sliding with lung rockets (multiple B lines → three or more in each field).

Anterior lung rockets associated with abolished lung sliding define the **B'-profile**. It is seen in inflammatory interstitial syndrome (pneumonia).

Unilateral rockets define the **A/B-profile**. This asymmetry of interstitial signs is also linked to pneumonia.

Anterior lung consolidation, regardless of number and size, defines the **C-profile**. In the BLUE protocol, the C-profile is associated with pneumonia. A shredded sign, irregular pleural line, alveolar opacity (tissue-like sign) and both dynamic and static air bronchograms suggest consolidation (pneumonia).

Anterior A lines associated with abolished lung sliding define the **A'-profile**. The A'-profile + the lung point defines a pneumothorax.

An A-profile without deep vein thrombosis (DVT) but with posterolateral alveolar and/or pleural syndrome (A-no-V-PLAPS profile) indicates pneumonia; an A-profile plus DVT indicates pulmonary embolism.

The FALLS protocol has been devised for rapidly diagnosing the cause of shock by echocardiogram and ultrasound (**Figure 5.6**).

FURTHER READING

1. Sikdar S, Das A, Panja A, et al. Lung ultrasound evaluation of diabetic patients with acute onset dyspnea and its relationship with established markers of heart failure. Indian Heart Journal 2018;70:S399–S402.
2. Lichtenstein D, Mezière G A. Relevance of lung ultrasound in the diagnosis of acute respiratory failure: The BLUE protocol. Chest 2008;134:117–125.
3. Lichtenstein D. FALLS-protocol: Lung ultrasound in haemodynamic assessment of shock. Heart, Lung and Vessels 2013;5(3):142–147.

6 Arterial Blood Gas

Swarup Paul and Sunandan Sikdar

Chapter 6 may be accessed online at: www.routledge.com/9780367462215

DOI: 10.1201/9781003027584-6

7 Approach to Electrolyte Abnormalities in CCU

Swarup Paul and Sunandan Sikdar

Chapter 7 may be accessed online at: www.routledge.com/9780367462215

DOI: 10.1201/9781003027584-7

8 Haemodynamics

Sunandan Sikdar and Swarup Paul

1. How do automated blood pressure cuffs work?

Automated blood pressure cuffs work on the basis of oscillometry. While traditional blood pressure cuffs determine the systolic and diastolic pressure from Korotkoff sounds, the automated cuff works on the principle that the amplitude of sensed oscillation is a maximum at mean blood pressure. Thus, *they measure mean blood pressure*. The systolic and diastolic blood pressures are not measured directly; they are derived from the rate of change in the oscillation amplitude based upon proprietary algorithms. Thus, measurement errors may occur in arrhythmia, very low or very high blood pressure, motion artefacts and a cuff of inappropriate size.

2. What factors affect the waveform recorded by the pressure monitoring system?

Like all waves, the pressure waveform (**Figure 8.1**) is a periodic fluctuation of force per unit area and can be resolved into waves of fundamental frequency (ff, cycles per second, at HR of 60/min, it is 60/60 or 1 Hz) along with its multiples (called harmonics, may be like 2, 3, 5 … Hz, etc.). The physiologic information is contained in the ff and its first 10 harmonics. Thus, at an HR of 120/min, the ff is 120/60, or 2 Hz and the 10th harmonic is 20 Hz.

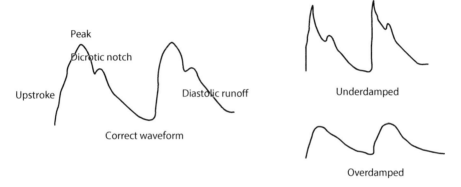

Figure 8.1 Waveforms on invasive monitor.

Three factors determine the crispness of the waveform: Natural frequency of the system, amplitude ratio and damping. These are of crucial importance in invasive arterial monitoring.

The natural frequency (nf) is the frequency at which a system (e.g. the components of a pressure transducer) naturally vibrates once it has been set into motion in the absence of friction. For a system to reproduce a distortion-free arterial pressure waveform with faithful reproduction of detail, when the heart rate is 120 beats/min, the transducer should have a frequency greater than the 10th harmonic of the waveform, i.e., 20 Hz. The larger the bore (increased radius) of the tubing and the shorter its length, less the compliance (no bubbles), less the density of the fluid (no blood) — higher the natural frequency of the system. When the nf of the system approaches the ff of the waveform, the output signal augments dramatically compared to the input signal. In order to maintain a proportional amplitude, a system of dissipation of energy is required, called damping. Optimal damping dissipates the energy of the vibration gradually and maintains a flat frequency response curve.

The amplitude ratio is the ratio of output vs input signal. It should be constant over a broad range of frequencies (also called frequency response – imagine if the ratio changes with HR, the waveform depicted in the monitor would get distorted). A stiff transducer membrane has a good frequency response. A flaccid membrane cannot pick up higher harmonics and distorts the waveform.

The dampening coefficient (must be ~0.5–0.6) quantifies the frictional forces that absorb energy and determine how quickly a signal decays back to baseline. An *underdamped* system overreacts to the pressure curve and gives rise to sharp/exaggerated systolic peaks and diastolic troughs. This leads to systolic and pulse pressure overestimation and diastolic pressure underestimation. Underdampening can be reduced by using longer and thinner tubing. An *overdamped* system, on the other hand, leads to loss of detail in the waveform and erroneously low systolic and pulse pressure.

DOI: **10.1201/9781003027584-8**

Overdampening occurs with additional tubing, stopcocks, air bubbles or blood clots in the system. To reduce the likelihood of overdamping, use of a short, stiff, non-compliant tubing and limiting the number of three-way valves are suggested.

However, in both overdamping and underdamping, the mean BP approximates to the actual mean BP.

3. What is a bedside flush test?

The valve of the continuous flush system must be pulled to generate a square wave on the output tracing. By releasing the valve, a variable number of undershot and overshot waves can be observed that will decay exponentially in accordance with the damping coefficient. Two measures are necessary:

Natural frequency = Paper speed (mm/sec)/Distance between successive peaks (mm)

of the return waves, e.g., 25 (mm/sec)/1.7 mm = 14.7 Hz

The damping coefficient can be derived by calculating the amplitude ratio (dividing the amplitude of the second oscillation by the first, damped/normal amplitude), e.g., 16 mm/22 mm = 0.72.

4. Where is the zero reference?

The axis is the reference or zero line corresponding to the middle point between the sternum and the back (5 cm below the sternum), at the left fourth intercostal space. The transducer should be positioned at the level of this space at the bedside. This is actually the level of the left ventricle and aorta in the supine position.

5. What haemodynamic information is obtained by changes in the arterial pressure waveform?

The pulse contour is the result of wave reflections from arterial bifurcations and high-resistance peripheral arterioles. The main point of reflection is the distal aorta. The more one goes to the periphery from the central aorta, the earlier the peak pressure is reached.

The normal waveform (**Figure 8.2A,B**) consists of a temporal sequence of systolic upstroke, systolic peak, systolic decline, a small hump of the reflected wave, dicrotic notch, diastolic runoff and end-diastolic pressure.

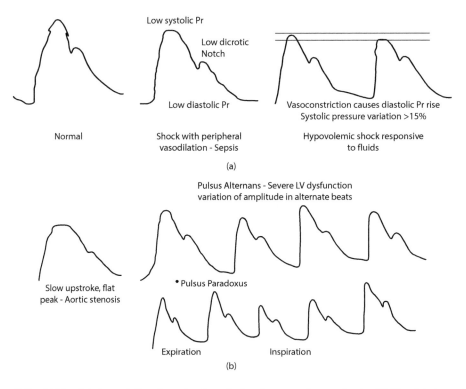

Figure 8.2 (a) Shock interpretation from tracings, 1. Sepsis versus hypovolemia. (b) Shock interpretation from tracings, 2. Alternans versus Paradoxus.

Increased pulse wave velocity and a prominent proximal hump of the reflected wave suggest arterial wall stiffening, as in ageing.

A rise in both systolic and diastolic pressures with a relatively early diastolic notch suggests vasoconstriction.

Reduced systolic and diastolic pressures and a delayed and low dicrotic notch suggest severe vasodilatation (e.g., sepsis, vasovagal reflex, nitrate administration), as a longer time is needed for the aortic pressure to exceed the ventricular pressure. However, if low pressure is associated with an early dicrotic notch, the possibility of volume loss with peripheral vasoconstriction should be kept in mind.

In cases of shock, except during acute inflammation, diastolic waves are often increased when hypotension is compensated for by peripheral vasoconstriction.

In aortic stenosis, the wave contour is rounded (pulsus parvus) due to the slow ejection and the dicrotic notch is less prominent. In aortic regurgitation, the reverse occurs – the waveform is characterized by a steep rise of the systolic upstroke, low diastolic and wide pulse pressure.

Alternation of beats with higher and lower pulse pressures is indicative of severe left ventricular dysfunction, called pulsus alternans. The augmented beat is due to the extra preload caused by excess blood remaining from the previous ejection.

In pulsus paradoxus, the rise of systolic blood pressure (SBP) in expiration and the fall in inspiration is exaggerated and is a characteristic feature of cardiac tamponade.

During positive pressure mechanical ventilation, the following changes occur: During inspiration due to increased pulmonary inflow into the left atrium (LA), left ventricle (LV) and reduced afterload, the stroke volume of LV, and hence the SBP, increases. During expiration due to pulmonary sequestration of blood, the SBP falls. If the difference of maximum SBP and the minimum SBP (called the systolic pressure variation) is more than 15%, provided there is no spontaneous breath or arrhythmia, a fluid challenge to treat hypotension is reasonable.

6. What are the uses of central venous pressure (CVP)?

Use of CVP has declined, but where it is being used it provides:

a. An idea of volume status; though this measurement has its pitfalls, response to fluid challenge and measurement during progressive hypotension does give some clues. CVP represents right atrium (RA) pressure and, by extension, right ventricle (RV) diastolic pressure in the absence of tricuspid stenosis.

b. The CVP waveforms have diagnostic value.

c. The line can be used to deliver fluids and drugs. It can be used to sample mixed venous O_2 saturation in those without a pulmonary catheter (ScVO$_2$). ScVO$_2$ >70% in septic shock is a useful target.

7. Where is the zero of CVP?

At the mid-point of the RA. A good approximation of this point is a vertical distance 5 cm below the sternal angle, where the second rib meets the sternum. This level is valid whether the subject is supine or sitting up. In practice, however, the transducer is levelled to the mid-thoracic position. This results in values ~3 mmHg higher than those based on the sternal angle, with the precise difference varying with chest size.

8. What are the waves of CVP?

The CVP tracing has three distinguishable upward waves:

a – atrial contraction

• *Significance*: Canon a wave – complete heart block

Tall a – Tricuspid stenosis

c – Bellowing up of tricuspid valve at onset of ventricular systole

v – RA filling

• *Significance*: Tall v wave – severe tricuspid regurgitation

The two downward waves are:

"x" – descent due to atrial relaxation

"y" – due to atrial emptying during the early phase of diastole

- *Significance*:
    - Prominent y descent – restrictive physiology
    - Absent y descent – cardiac tamponade

9. Where do you measure CVP?

In normal CVP, the a and v are large waves with a > v. The c wave is a minute deflection on the descending limb of the 'a' wave coinciding with the end of QRS on the ECG on the monitor. The CVP should be measured at the c wave in end expiration. An alternative is the base of the 'a' wave.

10. How do you interpret CVP?

In normal sitting subjects, CVP is sub-atmospheric, yet there is no need to give fluid. The value of CVP by itself is most useful in the negative sense. A high CVP indicates that fluid boluses are unlikely to be helpful. CVP measurements can assist in assessing the response to a fluid challenge. For practical purposes, the increase in CVP should be ≥2 mmHg on fluid bolus, as this can be readily identified on a monitor. If there is no inspiratory fall in CVP, it is unlikely that the patient will be fluid-responsive. Respiratory swings of CVP give an idea about inspiratory efforts and lung compliance.

11. What is a high CVP?

The plateau of the cardiac function curve usually occurs at values <10 mmHg (13–14 mmHg if using the mid-thoracic level). Without any measure of cardiac output, it is thus reasonable to target a CVP of 10 mmHg, as recommended in early goal-directed resuscitation protocols.

12. How does pulse oximetry work?

Oximetry is the measurement of oxyhaemoglobin in blood as a percentage of haemoglobin (Hb) species. The absorption of light is proportional to chromatophore concentration (Beer's law) and the thickness of the transmitting layer (Lambert's law). The differing absorption of light (emitted by two light-emitting diodes [LEDs] with wavelengths 660 nm red and 940 nm infrared) by two different species of Hb (oxy Hb and deoxy Hb) is measured by a photodiode. The transmitted and reflected signal is digitalized and the difference between systolic and diastolic measured to give a pulsatile component (ac) and non-pulsatile component (dc), therefore allowing for quantification of absorption due to tissue, venous blood and nail polish (this is the dc component). Finally, the ratio (R) is obtained as follows: (ac 660/ac 940)/(dc 940/dc 660). This R is then compared by the software to a standard table (SpO$_2$ of human volunteers breathing various known concentration of oxygen) to determine the SpO$_2$. Thus, SpO$_2$ is 94%, which means that 94% of the patients' haemoglobin is oxy Hb at that FiO$_2$ and oxygen flow. The probe calculates SpO$_2$ about 25 times/sec, rejects artefacts and determines the average of SpO$_2$ over 3–12 sec and updates the screen every 1–2 sec. Information about heart rate and pulse contour is also obtained.

13. What is the lag time for a drop in SpO$_2$ when FiO$_2$ is reduced?

The lag time is 10 sec for ear probes and 50 sec for finger probes.

14. What are the limitation of pulse oximeters?

a. Methaemoglobin (Met Hb) and carboxy Hb (COHb) cannot be determined, even though they may be producing hypoxia. Pulse oximeters read HbCO as mostly HbO$_2$ and over-read SO$_2$ by 1% for every 1% of COHb in the blood. For reading this, co-oximeters (using multiple wavelengths of light) are required.

b. Hypoperfusion reduces the accuracy of the SpO$_2$ measurement, and this is a common problem in the cardiac care unit (CCU) where patients are frequently on pressors.

c. They are insensitive to large changes in PaO_2 in the high PaO_2 range.

d. When the skin is cold or in presence of strong light, SpO_2 may be low.

e. Methylene blue and indocyanine green absorb red light, artificially lowering SpO_2.

f. MRI and cautery may interfere with SpO_2.

15. What are the markers of tissue hypoxia?

The ultimate common pathway of different aetiologies of shock is tissue hypoxia. It is defined as inadequate oxygen delivery compared to demand of metabolically active tissue. Normally in the presence of adequate oxygen, cellular glycolysis generates pyruvate, which enters mitochondria and participates in the Krebs cycle generating NADPH and FADH; these in turn generate adenosine triphosphate (ATP) by the electron transport chain using oxygen (36 ATP/cycle). When oxygen is inadequate, electron transport suffers, leading to mitochondrial dysfunction, and excess pyruvate is accumulated in the cell by anaerobic glycolysis (2 ATP/cycle). This pyruvate is converted to L-lactate by lactate dehydrogenase (D-lactate is found in intestinal flora). This lactate diffuses out of the cell and increases blood lactate levels (when haemodynamics are normal, part of it is taken up by the liver, and through the Cori cycle it is converted back to glucose – this beneficial mechanism is reduced in shock). Further in shock-like situations, oxygen extraction by capillaries becomes maximum, leading to decreased venous oxygen and widening of the arteriovenous oxygen difference.

Thus, the *markers of tissue hypoxia* are actually the markers of global hypoperfusion, as non-invasive measurement of tissue hypoxia is difficult in clinical practice:

a. $ScVO_2$ (venous saturation from central line) <70%

b. L-Lactate >3 mEq/L

c. P (v-a) CO_2 (veno-arterial CO_2 difference) >6 mmHg

16. What are the causes of increased lactate?

Anaerobic causes (Type A hyperlactataemia)

- Circulatory shock
- Microcirculatory shunting (sepsis)
- Carbon monoxide poisoning

Aerobic causes (Type B hyperlactataemia)

- Catecholamine (especially epinephrine)-induced stimulation of Na^+ and K^+ transporters
- Thiamine deficiency
- Sepsis
- Liver dysfunction (reduced clearance)
- Seizures
- Malignancy (Warburg effect – glycolysis under aerobic conditions)
- Drug induced – metformin, steroids, propofol, nucleoside reverse transcriptase inhibitors
- Toxins – methanol, ethylene glycol

17. What are the precautions of lactate sampling?

In leucocytosis and high haematocrit levels, lactate may be spuriously increased due to ongoing glycolysis. Analysis should be done within 15 min; otherwise, storage must be at <4°C or the use of fluoride oxalate tubes should be ensured.

18. What is the lactate-related target of resuscitation?

Reduction of lactate by 20% by the steps undertaken in **Figure 8.3**.

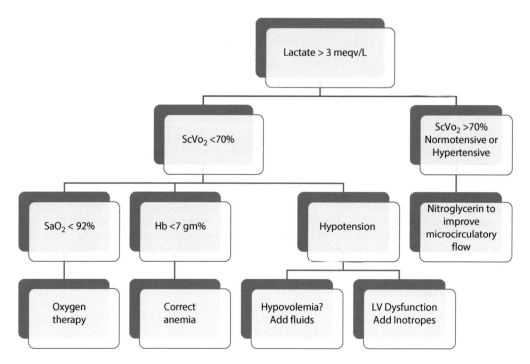

Figure 8.3 Lactate-guided management.

19. What raises the suspicion of ethylene glycol toxicity?

When this toxin is suspected, send one sample for arterial blood gas (ABG) sampling and another to the central lab. When point-of-care ABG shows increased lactate, but the central lab report does not, ethylene glycol toxicity is suspected.

FURTHER READING

1. Romagnoli S, Zagli G. Blood Pressure Monitoring in ICU, in Web A, Angus D, Feinfer S, et al. (eds) Oxford Textbook of Critical Care, 2nd Edition (2016): 609–612.
2. Jansen T C, Bakker J. Lactate Monitoring in ICU, in Web A, Angus D, Feinfer S, et al. (eds) Oxford Textbook of Critical Care, 2nd Edition (2016): 644–648.
3. Mocucci M, Grossman W. Pressure measurement, in Mosucci M (Ed): Grossman and Baims Cardiac Cathererization, Angiography and Intervention, 8th Edition (2014):223–244. Wolters Kluwer.

9 The Role and Interpretation of Biomarkers

Sunandan Sikdar, Barnik Chaudhuri, and Arijita Mukherjee

CLINICAL PEARL: CAN TROPONIN BE RAISED IN NORMAL INDIVIDUALS WITHOUT ISCHAEMIC HEART DISEASE?

As assays have become more and more sensitive, cardiac troponin can be detected even in normal population. In fact, sensitive assays can detect troponin in 20%–50% of the normal population, while highly sensitive assays can detect troponin in 50%–90% of healthy individuals. At what troponin level it will be labelled as pathological elevation is given as the 99th percentile of that particular assay by the respective manufacturer. This means that if the blood level exceeds that particular concentration only in one out of 100 individuals it will be false positive – that is a healthy person is misdiagnosed. Even with this cut-off it, is estimated that 20% of emergency room troponin-positive cases will *fail* to be finally labelled as acute coronary syndrome.

---

1. What is a biomarker?

A biomarker is noninvasive (usually body fluid-based) tool that reproducibly indicates the diagnosis or severity of one or more pathophysiological processes.

2. What are cardiac biomarkers?

Cardiac biomarkers are listed in **Table 9.1**.

Table 9.1: Biomarkers in Cardiovascular Disease

Parameter	Ischaemia	Heart Failure	Fibrosis/ Remodelling	Coagulation	Heart-Kidney Interaction	Aortic Dissection/ Aortitis
Standard	• Troponin I • Troponin T	• BNP • NT-Pro BNP	sST2	• D-dimer • Fibrinogen	• Creatinine • Cystatin C	D-dimer
Emerging	• Heart type Fatty acid binding protein	• Mid-regional pro-ANP • Copeptin (for severity)	Galectin 3	• Anti-thrombin • Protein C	NGAL	sST2
Less used now	• CPK-MB • Myoglobin					

---

3. What are the precautions during blood sampling for biomarkers?

Troponin values will depend on, if the sample is heparinized or not. A heparinized sample was used in the LITROP study for both hs-Trop T and Trop I. Brain natriuretic peptide (BNP) is usually collected in ethylenediaminetetraacetic acid (EDTA) vials, and they should be preserved with ice. BNP degrades quite rapidly and can give false-negative results. On the other hand, NT-Pro BNP is relatively stable.

4. What is troponin?

A contractile unit of sarcomere contains thick filaments (myosin) and thin filaments (actin). The troponin-tropomyosin complex localized on actin regulates the calcium-induced interaction of actin and myosin, which is the basis of heart muscle shortening. Troponin C binds calcium, troponin T is the link between tropomyosin and actin and troponin I inhibits cross-bridge formation when calcium is absent.

5. What are the non-cardiac causes of disproportionately raised troponin?

That pulmonary embolism, pulmonary hypertension and aortic dissection will cause raised levels is expected, but the more surprising among the list includes both hypothyroidism and

DOI: 10.1201/9781003027584-9

hyperthyroidism; any critical illness, including sepsis and burns; infiltrative diseases, including amyloidosis, sarcoidosis and scleroderma; cardiotoxic drugs (doxorubicin, 5-fluorouracil, trastuzumab); snake bite; endurance athletes; acute neurological events like stroke; and subarachnoid haemorrhage. So, in chest pain with ECG changes and raised troponin, each member of the big three – acute coronary syndrome (ACS), aortic dissection and pulmonary embolism – should be considered. Troponin is an organ-specific marker of myocardial injury, not a disease-specific marker. So, ECG, echocardiogram and symptoms should to be considered prior to a diagnosis of ACS.

6. What type of assay is used in measuring troponin?

Non-competitive enzyme-linked immunosorbent assays (ELISAs) based on the sandwich principle, using a capture antibody and a detection antibody (which attaches to a signal system). These antibodies bind the troponin fragments of the serum.

7. What is the advantage of hs-troponin over previous assays?

Introduction of hs-troponin has reduced the troponin-blind window while diagnosing myocardial infarction (MI). The rise is quite rapid, and serial measurement at 1 or 3 hours may suffice rather than waiting for 6 hours (**Figure 9.1**). Instead of considering troponin as a binary (positive or negative) biomarker, considering the absolute level and rate of rise is more appropriate. The larger the absolute level or the rate of rise, the more certain the diagnosis of ischaemia. However, if there is severe angina with ST elevation on the ECG, one must not wait for troponin, high sensitivity or otherwise.

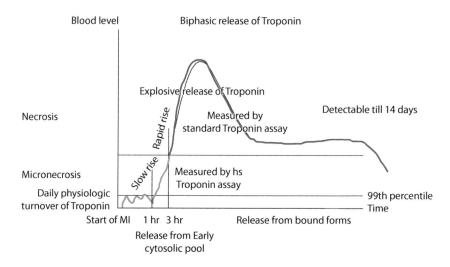

Figure 9.1 Troponin release kinetics and the importance of early detection by hs-troponin assays.

8. What are the disadvantages of the newer-generation assays?

By convention, the 99th percentile has been used as the cut-off based on a reference normal population. However, confusion arises as cTnI has different 99th percentile values from different manufacturers. Further, while evaluating acute chest pain, one in five patients will have discordant results between troponin T and troponin I.

9. What are the requirements for labelling a troponin assay as high sensitivity?

The coefficient of variation (CV) of troponin assays should be <10% at the 99th percentile upper reference limit in a normal population, and they need to measure concentrations above their limit of detection in >50% of a normal reference population. Sex-neutral cut-off of hs-troponin T is 14 ng/L and of hs-troponin I is 26 ng/mL (men have a higher cut-off than women). There is no circadian variation of levels of this marker.

10. What is the prognostic import of troponin?

Rise of troponin confers an adverse prognosis. In heart failure (HF), coronary artery disease, chronic kidney disease and pulmonary arterial hypertension, raised troponin signifies worse outcomes.

Rise of troponin in kidney disease may be due to both increased release and decreased clearance. Preoperative or postoperative rise of troponin in relation to non-cardiac surgery portends increased 30-day mortality. Nearly 90% of these patients have no chest pain, and this is usually a silent event. Thus, it may be prudent to get a preoperative and postoperative day 1 and day 2 troponin level in patients who are elderly (>65 years) or those with vascular risk factors.

11. What is the mechanism of release of troponin from cytosol?

There is a biphasic release of troponin (**Figures 9.1** and **9.2**) during ischaemia – the initial peak is due to release from the injured sarcomere's cytosolic pool (predominately free troponin T) and the later sustained phase from degradation of contractile apparatus (by the enzymes calpain, caspase and metalloproteinase). The latter phase indicates the extent of infarct. Thus after ischaemic insult, different forms of troponin are detected – free-form (4%–6%), binary and ternary forms.

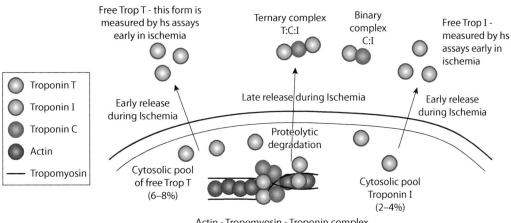

Figure 9.2 Concept of biphasic release of troponin.

12. What are the biomarkers for HF?

The natriuretic peptides are the established biomarkers for HF: BNP and NT-pro-BNP. The peptide is predominantly released from ventricular myocardium in response to stretch as a prohormone, pro-BNP. Half of this undergoes cleavage to active fragment BNP by neural endopeptidases and the other half cleaves to NT-pro-BNP. The BNP binds to the NPR-A receptor to counteract the renin-angiotensin and sympathetic system effects by cyclic guanosine monophosphate (cGMP). The NT-pro-BNP undergoes renal clearance. The BNP has a shorter half-life (20 min) compared with NT-pro-BNP (120 min).

13. What are the biological factors affecting natriuretic peptide levels?

Higher BNP levels are found in the elderly. Pathological states like renal failure and pulmonary hypertension/pulmonary embolism can cause raised BNP levels. In patients treated by the drug sacubitril-valsartan BNP levels may be falsely high, and NT-pro-BNP should be used to tailor therapy. In flash pulmonary oedema (1- to 2-hr symptom onset) and rarely in acute mitral regurgitation, the BNP level may be falsely low.

14. What are the normal cut-offs for natriuretic peptide measurements?

For the test, a 5-cc sample is taken in an EDTA (1 mg/mL) vial and measured by fluorescence immunoassay. BNP: <35 pg/mL (non-acute), <100 pg/mL (acute), NT-pro-BNP: <125 pg/mL (<75 years, non-acute), <450 pg/mL (>75 years, non-acute), <300 pg/mL (acute). In the BASEL study (2004) in acute dyspnoea in the emergency department (ED), the rule-out value of BNP for HF was <100 pg/mL and the rule-in value >500 pg/mL. In the PRIDE study (2005) the HF rule in cut-offs for NT-pro-BNP were >450 pg/mL for <50 years and >900 pg/mL for >50 years. The rule-out HF value for NT-pro-BNP is conventionally <300 pg/mL. For BNP values between 100 and 500 pg/mL right ventricular (RV) overload (pulmonary embolism and cor pulmonale) and renal failure should be considered apart from early/treated HF.

15. What are the non-cardiac causes of disproportionately raised BNP?

The more important causes are age, liver disease, sepsis, subarachnoid haemorrhage, stroke, trauma and anaemia.

16. What are the causes of disproportionately low BNP?

They include obesity and flash pulmonary oedema (1–2 hours). Pericardial diseases are characterized by dyspnoea with low BNP levels.

17. What are the diagnostic and prognostic import of BNP?

If the level of BNP/NT-pro-BNP is above the cut-off and symptoms/signs of HF are present, then echocardiography-guided left ventricular ejection fraction (LVEF) <40%, 40%–49% and >50% defines the entities of HF with reduced EF (HFrEF), HF with mildly reduced EF (HFmrEF) and HF with preserved EF (HFpEF), respectively. Raised BNP reliably predicts restrictive cardiomyopathy and rules out constrictive pericarditis. The level of BNP after treatment has been taken as a marker of clinical improvement across various studies.

18. What is the role of D-dimer?

Fibrinogen is converted by thrombin (**Figure 9.3**) to fibrin monomers, which undergo cross-linking to form polymers, a state that is stabilized by factor XIII. Plasmin degrades the fibrin network to generate D-dimers (two D subunits linked together). D-dimer is named from the D subunit of fibrinogen (fibrinogen has one D subunit flanking an E subunit, D-E-D).

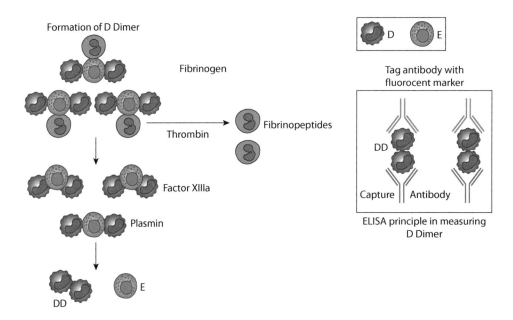

Figure 9.3 Formation of D-dimer and its measurement principle by ELISA.

19. What are the methods and cut-off values of D-dimer measurement?

D-dimer is measured by any of (1) whole-blood agglutination assays (semiquantitative positive/negative) – this has low sensitivity and should be avoided; (2) enzyme-linked immunosorbent (**Figure 9.3**) or immunofluorescent assays (ELISA and ELFA, respectively); and (3) latex agglutination assays (immunoturbidometric method). Often the numerical results of different methods/manufacturers are not comparable. D-dimer has high sensitivity but poor specificity for the detection of venous thromboembolism.

The normal cut-off is <500 mcg/L for <50 years; for age >50 years, the cut-off is 10 times the age (e.g., for 60 years, the cut-off is 600 mcg/L). For those with low pre-test probability, the more appropriate cut-off would be 1000 mcg/L.

20. What is the diagnostic importance of D-dimer?

It is predominately used in diagnosing venous thromboembolism (VTE), particularly in those with a low probability of VTE. It lacks specificity and can be raised in pregnancy, puerperium, chronic inflammatory conditions and hospital inpatients. Hence, in these conditions testing for D-dimer is rarely of value and imaging tests should be used.

However, it may also be of help in ruling out aortic dissection in low-risk patients (cut-off <500 mcg/L) and in disseminated intravascular coagulation (DIC).

In women with maintenance anticoagulation after an index VTE, a negative D-dimer can be used to decide when to stop anticoagulation after a proper time.

21. What are the biomarkers of aortic dissection?

Markers related to vascular smooth muscle (smooth muscle myosin), the interstitium (calponin), the elastic lamina (elastin), endothelial cells and blood-nonintima interactions (D-dimer) have been studied. D-dimer and an interleukin receptor family member, soluble ST2 (sST2), has been found to have clinical utility. A cut-off value of sST2 <34.6 ng/mL has been suggested to rule out aortic dissection in acute chest pain patients.

FURTHER READING

1. Park K C, Gaze D C, Collinson P O, et al. Cardiac Troponins: From Myocardial Infarction to Chronic Disease. Cardiovasc Res 2017;113:1708–1718.
2. Weitz J I, Fredenburgh J C, Eikelboom J W. A Test in Context: D-Dimer. J Am Coll Cardiol 2017;70:2411–2420.

10 Acute Chest Pain

Sunandan Sikdar and Mrinal Kanti Das

10.1 INTRODUCTION

Acute chest pain is a very important symptom in the cardiovascular system. A thorough clinical history and examinations at the emergency room (ER) can offer a lot of inputs regarding the aetiology. However, there is always the need for supporting investigations to clinch the cause. The following discussion in the format of questions is an attempt to arrive at the appropriate diagnosis of acute chest pain.

1. What are the characteristics of ischaemic chest pain?

Differentiating angina or ischaemic pain from non-ischaemic ones is of paramount importance in the cardiac care unit (CCU). However, in the elderly and in women, it is often difficult to differentiate. In diabetics the chest pain may be absent. The special characteristics of chest pain may be clarified using OLD CAAR mnemonic.

a. *Onset*: Sudden (acute coronary syndrome [ACS])/gradual (underlying chronic stable angina)

b. *Location*: Retrosternal

c. *Duration*: >20 min in the case of ACS, <10 min suggests relatively stable

d. *Character*: Deep and dull

e. *Aggravating factors*: At rest suggests ACS; on exertion suggest stable angina syndrome

f. *Associated symptoms*: Dyspnoea/sweating/syncope

g. *Radiation*: Arm

Chest pain should not be labelled as typical or atypical; rather, it should be labelled as cardiac, possibly cardiac or non-cardiac. In patients of 75 years of age or more, ACS should be suspected if there is dyspnoea, syncope or delirium along with pain (AHA 2021).

2. What is the differential diagnosis of acute chest pain and the identifying features?

The identifying features are shown in **Table 10.1**.

Table 10.1: Differential Diagnosis of Acute Chest Pain

Diagnosis	Presentation
Angina	• Retrosternal, deep, poorly localized chest pain radiating to neck, jaw, epigastrium • Duration ~2–10 min; triggered by stress, exercise, cold; often early morning; relieved by nitrates
Unstable angina	Angina at rest (usually >20 min)/severe pain, new onset (<1 mo)/crescendo pattern
Myocardial infarction	Sudden onset, angina-like, but more severe, duration >30 min, not relieved by nitrates
Aortic dissection	Sudden tearing pain with radiation to back, maximum at onset then may stabilize "Patient may not be able to continue holding a teacup"
Pulmonary embolism	Sudden onset, pleuritic pain, dyspnoea, sometimes associated with haemoptysis, often there is a history of immobilization, postoperative state, malignancy
Pneumothorax	• Pleuritic pain and dyspnoea. History of COPD/chest trauma/subclavian cannulation • Dyspnoea >> Pain
Pericarditis	• Positional ache, sharp stabbing pain • Relief on bending forward, increase on deep inspiration, occasional history of fever
Mitral valve prolapse	May occur at rest or exertion and can be associated with dizziness, hyperventilation, anxiety, depression, palpitations and fatigue
Pneumonia	Pleuritic pain, associated with fever, cough, dyspnoea, chills
Oesophageal rupture	• Constant retrosternal, epigastric pain • Often severe • History of inciting event, like vomiting/trauma

(Continued)

DOI: 10.1201/9781003027584-10

Table 10.1 (*Continued*): **Differential Diagnosis of Acute Chest Pain**

Diagnosis	Presentation
Musculoskeletal or chest wall pain syndromes	Highly localized, sharp chest pain and reproducible by light to moderate palpation, often related to movement/muscular action
GERD	Burning or gnawing, usually in the lower half of the chest and often accompanied by a brackish or acidic taste in the back of the mouth, pain precipitated by lying flat and relived by sitting up/antacids
Peptic ulcer disease	Postprandial, dull, boring pain located in the mid-epigastric region

3. What is Levine's sign?

When the patient clenches the fist in front of the sternum while describing the sensation (Levine's sign), it is classically described as ischaemic in origin.

4. What is the approach to a patient with cardiac chest pain?

Step 1. *Assess for haemodynamic stability*: In the case of haemodynamic instability, the possibility of ischaemic heart disease, aortic dissection, acute pulmonary embolism or cardiac tamponade must be ruled out rapidly. The nature of chest pain and the physical exam may be a clue, but for confirmation proceed to Step 2.

Step 2. *Four sequential tests are done in rapid succession*: This will give a diagnosis in most cases: ECG, echocardiography, troponin, chest X-ray (CXR). In all patients with chest pain, the ECG must be obtained within the first 10 minutes of arrival in the ER.

ECG confirms ST-segment elevated myocardial infarction (STEMI) or ACS. If suspicion is high but the ECG is not diagnostic, perform serial ECGs. Leads V7–V9 should be done to rule out posterior myocardial infarction (MI).

Echocardiography confirms cardiac tamponade and ischaemic heart disease. It can offer a clue about aortic dissection and pulmonary embolism.

Troponin: Very high values of troponin confirm ACS/STEMI. Moderate values can occur in pulmonary embolism.

CXR confirms a widened mediastinum and leads to suspicion of aortic dissection. It also rules out pneumothorax.

Based on Step 2, the next investigation is decided in Step 3.

Step 3. For suspected ACS or STEMI, one should proceed to coronary angiography. For suspected pulmonary embolism, the investigation of choice is contrast-enhanced CT scan of the chest. For aortic dissection, contrast CT of the chest/CT angiography suffices (**Figure 10.1**). CT scan of the chest will often surprise us with a diagnosis of pneumonia or pneumothorax, if they were missed in CXR.

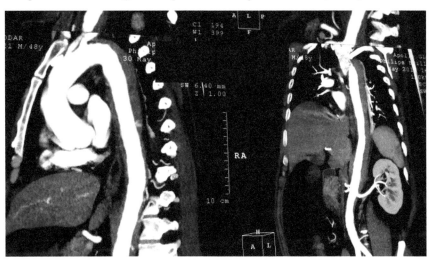

Figure 10.1 A middle-aged male patient presenting with severe chest, back pain and hypertensive crisis. CT aortic angiography shows Type B aortic dissection extending to the renal arteries.

Step 4. If the patient is haemodynamically stable, even then the tests mentioned in Step 2 are necessary. However, if no cause is found and gastrointestinal causes are suspected, appropriate referral is done, and endoscopy done after the patient is stabilized.

Using the treadmill test (TMT) as a predischarge workup is discussed later. The crux of the workup lies in the decision as to whether the patient can be discharged home.

Patients with normal troponin levels, no ECG abnormalities and a TIMI risk score of 0 or a HEART score of ≤3 have extremely low risk of adverse cardiovascular events and can be considered for discharge.

5. What are the elements of the TIMI risk score?

There are seven elements in the TIMI score, which is used to risk-stratify patients with ACS. The score is used to calculate risk of death/MI/revascularization at 14 days as given in **Table 10.2**.

Table 10.2: TIMI Score and Its Significance in Acute Coronary Syndrome

Parameters Counted (7) Each parameter 1 Point	Number of Parameters Positive	Death/MI/Revascularization at 14 Days (%)
Age >65 years	0–1	4.3
Risk factor for CAD >3	2	8.3
Aspirin use in past 7 days	3	13.2
Two or more episodes of angina in the past 24 hr	4	19.9
Troponin positive	5	26.2
≥0.5 mm deviation of the ST segment on ECG	6–7	40.9
Known coronary artery stenosis >50%		

Low risk: 0–2, intermediate risk 3–4, high risk: 5 and above.

6. Can the ECG be normal in an acute myocardial infarction (AMI)?

A normal ECG does not assure absence of ischaemic heart disease. AMI may still be present with a normal ECG in 4% of those with a history of coronary artery disease (CAD) and in 2% of those without such a history. A normal ECG has a negative predictive value of 90% for ruling out ischaemia in the case of acute chest pain.

7. What are the suggestive ECG findings in acute chest pain?

Though comparison with an older ECG is useful, they are often not available at the ER/CCU at the time of need. However, the following findings are of importance in diagnosing ACS

a. ST elevation >1 mm of new onset

b. ST depression of >0.05 mm that spontaneously resolves (dynamic ST change)

c. New Q wave

d. Fixed ST depression of recent onset

e. Conduction defect like left bundle branch block (LBBB) (or rarely right bundle branch block [RBBB]) of new onset.

The ECG may give a clue in the case of pericarditis (ST elevation with concavity up in multiple leads not fitting the MI pattern and with associated PR-segment depression) or in pulmonary embolism (sinus tachycardia, right axis, RBBB, T inversion in V1–V4, S1Q3T3 sign).

8. What is the frequency of doing troponin in the acute chest pain workup?

Troponin is done at presentation and at 3–6 hours after symptom onset. Due to the high sensitivity of troponin assays (some assays detect troponin even as low as <0.001 ng/mL), it may show biomarker positivity even in some without ACS. If the serial troponin measurement is negative, ACS can be ruled out with a high degree of certainty (negative predictive value [NPV] approaching 99%).

9. What is the role of the D-dimer test in the ER?

A negative D-dimer test rules out pulmonary embolism with an NPV of 99% and aortic dissection with an NPV of 96%.

10. What is the role of exercise ECG testing (treadmill test, TMT) in the ER?

For patients with low risk, with all the Step 2 tests normal, TMT has a strong NPV (99%) and poor positive predictive value (50%). It is a safe test, provided the modified Bruce protocol is used. Thus TMT can be considered as a part of the discharge pathway (negative TMT to discharge) in the following patients

a. Two sets of cardiac enzymes at 4-hour intervals – normal

b. ECG at admission and just before TMT – normal

c. Chest pain fully resolved before TMT/pain was not like angina

Contraindications are the standard contraindications of TMT: Changing ECG/rising biomarker/anginal pain. However, it is a fact that in the South Asian population with a high prevalence of triple-vessel disease, it is wise to be cautious while deciding whether to proceed with the TMT. Even if the three conditions are met, angina may be precipitated requiring emergent angiography. A wiser protocol may be to perform the test 1 or 2 days later in selected patients.

11. What is the role of imaging tests in acute chest pain?

Frequently patients with acute chest pain have comorbidities (osteoarthritis, costochondritis, chronic obstructive pulmonary disease [COPD], neurologic diseases) and non-interpretable ECGs (LBBB, left ventricular hypertrophy [LVH], Wolff-Parkinson-White [WPW] syndrome) that preclude advising a TMT. Three tests are available to help the clinician with their relative merits and demerits vis-a-vis one another:

a. *Radionuclide perfusion scan (thallium/technetium)*: While a stress imaging–induced myocardial perfusion defect implies provocable ischaemia, a defect at rest implies active ischemia or an old MI. This can be differentiated once pain subsides and the test is repeated. To correlate the chest pain with a perfusion defect, the imaging test must be performed during active pain or at least within 2 hours of chest pain resolution. A high-risk rest perfusion scan is an indication to proceed to coronary angiography. A low-risk rest perfusion scan predicts <2% of cardiac event rates in a month, and patients can be reassured.

b. *Stress echocardiography*: When wall motion abnormalities are present at rest, usually it is advisable to proceed to coronary angiography. However, if the chest pain is resolved and wall motion abnormalities are absent, dobutamine stress echocardiography (DSE) with its high sensitivity (85%) and specificity (90%) is a useful test. Risks of ischaemia and arrhythmia in this situation are obviously higher than standard DSE done in stable CAD. Patients with a normal DSE can be reassured.

c. *CT coronary angiography (CAG)*: CT-CAG has the virtue of being able to differentiate the "big three" of chest pain – ACS, pulmonary embolism and aortic dissection – in one go (triple rule-out). However, apart from ACS, the other two are very rare, and hence when cost, radiation exposure and contrast load are considered in balance, its intuitive advantage is not that clearly established in clinical practice. CT-CAG is recommended in patients of <65 years of age with a low or intermediate likelihood of obstructive CAD. CT-CAG gives a coronary calcium score and predicts advanced atherosclerosis and unstable plaques. Unstable plaques are characterized by positive remodelling of the vessel, i.e. dilatation, plaques with low attenuation <30 Hounsfield units, napkin ring sign and spotty calcium. However, being an anatomical test, it cannot predict ischaemia. That can be done by special software (CT-FFR [fractional flow reserve]) or by coupling it with positron emission tomography (PET) (PET-CT). But these are rarely available in the ER. CT-CAG, with a high sensitivity (90%) and moderate specificity (65%–90%), is a good rule-out test if normal. Utilizing this test in a low-risk population (TIMI risk score 2 or less) with a normal or indeterminate ECG and a normal biomarker, a higher proportion of patients can be discharged home confidently in a shorter time (**Figure 10.2**).

Place of cardiac MRI: If troponin-positive ACS is diagnosed and CAG does not show obstructive disease, cardiac MRI can be used to rule out myopericarditis.

12. What is the indication of CAG in the case of acute chest pain?

CAG is considered the gold standard for the diagnosis of CAD. Although the incidence of major complications is low (<2%), CAG has some risk, and hence being the final investigation of the chest

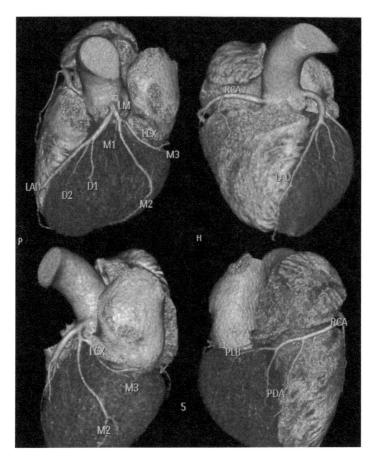

Figure 10.2 A CT-CAG showing normal coronaries has high negative predictive value for ruling out acute coronary syndrome during acute chest pain.

pain protocol, needs to be applied judiciously. It is imperative to avoid doing it in aortic dissection and pulmonary embolism, keeping in mind that dissection may mimic inferior wall MI with cardiogenic shock (dissection flap obstructing right coronary artery [RCA] ostium). Thus, a catastrophe may be avoided on the table. It is indicated in (1) STEMI <24 hr; (2) STEMI >24 hr with continuing pain, (3) ACS with moderate or more risk; (4) patients with markedly positive noninvasive tests; (5) patients with unstable or postinfarction angina; (6) patients with a contraindication to exercise or pharmacologic stress testing; and (7) patients with equivocal results on noninvasive stress testing when the diagnosis of CAD remains unclear.

10.2 CONCLUDING REMARKS

Triaging of the diagnostic pathway for any symptom or sign related to cardiovascular disease is as important as the decision pathway for management of the disease. Questions in tandem need to be asked to know the correct diagnosis, which ultimately leads to the success of appropriate therapy. This is more relevant in the case of acute chest pain.

FURTHER READING

1. Gulati M, Levy P D, Mukherjee D, et al. 2021 AHA/ACC/ASE/CHEST/SAEM/SCCT/SCMR Guideline for the Evaluation and Diagnosis of Chest Pain. *JACC* 2021;78:e187–e285.
2. NICE Guidelines on Chest Pain 2010.

11 Acute Coronary Syndrome

Sunandan Sikdar and Debabrata Roy

1. What are the points for clinical assessment of acute coronary syndrome (ACS)?

Confirming the diagnosis:

1. Angina at rest or angina equivalent (dyspnoea/epigastric pain).

2. *Cardiac biomarkers*: Raised hs-troponin. While T and I have nearly equal diagnostic accuracy, prognostic accuracy may be greater with troponin T. Quantitative value is available for Troponin I, but not with T. All patients must have a high-sensitivity troponin at arrival and repeated at 2 or 3 hours. Creatine phosphokinase (CPK) or CPK-MB is not recommended.

3. *ECG changes*: ST depression/T-wave inversion in multiple leads, dynamic ST changes (**Figures 11.1** and **11.2**).

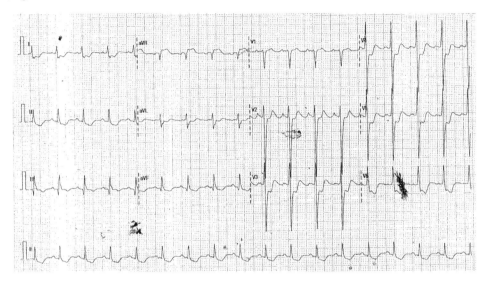

Figure 11.1 ACS – Dynamic changes in ECG.

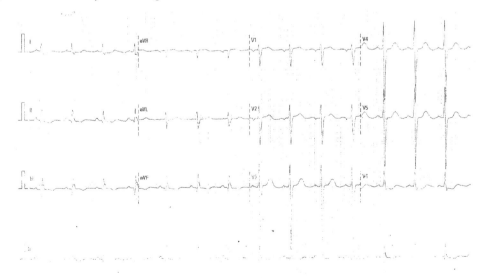

Figure 11.2 ACS – ECG normalization after heparin and nitroglycerin infusion in the same patient.

DOI: 10.1201/9781003027584-11

Nearly half of the ECG may have no clues for ischaemia. Ischaemia involving the circumflex territory or acute marginal branch of the right coronary artery may not show significant changes on the standard surface ECG leads.

Also look for pulse, saturation and blood pressure.

CT coronary angiography (CAG) can be used as a screening test if ECG, echocardiography and troponin are normal and the likelihood of coronary artery disease is low to intermediate.

2. What are the markers used for risk stratification?

TIMI risk score (c. 2000 Antmann et al.) is a handy method. One point each is assigned for age >65 yr, >3 coronary artery disease (CAD) risk factors, known CAD (>50% stenosis), prior aspirin use, >2 anginal episodes in the prior 24 hr, ST deviation >0.5 mm of the initial ECG and increased cardiac biomarkers.

Adverse cardiac events, (including death) at 2 weeks, occurred in roughly 5%–10% in low-risk (score 1–2), 10%–20% in moderate-risk (score 3–4) and 20%–40% in high-risk groups (score 5–7).

3. What are the types of plaque that result in ACS?

Optical coherence studies have shown coronary plaques (**Figures 11.3** and **11.4**) implicated in ACS are of three types (from most common to least): Plaques with rupture (lipid rich with a thin fibrous cap and macrophage-dominant inflammation – males usually), plaques with erosion (lipid poor, proteoglycan rich, low inflammation – females usually) and calcified nodules.

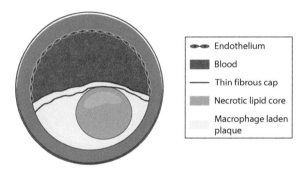

Figure 11.3   The vulnerable plaque in cross-section.

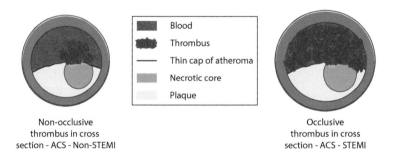

Figure 11.4   ACS spectrum.

4. What is the role of echocardiography in ACS?

Echocardiography is probably the most important test after ECG and is required for the following information: (1) Left ventricular function, (2) presence of regional wall motion abnormality, (3) presence of associated valvular pathology and (4) degree of pulmonary arterial hypertension.

5. What are the medications to use for ACS?

Antiplatelets: Aspirin should be loaded in aspirin-naive patients at 300 mg and continued in a maintenance dose at 75 mg once daily. Even if coronary artery bypass grafting (CABG) is recommended after CAG, aspirin should be continued.

Since ticagrelor is replacing clopidogrel in moderate to high ischaemic risk patients, it can be loaded as 180 mg followed by maintenance at 90 mg twice daily (contraindications include previous intracranial haemorrhage [ICH] or ongoing bleed). It has the advantage of being useful in both conservative and invasive strategies and also in renal failure. Ticagrelor has drug interactions with CYP3A inducers, and hence in patients receiving phenytoin or rifampicin, other antiplatelets are better used.

Prasugrel cannot be given unless the angiogram is complete, as it should only be used during and after percutaneous coronary intervention (PCI) and not in conservative therapies/CABG. The loading dose is 60 mg and the maintenance dose is 10 mg. Contraindications are weight <60 kg, age >75 years and renal failure. Prasugrel has been recommended for ACS patients proceeding for PCI (over ticagrelor) in the European Society for Cardiology (ESC) 2020 guideline.

Clopidogrel should be used in the elderly or if the bleeding risk is high and thrombotic risk low. Since only 15% of the drug is active after extensive metabolism and there are multiple interactions with cytochrome systems, clopidogrel is better avoided in diabetics, in cases with high thrombus burden or in complex PCI. The loading dose is 300–600 mg and the maintenance dose is 75 mg. We prefer the 600-mg loading dose for rapid and adequate antiplatelet effect.

For those patients who are selected for early invasive strategy and coronary anatomy is not known, preloading by a P2Y12 inhibitor is not advisable, as it does not decrease the ischaemic risk. It can be administered in the catheterization lab after CAG while proceeding for early PCI.

Anticoagulation: There is a preference for fondaparinux 2.5 mg SC once daily due to its low bleeding risk, but it has similar efficacy compared to the previous standard of enoxaparin 1 mg/kg SC twice daily (once daily if estimated glomerular filtration rate [eGFR] 15–30 mL/min/1.73 m^2, contraindicated if <15 mL/min). The only contraindication for fondaparinux is eGFR <20 mL/min/1.73 m^2. Fondaparinux has the advantage of once-daily dosing, no anti–Factor Xa level monitoring and does not cause heparin-induced thrombocytopenia. Anti–Xa level monitoring is required in GFR 15–30 mL/min or if body weight >100 kg, but this test is rarely available. For those with expected or reported low GFR, intravenous heparin 60–70 U/kg (max 5000 U) loading followed by 12–15 U/hr (max 1000 U/hr) can be considered. It is strongly recommended to measure activated partial thromboplastin time (aPTT) during heparin infusion (keep aPTT at 50–75 sec, 1.5–2 times upper limit of normal).

Oral anticoagulation: In patients with atrial fibrillation with a CHADVAS score of 2 or more or left ventricular (LV) thrombus or mechanical valve, oral anticoagulation is indicated. In the case of stenting with low bleeding risk, aspirin 75 mg, clopidogrel 75 mg and a novel oral anticoagulant (NOAC) (for non-valvular atrial fibrillation [AF])/vitamin K antagonist [VKA], for a mechanical valve) may be used for 1 month. In those with high bleeding risk, the combination is to be used for an even shorter time, 1 week. Following this, clopidogrel and a NOAC may be given the rest of the year. After 1 year, *only* anticoagulation is continued, preferably rivaroxaban or apixaban. If medical management is planned instead of stenting, only one antiplatelet (preferably clopidogrel) plus a NOAC may be used.

Statin: High-intensity statin therapy (low-density lipoprotein [LDL] reduction >50%) by either atorvastatin (40 mg or 80 mg) or rosuvastatin (40 mg) to reduce LDL <70 mg/dL is recommended. In spite of the maximum tolerated statin therapy, if this target is not achieved, then ezetimibe (10 mg) or a PCSK9 inhibitor (evolocumab) may be used.

Nitrates: IV nitroglycerin (NTG) (infusion pump 25 mg/50 mL at 0.6 mL/hr) is better than oral, especially in view of labile blood pressure. Prior intake of sildenafil (<24 hour) or tadalafil (<48 hour) is a contraindication to nitrate use. Persistent ischaemia, heart failure and hypertension are the niche areas where IV nitrates rapidly relieve symptoms. Often once failure and angina reduce, the pressure settles and it may be prudent to start tapering NTG.

Angiotensin-converting enzyme inhibitors (*ACEIs*): ACEIs (if not tolerated, an angiotensin receptor blocker [ARB]) should be used in ACS patients with LV systolic dysfunction, heart failure, hypertension or diabetes.

Beta-blockers: In the presence of heart failure, arrhythmia and LV dysfunction (left ventricular ejection fraction [LVEF] <40%) preferably bisoprolol, extended-release metoprolol, carvedilol or nebivolol may be used starting with lower doses.

Mineralocorticoid receptor antagonist therapy: Spironolactone or eplerenone may be used with careful monitoring of potassium levels in patients with LV dysfunction (LVEF <40%) or diabetes.

Diuretics: In patients with pulmonary oedema or decompensated heart failure, loop diuretics may use with intake-output monitoring.

6. What is the revascularization timing in ACS?

For convenience, the terminology used by the European guidelines for coronary angiography and revascularization is given here:

a. *Immediate invasive strategy (<2 hr)*: If there is refractory angina, heart failure, ventricular arrhythmias, recurrent ST-T changes/dynamic ST elevation or haemodynamic instability.

b. *Early invasive strategy (<24 hr)*: If there is a high-risk profile with GRACE score >140, dynamic ST changes or moderate and high risk based on TIMI score (>3). Though no mortality benefit could be demonstrated in early versus delayed invasive strategy, it is accepted that there is a reduction of recurrent ischaemic events and duration of hospital stay by following the invasive option.

c. *Invasive strategy (>72 hr)*: If there is at least an intermediate risk factor (diabetes mellitus, renal insufficiency, LVEF <40%, congestive heart failure, early post-infarction angina, recent PCI, prior CABG, GRACE risk score 109 and 140, recurrent symptoms).

d. *Selective invasive strategy*: For low-risk patients a stress test (preferably an imaging test) must be done. If reversible ischaemia is demonstrated, then this strategy should be used.

7. What are the revascularization options?

Based on CAG and the SYNTAX scores, either PCI or CABG is decided upon. PCI has the advantage of less bleeding, myocardial infarction (MI), stroke and renal injury, while CABG reduces the percentage of repeat revascularization.

8. What is the glycaemic target in diabetes?

Avoiding hypoglycaemic episodes is paramount. We keep a target of 180 mg/dL while using insulin and capillary blood glucose monitoring.

9. What strategy can be adopted in the case of ACS with cardiogenic shock?

After achieving haemodynamic stability with inotropes (or intra-aortic balloon pump [IABP] if required), CAG should be done after a frank discussion with relatives because outcomes are poor. This is even more true if mechanical complications or multivessel disease is present. A heart team approach with CABG may be required in some cases (**Figure 11.5**).

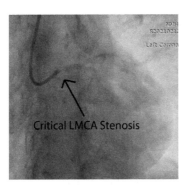 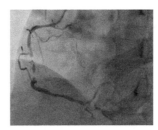

Figure 11.5 CAG in same patient as in Figure 11.1 – Left main coronary artery (LMCA) critical stenosis with triple-vessel disease. (Recovered after CABG.)

FURTHER READING

1. Collete J P, Thiele H, Barbato E, et al. 2020 ESC Guidelines for the management of acute coronary syndromes in patients presenting without persistent ST-segment elevation. European'l (2020) 00, 1–79.
2. Thygsen K, Alpert J S, Jaffe A S, et al. Fourth universal definition of myocardial infarction (2018). European Heart Journal (2019) 40, 237–269.
3. Antman EM, Cohen M, Bernink PJLM, et al. The TIMI risk score for unstable angina/non-ST elevation MI: A method for prognostication and therapeutic decision-making. JAMA(2000), 284:835–842.

12 ST Elevation Myocardial Infarction

Sunandan Sikdar and Saibal Mukhopadhyay

1. What is myocardial injury?

A rise in cardiac troponin (cTn) with one value above the 99th percentile of the upper reference limit (URL) indicates cardiac injury. A rise and fall implies acute injury. This can be classified into three categories:

A. Acute injury + Ischaemia = Acute myocardial infarction (MI)

B. Acute injury, no evidence of ischemia = Acute myocardial injury (e.g. myocarditis)

C. Stable but raised troponin value = Chronic myocardial injury (e.g. chronic kidney disease [CKD])

2. What is the definition of MI?

Acute myocardial injury, i.e. rise and/or fall of cTn values with at least one value above the 99th percentile of URL and *at least one* of the following:

1. **Symptoms** of myocardial ischaemia

2. New ischaemic **ECG** changes

3. Development of pathological **Q waves**

4. **Imaging** evidence of new loss of viable myocardium or new regional wall motion abnormality in a pattern consistent with an ischaemic aetiology

5. Identification of a coronary thrombus by **angiography** or **autopsy** (not for Type 2 or 3 MIs)

ECG changes in ST segment elevated myocardial infarction (STEMI) (**Figures 12.1–12.5**) are discussed in detail in the ECG chapter.

Frontal	Frontal augmented	Horizontal	Horizontal
I Lateral	aVR	V1 Septal	V4 Anterior
II Inferior	aVL Lateral	V2 Septal	V5 Lateral
III Inferior	aVF Inferior	V3 Anterior	V6 Lateral

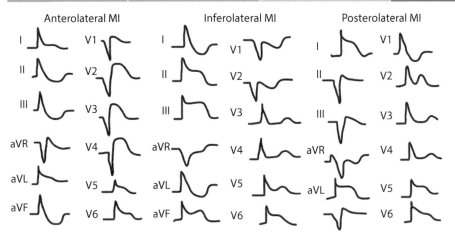

Figure 12.1 ECG patterns of STEMI.

DOI: 10.1201/9781003027584-12

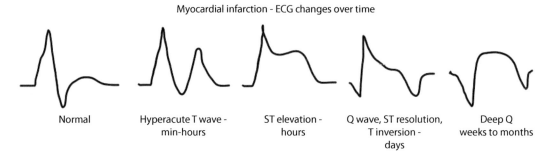

Figure 12.2 ECG guide to time of onset of MI.

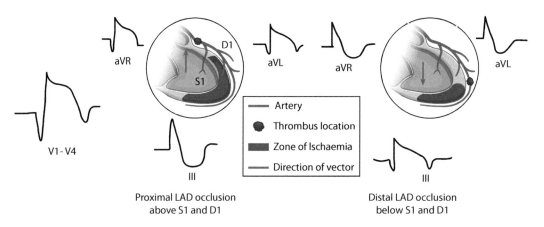

Figure 12.3 AWSTEMI – ECG localization of occlusion, proximal vs distal LAD, importance of III and aVR, aVL.

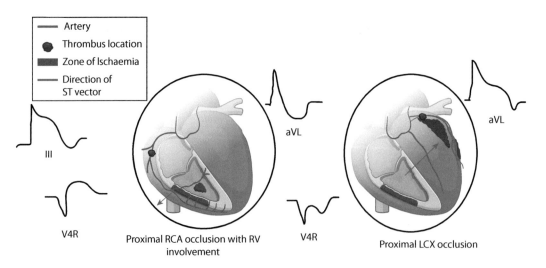

Figure 12.4 IWSTEMI (ST elevation in III common): ECG localization of occlusion RCA vs LCX, importance of aVL and V4R.

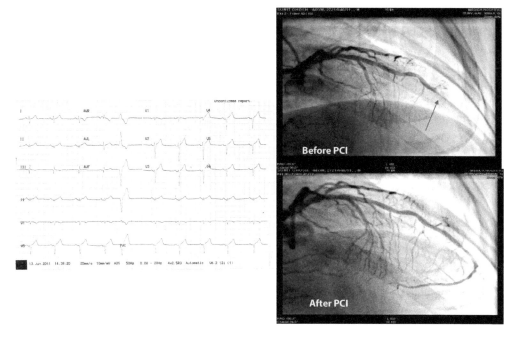

Figure 12.5 ST elevation in both the anterior and inferior walls: What may be the culprit artery? Distal LAD occlusion in wrap-around artery.

3. What are the types of MI?

The following types are as per the European Society for Cardiology (ESC) 4th Universal Definition of MI (2018) (**Table 12.1**).

Table 12.1: Types of Myocardial Infarction

Type	Definition of MI	Example/Categories	Comment
1	Spontaneous MI	Atherothrombotic plaque rupture/erosion/ulcer	Most common type
2	MI due to oxygen supply and demand mismatch	• Atherosclerotic disease + anaemia • Vasospasm/MINOCA • Spontaneous non-atherosclerotic coronary artery dissection • Coronary embolism • Tachyarrhythmia/bradyarrhythmia • Shock	STEMI in type 2 MI 3%–24%
3	Death due to suspected MI	• Death after documented VF or ischaemic ECG changes • Autopsy shows MI	Biomarker not available/too early to demonstrate rise
4a	Post-PCI MI (<48 hr)	Rise of cTn >5× 99th percentile URL if baseline was normal or >20% increase if baseline was raised but stable	Apart from new ECG/echocardiography changes, CAG evidence of dissection/occlusion and slow flow required
4b	Stent thrombosis–related MI	Timeline from PCI: • Acute <1 day • Subacute 1 day to -1month • Late 1 month to 1 year • Very late >1 year	Documentation by CAG/autopsy
4c	Restenosis-related MI	Focal or diffuse restenosis + rise/fall of cTn	Documentation by CAG
5	Post-CABG MI	• Rise cTn >10× 99th percentile URL if baseline was normal or >20% increase if baseline was raised but stable • absolute value must be more than 10 times	Documentation by CAG of occluded graft/native artery

4. What is the pathophysiology of MI?

There are two components in pathophysiology, which interact to create thrombotic occlusion of the vessel.

A. *The vulnerable plaque*: Four different types of events related to coronary plaque occur in different patient subsets, all of which lead to a similar manifestation – acute coronary syndrome (ACS)

    a. *Plaque fissure with systemic inflammation*: There is discontinuity of a fibrous cap with some unique features.

        i. Widespread inflammation in different plaques in different coronary arteries simultaneously

        ii. *Activation of innate immunity*: Monocyte macrophage system overexpressing toll-like receptors activates inflammatory cytokine and matrix metalloproteinase that cause the fibrin cap to become unstable

        iii. *Activation of adaptive immunity*: Defective T-cell regulation leading to unstable plaques

    b. *Plaque fissure without systemic inflammation*: Sympathetic overactivity/coronary vasoconstriction are triggers.

    c. *Plaque erosion*: Here the fibrous cap is intact, but the endothelium is denuded with a predominance of myeloperoxidase-positive neutrophil and hyaluronic acid. Inflammation is lower grade compared to fissure and macrophage is sparse.

    d. *Smooth plaque with coronary vasospasm* (microcirculatory alteration).

B. *The thrombotic blood*: Two basic events shape the thrombogenicity when the endothelium of the plaque is denuded, exposing the collagen underneath

    a. *Activation of the coagulation system*

        i. Contact activation of factor XII and triggering the intrinsic coagulation pathway

        ii. Tissue factors release from the sub-endothelium activates factor VII, triggering the extrinsic pathway

    b. *Activation of platelets*

        i. *Adhesion*: By GP I receptor

        ii. *Activation*: By GP VI receptor

        iii. *Release: From membrane* – Thromboxane-positive feedback on activation

From dense granules – Adenosine diphosphate (ADP) causes activation of P2Y12 receptors, which in turn activates GP IIb/IIa receptors on the platelet membrane. Activation of GP IIb/IIIa leads to platelet-platelet interactions via von Willebrand factor and is the crucial event in the aggregatory response.

From alpha granules – P selectin – causes platelet-leucocyte aggregation and proinflammatory response.

5. What are the options for STEMI treatment during the first 24 hr?

STEMI diagnosis and preferred management strategy are presented in **Table 12.2**.

Table 12.2: Management Strategy on the Basis of Presentation

Time from Symptom Onset to Hospital Triage	Modifiers	Strategy	Comment
<12 hr	Time to primary PCI <120 min	Primary PCI	<3 hr and anterior wall MI, rapidity of revascularization may be more important than strategy used
<12 hr	Time to primary PCI >120 min and no contraindications to fibrinolytics	Fibrinolysis	>3 hr lesser benefit of fibrinolysis

(Continued)

Table 12.2 (*Continued*): Management Strategy on the Basis of Presentation

Time from Symptom Onset to Hospital Triage	Modifiers	Strategy	Comment
12–48 hr	Symptoms/haemodynamic instability present	Primary PCI	• Benefit reduces with passing time • Anterior wall MI to have lower threshold for PCI
3–28 days	No symptoms	Medical therapy	OAT trial

6. What is the checklist for thrombolysis?

Contraindications to fibrinolytics given by European Society of Cardiology (ESC) are listed in **Table 12.3**.

Table 12.3: Contraindication of Fibrinolysis

Absolute	Relative
Previous ICH/Unknown stroke at any time	TIA 6 months or less
Ischemic stroke 6 months or less	Oral anticoagulation
CNS neoplasm/AV malformation	Pregnancy/Postpartum 1 week
Trauma/Surgery/Head injury 1 month or less	SBP >180 mmHg, DBP >110 mmHg
GI bleed 1 month or less	Advanced liver disease
Known bleeding disorder (not menses)	Infective endocarditis
Aortic dissection	Active peptic ulcer
Non-compressible puncture <24 hr (internal organ biopsy/spinal anaesthesia)	Prolonged traumatic resuscitation

7. What are the thrombolytics?

Thrombolytic regimen is given in below **Table 12.4**.

Table 12.4: Thrombolytic Regimen and Dose

Drug	Dose	Comment
Streptokinase	1.5 million units in 30–60 min	Contraindicated in previous treatment with streptokinase
rtPA	• 15 mg IV bolus • 0.75 mg/kg over 30 min (max 50 mg) • 0.5 mg/kg over 60 min (max 35 mg)	
Tenecteplase (TNK)	• 30 mg if <60 kg • 35 mg if 60–70 kg • 40 mg if 70–80 kg • 45 mg if 80–90 kg • 50 mg if >90 kg • If age >75 yr, use half-dose TNK	
Reteplase	10 + 10 U IV 30 min apart	

8. What are the antiplatelet doses in STEMI?

Table 12.5: Antiplatelet Doses in STEMI

Drug	Fibrinolysis	Primary PCI
Aspirin	• Loading 300 mg • Maintenance 75 mg	Loading 300 mg Maintenance 75 mg once daily
Clopidogrel	• Loading 300 mg • Maintenance 75 mg • *If age > 75 yr, no loading dose*	• Loading 600 mg • Maintenance 75 mg

Table 12.5 (*Continued*): Antiplatelet Doses in STEMI

Drug	Fibrinolysis	Primary PCI
Ticagrelor	• No recommendation but TREAT trial used standard dose • Ticagrelor should be started 48 hr after fibrinolysis, if at all	• Loading 180 mg • Maintenance 90 mg twice daily
Prasugrel	Not recommended	• Loading 60 mg • Maintenance 10 mg • Contraindicated in age >75 yr, wt <60 kg, previous stroke, avoid in renal failure • If at all used in <60 kg, use maintenance 5 mg

9. What are the options for STEMI treatment?

Table 12.6: Categories of PCI and Its Definitions

Category	Term	Explanation
1	Primary PCI (**Figure 12.6**)	Emergent PCI of infarct-related artery
2	Rescue PCI	Emergent PCI in case of failed thrombolysis
3	Routine early PCI	PCI in 3–24 hr of successful fibrinolysis
4	Pharmacoinvasive strategy	Categories 2 and 3

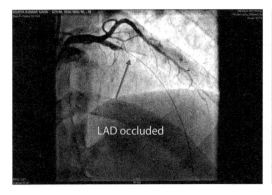
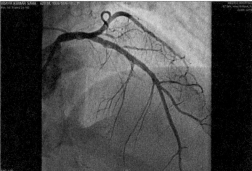

Figure 12.6 Primary PCI: Anterior wall MI.

10. What are the options for STEMI with multivessel disease (MVD)?

MVD occurs in 50% of STEMI cases. If a patient is in cardiogenic shock, the non-infarct–related artery (IRA) with critical stenosis may be attempted as per guidelines during the index procedure. However, this decision has to be individualized. If the presumed cause of cardiogenic shock is ischaemia of the non-IRA vessel, it must be attempted. But there is a real risk of having a slow flow in the non-IRA territory and further worsening of the haemodynamics. This is especially true if mechanical circulatory support is not available. We often attempt a non-IRA vessel in case of inferior wall MI with a critical proximal/mid–left anterior descending artery (LAD) lesion during the index procedure.

In cases of MVD STEMI and no shock, the IRA approach during the index procedure and percutaneous coronary intervention (PCI) of non-IRA vessels is recommended before discharge.

11. How is STEMI with cardiogenic shock diagnosed?

Cardiogenic shock is defined as systolic blood pressure (SBP) <90 mmHg for a prolonged period with clinical features of hypotension (cool extremities, resting tachycardia, mental obtundation, urine <20 mL/hr) despite adequate filling pressure (pulmonary capillary wedge pressure [PCWP] >18 mmHg) and a cardiac output <2.2 L/min/m^2.

In the best of centres the mortality from cardiogenic shock approaches 50% or more. Since almost half of these subset patients progress to cardiogenic shock nearly *6 hr after* hospital admission, it is imperative to communicate this possibility at the earliest. Late presentation, elderly, severe left ventricular (LV) systolic dysfunction, anuria, history of cardiac arrest and severe metabolic acidosis on presentation are important predictors of mortality even if promptly revascularized by primary PCI after hospital admission (**Table 12.7**).

Table 12.7: Classification of Heart Failure

Clinical Class	Killip Presentation	Subset	Haemodynamic Presentation
I	No clinical signs of heart failure	I (normal)	PCWP <18, CI >2.2
II	Crackles in lung, S3 gallop, elevated JVP	II (pulmonary congestion)	PCWP >18, CI >2.2
III	Frank pulmonary oedema	III (hypoperfusion)	PCWP<18, CI <2.2
IV	Shock with hypoperfusion	IV (shock with pulmonary congestion)	PCWP >18, CI >2.2

12. What are the causes of STEMI with shock?

The causes include (**Box 12.1**)
Reversible and mechanical causes

BOX 12.1 CARDIOGENIC SHOCK IN MI

REVERSIBLE CAUSES

i. Hypovolemia
ii. Drug induced hypotension (e.g nitrate in IWM)
iii. Arrhythmias
iv. Ischaemia in non-IRA territory (in multivessel disease)
v. RVMI (improves with revascularization)

MECHANICAL CAUSES

i. Pump failure
ii. Mitral regurgitation
iii. Ventricular septal rupture
iv. Free-wall rupture

It is extremely important to detect the reversible causes, as correction of these factors leads to rapid haemodynamic stabilization.

13. What is the initial management for STEMI with cardiogenic shock?

After the reversible factors are taken care of, look at the arterial blood gas (ABG) and invasive arterial monitor (mean arterial pressure [MAP]). Before being shifted to the catheterization lab, a minimum haemodynamic stability should be ensured. If there is pulmonary oedema leading to severe hypoxia plus severe metabolic acidosis, it may be wise to go for early mechanical ventilation after starting on noradrenaline (4/50 concentration) in an appropriate dose to keep MAP >70 mmHg. The objective is to ensure tissue perfusion and maintain urine output. Once anuric for a few hours, only a few survive. Next is the decision whether to use an intra-aortic balloon pump (IABP). Though the IABP SHOCK trial failed to show a mortality benefit, it may be beneficial in a very select subset. We use it if the noradrenaline dose requirement is very high. IABP allows us to taper the dose of noradrenaline to potentially reduce organ damage. The patient is then shifted to the catheterization lab for revascularization. If the coronary angiogram (CAG) shows high-risk anatomy, that is also an indication for IABP insertion in the lab. Once revascularization is done, close monitoring with ABG is necessary, often because acidosis worsens due to various factors. Electrolyte (especially potassium) correction is paramount. For extubation, it is imperative that (1) the noradrenaline dose has been reduced to a minimum (though on IABP), (2) the ABG is satisfactory and there is no acidosis or hypoxia and (3) urine output is adequate. If the parameters improve gradually, the timing of extubation is individualized.

14. How do you use inotropes in MI?

Among the vasopressors, though there is no randomized trial to support one vasopressor over another, there is general agreement that:

a. Noradrenaline is the first-line vasopressor agent because its α1 and β1 actions increase MAP (maintains end-organ perfusion) and the cardiac index without a significant increase in heart rate and oxygen consumption. Compared to dopamine, the increase in lactate is far lesser. In smaller studies dopamine has been found to increase arrhythmic events compared to noradrenaline but there was no difference in mortality. Noradrenaline should be started at a low dose (0.1 mg/kg/min) and increased to obtain a MAP at about 65–70 mmHg. After having stabilized arterial pressure, evaluate if noradrenaline alone was able to reverse the signs of hypoperfusion (low cardiac output, low SvO_2, hyperlactataemia, mottling, oliguria). If MAP is stabilized but signs of low stroke volume/hypoperfusion persist, start inotropes. But if the MAP target is not achieved, add IABP.

b. Dobutamine is the inotrope of choice because of its predominant agonist action on β1 receptors (weak α1 and β2). In cardiogenic shock, dobutamine has been shown to significantly increase heart rate, cardiac index and SvO_2 while decreasing both pulmonary artery wedge pressure and lactate. The therapeutic dose is 2–20 micrograms /kg/min. Thus noradrenaline and dobutamine are a useful second-line combination *if noradrenaline alone is not sufficient.*

c. Levosimendan is an inotrope and calcium-sensitizing agent that binds to cardiac troponin C in a calcium-dependent manner. It also has a vasodilatory effect in vascular smooth muscle by opening adenosine triphosphate–sensitive potassium channels. It is used in patients already on beta-blockers where dobutamine has reduced efficacy. Unlike traditional inotropes, such as dobutamine, levosimendan neither increases myocardial oxygen consumption nor impairs diastolic function and has no pro-arrhythmic effects. Being a long-acting agent, it can be used for first the 24 hr with effects persisting for 7–9 days.

15. How do you diagnose and treat STEMI with RVMI?

One-third to one-half of inferior wall (IW) STEMI cases present with evidence of RVMI, but only half of this subset develop haemodynamic derangement due to the said pathology. The right ventricle (RV) is a thin-walled, pyramidal, volume pump having a dual right coronary artery (RCA) and left circumflex artery (LCX) supply. It can rapidly develop collaterals during ischemic insult, and *if the acute period is over,* recovery starts at 3–10 days. Hence early treatment and tiding over the crisis are of paramount importance. Acute RV dilation leads to septal shift and underfilling of the LV, as both are encased in a stiff pericardial sac. Reduced RV stroke volume and LV underfilling are the cause of shock in RVMI. If there is an associated right atrium (RA) infarct, RV output falls further.

The clinical characteristics of RVMI are a triad of hypotension, clear lung fields and raised jugular venous pressure (JVP) (prominent a wave with a sharp "x" descent due to a hypercontractile RA and blunted "y" descent – the W pattern). Kussmaul sign (increase in JVP on deep inspiration) in the setting of IWSTEMI predicts RVMI. Pulsus paradoxus (inspiratory drop of SBP >10 mmHg) may also occur. A blunted a wave in the JVP suggests an RA infarct (M pattern).

Diagnosis: ECG: IWSTEMI plus lead V4R showing:

■ ST elevation > 1 mm V4R with +ve T: Proximal RCA occlusion – significant RVMI

■ No ST elevation but + T wave: Distal RCA occlusion – RVMI uncommon

■ ST-segment depression >1 mm and –ve T wave: LCX occlusion – RVMI uncommon in this situation

■ Sometimes IWMI + RVMI may present with ST elevation in V1–V4 (rightward axis of ST elevation distinguishes it from anterior wall MI)

Echocardiography: RV free wall (RVFW) hypokinesia with reduced tricuspid annular pulmonary systolic excursion (TAPSE).

Contraindications: Avoid nitrates, morphine, diuretics

Treatment

a. IV fluids up to 1 litre are necessary. If SBP does not recover, invasive monitoring of RV pressures is required. Maintain central venous pressure (CVP) at 15 mmHg. Excessive fluid may induce septal shift and systemic congestion.

b. *Dobutamine*: Dobutamine may increase RV output by increasing septal contraction.

c. *Malignant ventricular arrhythmias*: A dilated RV and peri-infarct denervation are the cause of the trimodal pattern of arrhythmia: During occlusion, during reperfusion and during recovery.

d. Severe bradycardia due to vagal-mediated sinus bradycardia or atrioventricular (AV) block may progress to haemodynamic deterioration and require AV sequential pacing (preferred, as it restores atrial kick) or RV pacing. If during initial stabilization atropine fails to improve heart rate, aminophylline may be used.

e. Early revascularization, preferably by primary PCI.

16. How do you manage STEMI with pulmonary oedema?

Pulmonary oedema is a common complication of anterior wall STEMI and requires rapid management to avoid tissue hypoxia.

a. *Control of Hypoxia*: Routine O_2 inhalation is not necessary unless SaO_2 <90% (in non-hypoxic patients O_2 may increase systemic vascular resistance and promote coronary vasoconstriction). Non-invasive ventilation may be considered if still hypoxic even after O_2 by face mask.

b. *Control of Angina*: Injectable morphine 4 mg may be used and repeated after 5–15 minutes provided there is no hypotension, vomiting and depressed respiration. As an alternative injectable fentanyl may be given. Control of angina is a crucial step in reducing the hyperadrenergic state, arrhythmia and heart failure. Use of nitroglycerin (GTN) infusion (titrated to SBP) is a common and time-tested practice, provided a history of sildenafil use, hypotension and RVMI are excluded, and continuous monitoring of vitals is done. This promotes coronary vasodilation and reduces preload. Even a small dose of sublingual GTN may cause hypotension and bradycardia, which can be reversed with atropine. Hence, sublingual GTN can be cautiously given in sitting position if hypotension is excluded, but GTN infusion is always preferred over sublingual formulation.

c. *Control of Hyperadrenergic State*: Angina, anxiety and heart failure create a hyperadrenergic state. Routine administration of i.v beta-blocker increases the risk of cardiogenic shock. They may be given if tachycardia and hypertension persist even after initiation of the earlier measures and there is ongoing ischaemia. Though three boluses of 5 mg metoprolol at >5-min intervals may be used if HR >60/min and SBP >120 mmHg after every dose, it may be prudent to wait sometime after the next dose is initiated. In the days of rapid primary PCI, often oral therapy suffices after revascularization is over and use of i.v metoprolol is extremely rare. Often after the initial chest pain and pulmonary oedema are settled after revascularization, the SBP comes down – often noradrenaline is required at this stage. So, using i.v metoprolol prior to primary PCI may be a disadvantage. Oral metoprolol (short acting) 25 mg twice daily is started early and the dose is titrated upward as tolerated in 2–3 days.

A mild tranquillizer (usually a benzodiazepine) may be used in very anxious patients, provided hypoxia has been corrected and patient is not on bilevel positive airway pressure (BIPAP). It is better not to sedate a patient on BIPAP.

17. How do you manage CKD with MI?

Renal dysfunction (estimated glomerular filtration rate [eGFR] <30 mL/min/m²) may be present in 30% of elderly ACS patients and is often diagnosed after admission and sometimes after primary PCI is over. In the case of diabetic nephropathy patients, symptoms are often not evident. In case of suspicion, it is wise to properly hydrate before, during and after primary PCI. Use of N-acetylcysteine has an insufficient evidence base. The bleeding risk is higher. Unfractionated heparin (UFH) is the preferred anticoagulant. Fondaparinux is contraindicated. Drugs should be used as per the eGFR.

18. What are the presentation and management of STEMI in diabetes?

Diabetes constitutes 20% or more of the acute infarct population. A few special characteristics occur with diabetic subsets.

a. More frequency of atypical chest pain or silent ischaemia.

b. Delayed presentation.

c. Multivessel and diffusely diseased vessel and increased risk of PCI-related complications. Increased risk of renal dysfunction.

d. Higher risk of cardiogenic shock and poorer outcomes.

e. If diabetic ketoacidosis (DKA) and MI coexist or if a combination of STEMI, shock, metabolic acidosis and urinary ketones is present, cautious fluid repletion, vasopressor and electrolyte correction are required prior to initiation of PCI. Outcomes are universally poor.

f. Insulin infusion (along with potassium correction if necessary) is instituted to keep capillary blood glucose (CBG) <180 mg/dL. Once CBG reaches <250 mg/dL the infusion is stopped and a regimen of basal insulin + premeal bolus may be considered as per a sliding scale. Avoid hypoglycaemia (CBG <70 mg/dL) at all costs.

g. Use of an SGLT2 inhibitor may be considered once the patient is stabilized and is near discharge.

h. Usually, a potent antiplatelet like ticagrelor/prasugrel should be used instead of clopidogrel.

19. How do you manage MI with non-haemorrhagic stroke?

Acute MI has been considered a cause for ischaemic stroke only if it occurs within 1 month of the stroke. But there are studies documenting heightened risks up to 3 months post-MI. The pathogenesis may be increased thrombotic tendency, new-onset atrial fibrillation or LV thrombus. Fibrinolysis is contraindicated. Fibrinolysis-related haemorrhagic stroke or haemorrhagic transformation of ischaemic stroke has a poor prognosis, especially if involving the dominant hemisphere. Primary PCI is the modality of choice. Regarding stroke thrombolysis in this situation, evidence-based recommendations are not available.

20. What is the recommended diet in post-STEMI care during home discharge?

The recommended diet during discharge after STEMI includes the following.

a. Less than 10% of total energy intake from saturated fat, by replacing it with polyunsaturated fatty acids and as little as possible of trans fatty acids

b. Salt intake of <5 g per day

c. 30–45 g fibre per day

d. >200 g fruits and 200 g vegetables per day

e. Fish 1–2 times per week (especially oily varieties)

f. 30 g unsalted nuts daily

g. Limited alcohol intake

21. What is the maintenance regimen for antiplatelets in STEMI at discharge?

As per current guidelines, antiplatelets at discharge can be of different regimens (**Table 12.8**).

Table 12.8: Antiplatelets Post-PCI Preferred Strategy

Indication/Subset	Antiplatelet Regimen	Duration
Post–Primary PCI, normal bleeding risk, normal thrombotic risk	Aspirin 75 mg + ticagrelor 90 mg twice daily or prasugrel 10 mg once daily	12 months
Post–Primary PCI, normal bleeding risk, increased thrombotic risk	Aspirin 75 mg + ticagrelor 90 mg twice daily	12 months
• Age >65 years, diabetes, multivessel, prior spontaneous MI, CKD	*After 12 months*: Aspirin 75 mg + ticagrelor *60 mg* twice daily	3 years
Post–primary PCI high bleeding risk	Aspirin 75 mg + clopidogrel 75 mg OD or ticagrelor 90 mg BD	6 months
	After 6 months: Only aspirin 75 mg or clopidogrel 75 mg (if GI bleed risk)	Continue
In STEMI on medical therapy, no PCI, normal bleeding risk	DAPT	12 months
STEMI, low bleeding risk with LV thrombus	Aspirin + clopidogrel + anticoagulation (Apixaban/Rivaroxaban)	DAPT + anticoagulation for 6 months then DAPT continues

22. What are the post-procedure and discharge medications in MI?

Table 12.9: Discharge Medications

Drug	Indication
ACEI/Valsartan	In STEMI with HF, LVEF <40%, anterior infarct, diabetes
Beta-blocker	• In STEMI with HF/LVEF < 40% if no contraindication, initiated in hospital in first 24 hr • Benefit marginal in primary PCI • No guideline recommendation about how long to continue
Spironolactone/Eplerenone	In STEMI with LVEF <40% with HF or diabetes if already on ACEI + BB

High-intensity statin
Atorvastatin (40–80 mg)
Rosuvastatin (20–40 mg)
	• Goal LDL <70 mg/dL or >50% reduction
	• If goal not reached even after high-intensity statin, then consider:
	  • Ezetimibe 10 mg
	  • Evolocumab (PCSK-9 inhibitor) injection – though no mortality benefit

Proton pump inhibitors	Those who have high GI bleeding risk

23. What is the role of an angiotensin receptor/neprilysin inhibitor (ARNI) in STEMI?

The role of sacubitril/valsartan in post-MI situation is under investigation. There is a possibility of improvement in LV remodelling after infarct/reperfusion-related injuries in a rabbit model. In PARADISE MI (2021) trial ARNI was not superior to ramipril in reducing death from cardiovascular causes or from heart failure in post MI situation.

24. How do you manage MI in octogenarians?

The elderly often present with atypical symptoms and hence have a delay in diagnosis and treatment. They have multiple comorbidities and higher bleeding and stroke risk. Primary PCI with radial access is favoured, but because of calcified arteries and multivessel involvement, results and outcomes may not be as in younger age groups. Because of tortuous arteries, both in radial and femoral routes, catheter manipulation may be difficult. An effort must be made for an early discharge, as nosocomial infections are common and recovery at home with good nursing care is not unusual.

25. How do you manage STEMI in a post-CABG case?

STEMI after CABG, though uncommon, is an event that has adverse outcomes. In the case of thrombosis in a vein graft, primary PCI is quite challenging given the difficulty in graft cannulation and tackling the large thrombus burden (usually with GP IIb/IIIa and aspiration devices). Data from an analysis of the APEX MI trial showed that these patients were elderly and had multiple comorbidities. The graft vessel was involved as frequently as the native arteries. The outcome was worse in the case of primary PCI of the graft vessel. However, in the ACS–Israeli Survey (2000–2008) this subset of patients who were subjected to primary PCI had similar outcomes as those with native-vessel STEMI. Their 30-day mortality was 5.9% and the major adverse cardiac event (MACE) rate was 17% in post-CABG patients.

26. What is the management of MI in a post-PCI patient?

STEMI post-PCI may be either an occlusion of a nonstented vessel (Type 1) or a stented vessel (Type 4b). Acute stent thrombosis (<1 day) or subacute stent thrombosis (one day to one month) has a high mortality. It may be related to procedural factors (dissected vessel, thrombus migration, bifurcation stenting or under deployed stent), especially in the case of acute thrombosis, or due to patient-related factors (discontinuation of antiplatelets, smoking) in the case of subacute stent thrombosis. Rapidly shifting to catheterization lab and reperfusing the vessel is the top priority. If the patient was on clopidogrel, it would be wise to shift to ticagrelor/prasugrel after such an event.

27. How do you manage arrhythmia after STEMI?

Tachy and brady arrhythmia often are the cause of sudden worsening post MI (Table 12.10 and 12.11).

Table 12.10: Tachyarrhythmia Post-STEMI

Arrhythmia	Characteristics	Comment/Treatment
Premature ventricular contraction (PVC)	• Common • R on T may occur but VF rare	Beta-blocker as per standard protocol
Atrial fibrillation	Increased risk of AF in AWSTEMI due to increased sympathetic tone and LV dysfunction	• *Acutely*: DC cardioversion if hypotensive • Consider amiodarone infusion if stable • *Maintenance*: Beta-blocker, amiodarone • Individualize anticoagulation
Accelerated idioventricular rhythm	• Initial few days of MI • Follows successful reperfusion both in anterior and inferior infarction (frequently found during primary PCI)	Prognosis good
Ventricular tachycardia	More common late in the course when LV dysfunction has set in	• Echocardiography to look for scar • Maintain target values of serum potassium and magnesium, >4 mEq/L and >2 mEq/L • Start amiodarone ± lidocaine • Consider AICD if recurrent episodes on antiarrhythmics and no reversible cause found
Ventricular fibrillation	• VF may occur in the acute ischaemic phase (<48 hr) • Also, later (>48 hr) – ischemic injury to papillary muscle	• If VF occurs <48 hr after onset of MI, revascularization should be considered first • Maintain target values of serum potassium and magnesium, >4 mEq/L and >2 mEq/L • Amiodarone ± lidocaine infusion continued • If VF occurs >48 hr after onset of MI and patient already on antiaarrhythmic and revascularized – AICD indicated

Table 12.11: Bradyarrhythmia Post-STEMI

Block	Characteristics	Treatment
Sinus bradycardia	Often IWSTEMI	Atropine if HR <40/min plus hypotension
First-degree heart block	In IWSTEMI	• Monitoring • Stop beta-blocker if PR >0.24 sec
Second-degree heart block	• Mobitz I in IWSTEMI • Mobitz II in IWSTEMI/AWSTEMI	Temporary pacing if related to AWSTEMI
Third-degree AV block if related to intranodal location	• More common in IWSTEMI • Usually transient (2–3 days) • Stable escape >40 min • Narrow QRS escape rhythm	• Temporary less common (if severe bradycardia + hypotension) • Permanent requirement rare
Third-degree AV block if related to infranodal location	• More common in AWSTEMI due to septal perforators of LAD • Usually transient, but some conduction defect may persist Unstable escape <40 min • Wide QRS escape rhythm • May progress to asystole	• Temporary pacing if third-degree AV block or in acute onset bi-fascicular block (large MI) • Permanent pacing if complete heart block persists during admission

28. What is the protocol for STEMI patients who are on oral anticoagulation?

Oral anticoagulation is a relative contraindication for fibrinolysis, and patients should be triaged for primary PCI strategy, regardless of the anticipated time to PCI-mediated reperfusion. The P2Y12 inhibitor of choice in this case is clopidogrel (loading dose 600 mg) and a GP IIb/IIIa inhibitor should not be used during PCI. Post-discharge aspirin, clopidogrel and a novel oral anticoagulant

(NOAC) (preferably apixaban or rivaroxaban) should be used for 1 week (from the time of primary PCI) after which clopidogrel and the NOAC can continue up to 1 year. The dose of the NOAC is reviewed in detail in the chapter on NOACs. The indication and bleeding risk related to NOAC should be assessed regularly.

29. What are STEMI-related mechanical complications and their management?

STEMI-related mechanical complications (**Table 12.12**) are not common but may be of supreme importance to recognize, because the post-PCI outcome may be grim and needs discussion with all stakeholders, including relatives and cardiac surgeons. *Auscultation is thus very important in all cases of late presentation of STEMI to pick up the systolic murmur of mitral regurgitation (MR) and ventricular apetal defect (VSD).*

Table 12.12: Mechanical Complications Post-STEMI

Feature	Acute MR (Papillary Muscle Rupture)	Ventricular Septal Rupture	Free Wall Rupture
Defining feature	IWSTEMI (posteromedial papillary muscle [PMPM] rupture) more common	• AWSTEMI–apical VSR • IWSTEMI-basal VSR (worse prognosis)	Primary PCI reduce risk, free wall rupture often causes PEA/sudden death
Time	Within 2 weeks	Within 2 weeks	Within 2 weeks
Presentation	Acute-onset dyspnoea	Chest pain, hypotension	Sudden chest pain and death
Echocardiogram	Acute MR, torn PMPM	Left-to-right shunt, often serpiginious defect	Pericardial effusion (often >5 mm)
Treatment	IABP + Urgent surgery	Surgery/Device	Surgery often not possible

30. How do you diagnose and manage post-MI pericarditis?

Post-MI pericarditis often occurs in late presenters of STEMI who have not been thrombolysed. The characteristic of the pain is increased pain on deep inspiration or on lying down, which is referred to the trapezius ridge, usually in the period from the first 1–8 weeks. Post-MI pericarditis sometimes occurs due to pericardial inflammation from a transmural infarct and is called pericarditis epistenocardia. Aspirin and paracetamol are the treatment of choice.

Another subset of post-MI pericarditis is Dressler syndrome, in which immune-mediated mechanism is the cause. It occurs between 1 and 8 weeks. Patients have malaise, fever, chest discomfort, raised erythrocytre sedimentation rate (ESR) and leucocytosis. Aspirin is the treatment of choice.

31. What is an LV aneurysm?

An LV aneurysm is a focal dyskinetic area of the LV that bulges out during systole with a wide neck (see the echocardiography chapter for the differential diagnosis). It is made of fibrous tissues and requires a few weeks for development. Because of a lack of reperfusion, the ECG leads pertaining to the territory show persistent ST elevation. LV aneurysms have become rare (5%) due to early reperfusion strategies. An apical aneurysm due to an occluded LAD after AWSTEMI is more common than a basal aneurysm due to an occluded RCA after IWSTEMI. Because of the loss of contracting myocardium, heart failure is the presenting feature. Ventricular tachycardia (due to scar) and thrombus formation may also occur. Surgical resection may be of benefit if there is worsening angina or heart failure, provided the rest of the viable contracting myocardium is adequate. Percutaneous use of a parachute device to exclude the aneurysm may be a promising approach in the future.

FURTHER READING
1. Ibanez B, James S, Agewall S et al. 2017 ESC Guidelines for the management of acute myocardial infarction in patients presenting with ST-segment elevation European Heart Journal (2018) 39, 119–177.

13 Post-Procedure Management in the CCU

Sunandan Sikdar, Devendra Shrimal, and Simarjot Singh Sarin

1. What are the different aspects of post Percutaneous Coronary Intervention (PCI) care in the cardiac care unit (CCU)?

There may be a difference of opinion whether CCU monitoring post-PCI may be avoided in some cases (e.g. in the case of radial angioplasty in stable patients with type A lesions), but it is a fact that many patients do require CCU care. The intensity of monitoring will depend on the following factors:

a. Haemodynamic stability

b. Presence of heart failure

c. Presence of acute coronary syndrome

d. *Presence of comorbidities*: Diabetes, chronic obstructive pulmonary disease (COPD), chronic kidney disease (CKD), hypertension

e. Vascular access issues

f. Complexity of the PCI

g. Possibility/presence of complications related to the procedure

2. What are the steps of CCU care in post-PCI patients?

After the patients enter the CCU from catheterization lab, the following can be considered with institutional modifications:

a. *Measurements of vitals and physical exam*: Pulse, BP, SpO_2, site of vascular access especially if femoral (particularly for prolonged procedure/large dose of heparin/patient is restless).

b. ECG

c. Check whether continuation of IV fluids is necessary. In the case of raised creatinine, adequate hydration is required (see the chapter on cardiorenal syndrome and heart-kidney interactions).

d. If a femoral sheath is present, activated clotting time (ACT) is required. Once ACT falls below 160 sec, the sheath must be removed. If manual compression is used, care must be taken to compress at and above the puncture site of the common femoral artery and not at the skin entry site.

e. During manual compression, the neurocardiogenic/vagal reflex is activated in response to pain. IV fluids must be increased, and atropine must be ready.

f. After compression is over, proper bandaging is necessary and is a crucial step to avoid haematoma and blood loss. Before bandaging ensure that there is no bleeding even after coughing.

g. Ensuring immobility of the limb is a vital step. The next day palpate the site and check for the continuous murmur of a pseudoaneurysm by auscultation. For the radial site, checking the radial pulse is essential. If absent, check for the plethysmographic waveform displayed by the oximeter placed on the thumb.

3. What are the causes of new-onset hypotension post-PCI?

The causes of new-onset (i.e., non-pre-existing) hypotension post-PCI include:

a. Blood loss during PCI

b. Haematoma (including retroperitoneal haematoma)

c. Periprocedure myocardial infarction (MI) (e.g. due to branch occlusion/slow flow)

d. Overdose of drugs used – Nitroglycerin, fentanyl, midazolam

e. Acidosis/Hypoxia

f. Anaphylaxis to contrast/Drugs

DOI: 10.1201/9781003027584-13

4. What is the cause of desaturation post-PCI?

Before confirming desaturation, check carefully the sensor, whether it is snugly fitting the finger and the plethysmography curve is satisfactory. The causes of desaturation post-PCI include:

a. Pulmonary oedema

b. Hypotension and improper reading (arterial blood gas [ABG] may be better)

c. Oversedation and hypoventilation

d. Sensor on right thumb in a radial procedure, where the bandage over the puncture site is too tight

5. What is the cause of altered sensorium post-PCI?

The causes of altered sensorium post-PCI include:

a. Periprocedure/Post-thrombolysis stroke (infarct/bleed) (**Figure 13.1**)

b. Hypoglycaemia, especially in diabetics/fasting

c. Hypoxia/Hypotension

d. Dyselectrolytaemia

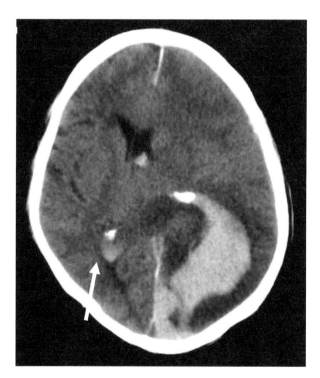

Figure 13.1 Patient presented in emergency room (ER) with altered sensorium with hypertension. Intracranial haemorrhage after streptokinase for AWSTEMI. Notice the midline shift and intraventricular extension of the bleed *(arrow).*

6. How do you grade haematoma post-PCI?

Femoral access haematomas are more common in the obese, prolonged procedures with more heparin, females (especially small sized), hypertension, those who received glycoprotein IIb/IIIa and those with kidney disease.

- *Small haematoma*: <1 cm

- *Medium haematoma*: 1–5 cm

- *Large haematoma*: >5 cm

While small and medium haematomas resolve with compression and immobilization, a large hae-matoma may require surgical removal. While manually compressing a haematoma, it is critically important to compress on the sheath entry site in the artery (more toward the inguinal crease) rather than the skin puncture site.

7. What is the time for femoral sheath removal?

For procedures like angiogram (without anticoagulation or heparin <2500 units), the sheath should to be removed immediately. For angioplasty, sheath removal should be done when ACT <160 sec, for patients on enoxaparin 6–8 hr, for those on bivalirudin >2 hr and if a fibrinolytic is used when fibrinogen >150 mg/dL. For those on full anticoagulation, a vascular closure device is better.

8. What are the precautions for manual compression during sheath removal?

The following are salient points about manual compression, which is the most widely used and the gold standard technique:

1. The duration of compression is 5 min for each French (Fr) sheath size above 6F (6Fr = 30 min) for a therapeutic (angioplasty) procedure.

2. The time of immobilization is 1 hr for each French sheath size (6Fr = 6 hr).

3. Use three finger-widths of a roll of gauze at the sheath entry site.

4. The arterial sheath must be removed before the venous sheath. Remove the venous sheath 5 min later (prevents fistula formation) and then continue compression as before.

5. Lower the bed height and bring the patient to the edge of the bed for better compression. Lock the elbows for better pressure.

6. Always watch out for signs of the vasovagal response. It is useful to infiltrate local anaesthetic around the site before beginning compression.

9. How do you manage a pseudoaneurysm?

A pseudoaneurysm is a sac-like structure caused by rupture of the layers of the vessel wall con-tained by the overlying fibromuscular tissue with a communicating neck. The pseudoaneurysm is characterized by initially painless and later painful pulsatile swelling (as the sac expands) with a continuous bruit. Risk factors for pseudoaneurysm include low puncture and improper man-ual compression. Diagnosis is confirmed by Doppler ultrasound. *Every patient must have his or her groin auscultated in the CCU the day after a femoral procedure.* A bruit which is heard in both systole and diastole is an early clue, when ultrasound-guided manual compression is of immense value. A pseudoaneurysm <2 cm in diameter can be treated by manual compression. If ultrasound-guided compression for half an hour fails, repeat the manoeuvre. In refractory cases, ultrasound-guided thrombin injection in the sac or surgical evacuation is required.

10. What is the management of retroperitoneal haemorrhage?

Due to the high-up femoral puncture above the inguinal ligament, often with a posterior punc-ture this rare but near-fatal complication may occur. There may not be a visible haematoma in the groin, but discolouration in the flanks (Cullen sign) or around the umbilicus (Gray-Turner sign) with hypotension, diffuse abdominal pain and sweating post-procedure. The test of choice is a CT pelvis without contrast (or if the femoral sheath is in place, an arteriography shows dye extrava-sation). Immediate resuscitation with fluids and packed cell transfusion and early transfer to the catheterization lab is lifesaving. Often due to surgical reluctance (due to heparinized status), taking a contralateral femoral access, taking a balloon in the iliac artery proximal to the leakage site and inflating it to achieve occlusion of the vessel are lifesaving. Alternatively if the leakage persists even after balloon tamponade for an adequate time, a covered stent may be the best option.

11. What is the management of limb artery occlusion?

This catastrophe can often be avoided by meticulous sheath management. If a femoral sheath is required to be kept in place, always connect to an invasive arterial monitor. Proper and timely (may be hourly) flushing is a must. Though heparinization may be done, it often causes local haematoma and so must be considered on merit. An arterial sheath left undetected in the groin, under the bed-sheet, is a sure recipe for future arterial occlusion. Remove a sheath whenever it is not needed. Even though radial artery occlusion seldom causes symptoms, it can be prevented by timely release of the radial bandage and adequate heparinization (3.000–8,000 units) during the procedure. This complication precludes future access. A small artery, peripheral artery disease, larger sheath, low puncture (superficial femoral artery/profunda femoris) and use of closure devices are the risk factors. The five Ps: Pain, pallor, paraesthesia, pulselessness and paralysis are frequent, especially in large artery complications. The diagnostic test is colour Doppler, confirmed by arteriography. Catheter-directed fibrinolysis (see acute limb occlusion) from the contralateral side or thrombectomy is usually used. Surgical thrombectomy is rarely used.

12. What is the management of an arteriovenous fistula?

An arteriovenous fistula may not be as commonly detected in the CCU, as it may occur later. Puncture of the artery through a vein and multiple puncture attempts are predisposing factors. It may present with increased cardiac output/limb ischemia and a bruit on physical examination. The diagnosis is confirmed by Doppler and arteriography. Ultrasound-guided compression often suffices.

13. How do you manage contrast allergy?

Contrast allergy (**Figure 13.2**) is uncommon. In the era of ionic, high-osmolar contrast agents for angiography, the incidence of contrast-related adverse effects was 15%. Nowadays because low or iso-osmolar contrast agents are being used in most centres, the incidence has reduced to less than 3%. Severe or prolonged contrast-related adverse effects are even rarer – 0.2%–2%, nearly 1 out of 55,000 procedures. Risk factors related to contrast allergy are previous reaction history, atopy/ allergy and female sex. There are two different types of reactions:

a. *Anaphylactoid reaction*: It is an IgE-independent reaction which may occur even on first exposure. It presents with rash, hives, bronchial or laryngeal spasms, nausea/vomiting, hypotension and, rarely, shock.

b. *Chemotoxic reaction*: This reaction is due to the toxic effect of the agent. Manifestations include warmth, flushing, vasovagal changes and renal toxicity. Properties like osmolality and the infusion rate of the media highly influence these reactions.

For those with a history of contrast allergy, the following premedication can be used: Prednisolone 1 mg/kg mg at 13, 7 and 1 hr prior to contrast exposure plus diphenhydramine 50 mg intramuscular (i.m) 1 hr before the procedure. Ranitidine 300 mg orally or 50 mg intravenous may be used along with the previously noted regimen.

If a desensitization protocol is to be used, it is started about 2 hr before the catheterization lab entry. If the agent chosen is iso-osmolar (Visipaque), which is often the case, escalating concentration of the diluted contrast is used. Any sign of reaction is promptly treated with diphenhydramine, methylprednisolone and epinephrine.

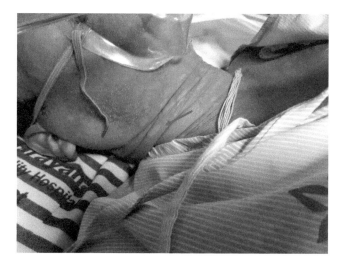

Figure 13.2 Contrast allergy post-CAG.

A full-blown contrast reaction is treated with i.m epinephrine, diphenhydramine 50 mg i.v (or slow IV over 2 min) and IV hydrocortisone. Always preserve IV access and rapidly infuse normal saline (about 1 litre) if hypotension is already underway.

If (1) laryngeal oedema or (2) bronchospasm or (3) hypotension and tachycardia is occurring (systolic blood pressure [SBP] <90 mmHg, HR >100), IV epinephrine 1 mL of a 1:10,000 dilution (0.1 mg) may be administered through a running IV infusion set. This dose can be repeated as required up to a total of 10 mL (1 mg). If using the IM route, then 0.3 mL of a *1:1000* dilution epinephrine is used (0.3 mg) up to a total dose of 1 mg. However, the IV route is preferred in emergency situations. Salbutamol nebulization is also helpful in bronchospasm.

In hypoglycaemia 50% dextrose is administered (glucagon 1 mg i.m is used if refractory).

If a vasovagal-type reaction occurs with hypotension and bradycardia, then atropine 0.6 mg IV may be infused into a running drip to a maximum of 3 mg.

If hypertensive crisis occurs after IV contrast, labetalol (20 mg IV) or nitroglycerin infusion is the treatment of choice.

Most of the contrast-related reactions usually settle by hydrocortisone and H1 blockers when given sufficient time.

14. How do you manage shivering post–catheterization lab procedure?

This is a common occurrence, especially if reused hardware is used (even if ethylene oxide (ETO) sterilized). Apart from giving warmers, the best way is to apply injectable fentanyl 25 mg or morphine 1–3 mg. Because of the possibility of vomiting, injectable ondansetron 4 mg IV may be given as premedication.

15. What are the postoperative complications of pacing that need to be monitored?

The common complications in the immediate postoperative period includes:

a. *Pneumothorax*: Always auscultate the back of the chest, infrascapular, interscapular and infraaxillary areas. Breath sounds are markedly diminished in these areas, compared to the other side (normally it is slightly diminished due to reduced chest excursion caused by pain from the local site) if this complication has taken place. Chest X-ray the next day, done in the erect position in full inspiration (**Figure 13.3**), will show the collapsed lung margin. A small pneumothorax shows up above the clavicle. The larger one will show up lateral to the collapsed lung margin. Always drain an iatrogenic pneumothorax for sure and rapid relief.

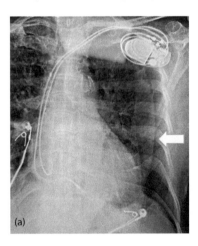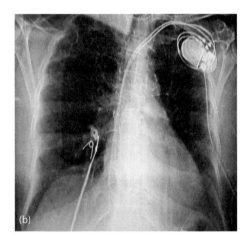

Figure 13.3   Post-pacing pneumothorax – Notice the margin of (a) collapsed lung *(arrow)* and (b) resolution after intercostal drain.

b. Haemothorax (**Figures 13.4** and **13.5**) is a rare but very troubling complication. This needs to be drained, and surgical intervention may be required.

c. *Swelling over pacemaker site*: It is wise not to drain.

d. Lead dislodgement and loss of pacing.

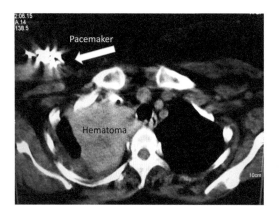
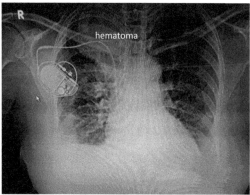

Figure 13.4   Post-pacing intrathoracic haematoma caused by slow oozing from the venous puncture site in a patient with complete heart block, shock liver and deranged coagulation.

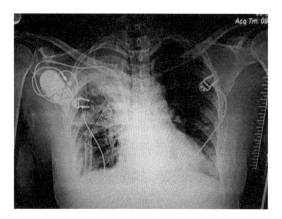
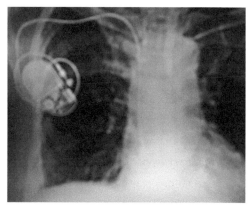

Figure 13.5   Same patient. Before and after haematoma removal by video-assisted thoracoscopy.

FURTHER READING

1. Sripal Bangalore. Vascular Access and Closure. In Bhatt D L (Ed) Cardiovascular Intervention: A Companion to Braunwald's Heart Disease. (2016), pp 20–51.

14 Cardiogenic Shock and Management of Hypotension

Sunandan Sikdar, Amit Mittal, and Umesh Kohli

1. How do you define cardiogenic shock (CS)?

This is defined based on clinical and haemodynamic parameters, as given in **Table 14.1**.

Table 14.1: Definition of Cardiogenic Shock	
Clinical Criteria	**Haemodynamic Criteria**
Hypotension	Cardiac output <2.2 L/min/m²
SBP <90 mmHg for 30 min or requires vasopressors/support to maintain SBP above that level	PCWP >15 mmHg
End-Organ Hypoperfusion	
Urine output <30 mL/hr	
HR >100/min	
Cool extremities	

2. What are the causes of CS?

Myocardial infarction (MI) accounts for 80% of cases of CS. The common causes include:

1. MI and its complications
2. Cardiac tamponade
3. Pulmonary embolism
4. Pump failure in a case of severe left ventricular (LV) dysfunction
5. Tachyarrhythmia or bradyarrhythmias
6. Acute myocarditis
7. Acute aortic or mitral regurgitation
8. Postcardiotomy cardiogenic shock

3. What is the pathophysiology of CS?

CS involves not only low cardiac output but also an inflammatory response triggered by it. Both of these factors are responsible for the multiorgan dysfunction (**Figure 14.1**).

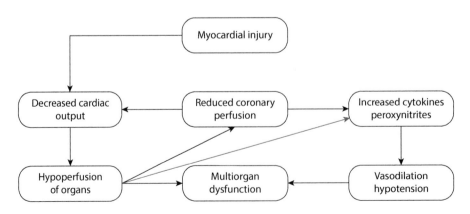

Figure 14.1 Pathophysiology of cardiogenic shock.

DOI: 10.1201/9781003027584-14

4. Why is haemodynamic data important?

Often the MI patients subtly slide into shock unnoticed, a stage where active management of shock (pre- or post-percutaneous coronary intervention [PCI]) is rewarding. Further, up to 25% of patients presenting with CS owing to LV failure in the setting of acute MI (AMI) do not present with the classic symptoms in the emergency room (ER), instead displaying isolated hypoperfusion in the absence of pulmonary congestion, despite high pulmonary capillary wedge pressure (PCWP).

5. What are the normal haemodynamic parameters?

Normal haemodynamic parameters are given in **Table 14.2**.

Table 14.2: Shock-Related Parameters

Parameter	Definition	Normal Values
Blood pressure	$CO \times SVR$	100–140/70–90 mmHg
Cardiac output	$= \text{Stroke volume} \times HR$ $\dfrac{135 \text{ mL/min/m}^2 \times BSA}{13.4 \times Hb \times (SaO_2 - SvO_2)}$	4–7 L/min
Cardiac index	CO/BSA	2.8–3.6 L/min/m^2
SVR	$[MAP - CVP/CO] \times 80$	800–1200 dynes/s/cm^{-5}
PVR	$[PAM - PCWP/CO]$	1–2 Wood units
Mean systemic BP	$(SBP + 2 \times DBP)/3$	80–100 mmHg
Mean pulmonary pressure	$(PASP + 2 \times PAEDP)/3$	15–20 mmHg
Central venous pressure		2–6 mmHg
Mixed venous O$_2$ saturation		70%–75%
Arterial O$_2$ saturation		95%–100%
Pulmonary capillary wedge pressure		8–12 mmHg

Table 14.3: Diamond Forrester Classification of Cardiogenic Shock in MI

Class	Cardiac Index	PCWP	Mortality (%)
I	>2	<18	3
II	>2	>18	9
III	<2	<18	23
IV	<2	>18	51

6. What are the mortality rates of CS due to MI?

Randomized clinical trials report mortality rates between 40% and 60% for patients with MI and shock. In the SHOCK trial (1999), the corresponding mortality rates for those over 75 years of age was 75%.

7. How can haemodynamic data be used for classifying shock?

Haemodynamic data may help to have an idea about the aetiology of shock (**Table 14.4**).

Table 14.4: Diagnosing Shock by Haemodynamic Data

Parameter	Cardiogenic	Septic	Hypovolemic	Neurogenic (Injury above C6)
CI	Decreased	Normal/Increased	Decreased	Normal/Decreased (if bradycardia)
SVR	Increased	Decreased	Increased	Decreased
RA pressure	Increased	Decreased	Decreased	Decreased
PCWP	Increased	Decreased	Decreased	Decreased
SvO$_2$	Decreased	Increased	Increased	Decreased

8. What is the Society of Coronary Angiography and Intervention (SCAI) classification (2019) of CS?

The SCAI has published a convenient clinical classification of CS (**Table 14.5**).

Table 14.5: SCAI Classification (2019) of Cardiogenic Shock

Stage	Definition	Findings	Biochemical Parameters	Haemodynamics
A	**At risk**	• Good pulse, normal JVP • Clear lungs	• Normal labs • Normal renal function • Normal lactic acid	• CI >2.5 • SBP >100 mmHg • CVP <10 mmHg • PA sat >65%
B	**Beginning CS**	Good pulse, raised JVP, lung crepitations	• Mild renal dysfunction • Normal lactate <2 mmol/L • Raised BNP	• CI: 2.2–2.5 • SBP <90 mmHg MAP >60 mmHg or >30 mmHg drop • HR >100/min • PA sat >65%
C	**Classic CS**	• Cold, pulse volume low • Crepitations • Low urine output <30 mL/hr	• Doubling of creatinine/>50% drop in GFR • Deranged LFT • Lactate 2–5 mmol/L	• MAP <60 mmHg/drugs/device to maintain these targets • SBP <90 mmHg • PCWP >15 mmHg • RAP/PCWP >0.8 • PAPI <1.85 • Cardiac power <0.6 W
D	**Deteriorating doom**	As earlier	As earlier	Requires multiple pressors/MCS
E	**Extremis**	Pulseless, arrest/Defibrillated	pH <7.2 Lactate >5 mmol/L	• No SBP without CPR • PEA • Hypotension despite maximal support

9. What are the predictors of in-hospital mortality in AMI-CS?

Predictors of in-hospital mortality include age >70 years, creatinine >2.0, lactate >4.0 and cardiac power output <0.6 W.

10. What is the protocol of treatment of CS?

Step 1. *Confirm CS*: Systolic blood pressure (SBP) <90 mmHg for >30 min or requires inotropes/vasopressor for SBP >90 mmHg, cool extremities, urine <30 mL/hr, check ECG to rule out MI, echocardiography for left ventricle/right ventricle (LV/RV) function and inferior vena cava (IVC).

Step 2. *Get blood gas data*: Obtain arterial blood gas (ABG) for pH, SaO_2, lactate. Lactate >2 moles/L. Proceed to Step 3.

Step 3. If MI is suspected, proceed for *cardiac catheterization*: Right heart catheterization and coronary angiography. Obtain SvO_2 value and proceed to Step 4.

Step 4. Calculate cardiac index (CI) by the Fick equation:

- $$CI \ (Fick) = \frac{135 \ mL/min/m^2}{13.4 \times Hb \times (SaO_2 - SvO_2)}$$

Step 5. *Interpretation*: If CI <1.8 L/min/m^2 without or <2.0–2.2 L/min/m^2 with supportive measures and adequate or elevated filling pressure (e.g., LV end-diastolic pressure [LVEDP] >15 mmHg or RV end-diastolic pressure [RVEDP] greater than 10–15 mmHg). Check if Pulmonary Artery Pulsatility Index (PAPI) <1.0 and cardiac power output <0.6. If haemodynamic criteria are met, mechanical circulatory support (MCS) is required. Since intra-aortic balloon pump (IABP) is widely available, it should be utilized prior to revascularization (as early as possible). However, the Impella device may provide a higher stroke volume. If the patient is in shock with pulmonary oedema, it may be wise to ventilate before starting PCI.

Step 6. Revascularize as completely and as quickly as possible. If acute decompensated heart failure (ADHF) is due to a non-coronary cause like myocarditis, appropriate therapy should be started.

Step 7. Daily monitoring of MCS device.

a. Peripheral pulse for IABP by Doppler probe in the respective limb

b. Echocardiography

c. ABG and lactate

d. Monitoring of anticoagulation by activated partial thromboplastin time (aPTT)

e. Tailoring of vasopressors as per MAP

f. Daily inspect insertion site of device

g. Daily assess urine output and ventilatory parameters

11. What is PAPI?

PAPI is a novel index of RV function, which is defined as pulmonary pulse pressure (pulmonary artery systolic pressure [PASP] minus pulmonary artery diastolic pressure [PADP]) divided by right atrial pressure [RAP]: PASP – PADP/RAP. It predicts severe RV dysfunction in inferior wall MI, and PAPI <1.0 is a criteria in CS.

12. What is cardiac power output (CPO)?

Traditional haemodynamic measurements obtained from a pulmonary artery catheter, such as cardiac output (CO), do not fully describe the fundamental state of the cardiovascular system in the setting of severe illness. In particular, because of its critical dependence on preload and afterload, measured CO provides a limited estimation of ventricular function. CPO is a novel haemodynamic measure that is the product of simultaneously measured CO and mean arterial pressure (MAP). By incorporating both the pressure and flow domains of the cardiovascular system, CPO is an integrative measure of cardiac hydraulic pumping ability. CPO has been shown to be a powerful predictor of mortality in patients with chronic heart failure (HF) and in those with CS. CPO is (CO × MAP)/451. Previously, the SHOCK investigators determined that the cut-off value of CPO that most accurately predicted in-hospital mortality in their patient cohort was 0.53 W.

13. What is postcardiotomy CS?

Two to six percent cases of cardiothoracic surgery are characterized by development of low CO and hypoperfusion in the early postoperative period. Factors predisposing patients to the development of postcardiotomy low-output syndrome include LV ejection fraction <20%, reoperative or emergency surgery, age >70 years, diabetes mellitus, triple-vessel or left main disease and recent MI. Mortality for postcardiotomy CS is 50%–80%. Surgically implanted extracorporeal centrifugal pumps may be used to treat postcardiotomy shock.

14. How do different inotropes and vasopressors compare?

Comparison between different inotropes and vasopressors are given in **Table 14.6**.

Table 14.6: Vasopressor and Inotropes in Use in the CCU

Drug	Mechanism/ Receptor	MAP	HR	CO	Dose	Comment
Noradrenaline	α1 >> β1> β2	Increase	Increase/ Decrease	Increase	0.05–1 mcg/kg/ min	Useful for haemodynamics
Dobutamine	β1 >> β2	Decrease	Increase	Increase	2–20 mcg/kg/min	Useful in SBP 80–90, in addition to NE
Levosimendan	Ca sensitizer	Decrease	Increase	Increase	0.5–2 mcg/kg/min	Useful if history of beta-blocker usage
Enoximone	PDE-3 inhibitor	Decrease	Increase	Increase	0.12—0.75 mcg / kg/min	In cardiothoracic ICU

(Continued)

Table 14.6 (*Continued*): Vasopressor and Inotropes in Use in the CCU

Drug	Mechanism/ Receptor	MAP	HR	CO	Dose	Comment
Adrenaline	$\alpha1 \gg \beta1 > \beta2$	Increase	Increase	Increase	0.1–1 mcg/kg/min	Useful in selected cases
Dopamine	DA, $\beta1 \gg \alpha1$	Increase	Increase	Increase	5–20 mcg/kg/min	• Arrhythmia risk (AF) • Usually used if bradycardia is a concern
Vasopressin	V1	Increase	Decrease	Decrease	0.01–0.04 U/min	If sepsis-related hypotension suspected, not favoured
Mephentermine	$\beta1$	Increase	Decrease	Variable	30- to 50-mg bolus	To tide over sudden profound hypotension

15. Who are the candidates for permanent circulatory support?

Inclusion criteria

American Heart Association (AHA) stage D heart failure

VO_2 max <14 mL/kg/min, <50% attainment of respiratory anaerobic threshold

New York Heart Association (NYHA) functional class III–IV for 3 months on optimal medical therapy

16. How do the different mechanical circulatory support (MCS) systems compare?

Comparison between different MCS systems (**Figure 14.2**) is given in **Table 14.7**.

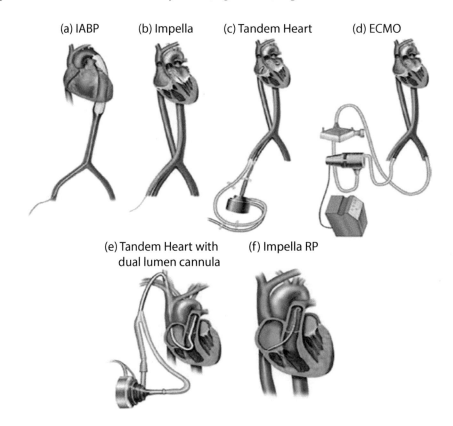

Figure 14.2 Mechanical circulatory support. (With permission from [1].)

Table 14.7: Mechanical Circulatory Support

Parameter	IABP	Impella 2.5	Impella CP	Tandem Heart	ECMO
Mechanism	Pneumatic	Axial	Axial	Centrifugal	Centrifugal
Flow augmentation	Variable, dependent on intrinsic function	2.5 L/min	2.5–3.5 L/min	4–5 L/min	Variable, can give full support
Cardiac index and MAP	Increased mildly	Increased mildly	Increased significantly	Increased significantly	Increased significantly
Coronary perfusion	Increased	Increased	Increased	Increased	Variable, may decrease –addition of IABP may be considered
Myocardial wall stress and work	Decreased	Decreased	Decreased	Decreased	May be increased
Arterial access	7–8F	13F	14F	15–19F	15–17F
Venous access	None	None	None	Trans-septal access	19–25F
Contraindication	Peripheral vascular disease	Peripheral vascular disease, AR, LV thrombus	Peripheral vascular disease, AR, LV thrombus	Peripheral vascular disease, RV failure	Peripheral vascular disease

17. What is the benefit of IABP?

The IABP can decrease myocardial oxygen consumption, increase coronary artery perfusion, enhance CO by augmenting diastolic arterial pressure and coronary blood flow during the balloon inflation phase and increase LV stroke volume by lowering LV afterload.

CASE STUDY 14.1

A 42-year-old male smoker, diabetic, with chest pain for 2 hr, presented with vomiting and restlessness. Radial pulse was not palpable, femoral pulse was feeble and BP was not recordable. ECG showed ST elevation in inferior leads with AV dissociation. Echo showed dilated LV cavity, akinetic basal inferoseptal wall, hypokinesia in mid and apical anteroseptum, apex and RV dysfunction (TAPSE 10) and LVEF 22%. ABG on admission (ER) pH 6.99, pCO_2 50 mmHg, pO_2 60 mmHg, lactate 15 mmol/L.

■ *Question*: *Should we intubate first or IABP first?*
Temporary pacing implantation (TPI) and arterial access from right groin, IABP from left groin. Next intubated – ventilated. On noradrenaline + insulin infusion (CBG 486 mg/dL), BP now 116 (augmented) 70/40/50 mmHg. IABP-assisted CAG showed an occluded RCA and occluded mid-LAD.

■ *Question: Which should be opened first? RCA or LAD?*
PCI to RCA was done, as this was the culprit vessel by ECG. Persistent acidosis continued but pH 7.1 and then 7.2 by the next day, urine output was good. On the second day, the pH normalized

■ *Question: IABP or ventilation, which one to remove first?*
On the third day, we extubated him, keeping IABP. On bilevel positive airway pressure (BIPAP) we started tapering noradrenaline from 12 mL/hr. On the fifth day, Noradr (4/50) @ 6 mL/hr.
When IABP support reduced to 1:4, SBP fell to 60 mmHg and MAP to 50 mmHg.

■ *Question: What is the solution?*
Adrenaline (4/50) @ 3 mL/hr. IABP removed, then vasopressors tapered off. Had an episode of LVF, managed with BIPAP. Discharged on 10th day with BIPAP sos at home.

However in spite of its widespread use, the IABP SHOCK trial and IABP SHOCK II trial failed to show evidence that IABP improved mortality in CS with or without associated PCI even in ST-segment elevated MI (STEMI) situations. But because in most centres Impella or venoarterial extracorporeal membrane oxygenation (VA ECMO) is out of reach for patients requiring them, IABP, in spite of its questionable efficacy, plays a pivotal role as the only available MCS even today in many centres.

FURTHER READING

1. Rao S V, Mandawat A. Percutaneous Mechanical Circulatory Support Devices in Cardiogenic Shock. Circ Cardiovasc Interv 2017;10:e004337.
2. Doll J A, Ohman E M, Patel M R, et al. A Team-Based Approach to Patients in Cardiogenic Shock. Catheter Cardiovasc Interv 2016;88(3):424–433.

15 Inotropes and Vasopressors

Sunandan Sikdar and Aman Makhija

Chapter 15 may be accessed online at: www.routledge.com/9780367462215

DOI: 10.1201/9781003027584-15

16 Antiplatelets and Anticoagulants

Perioperative Issues

Sunandan Sikdar and Dipankar Ghosh Dastidar

1. What is the mechanism of action of aspirin?

Aspirin blocks production of thromboxane A2 (a platelet aggregator and vasoconstrictor) by acetylating a serine residue near the active site of the platelet COX-1 receptor (**Figure 16.1**). Because platelets do not synthesize new proteins, the action of aspirin on platelet COX-1 is permanent, lasting for the lifetime of the platelet (7–10 days). Thus, repeated doses of aspirin produce a cumulative effect on platelet function. Complete inactivation of platelet COX-1 is achieved with a daily aspirin dose of 75 mg. Therefore, aspirin is maximally effective as an antithrombotic agent at doses much lower than those required for other actions of the drug.

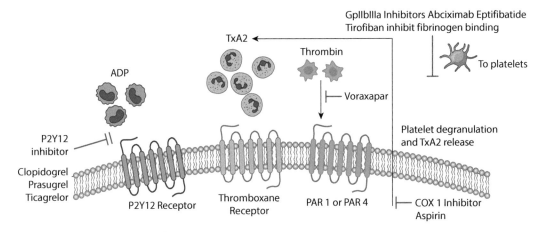

Figure 16.1 Antiplatelets and their basic mechanism of action.

2. What are the side effects of aspirin?

Higher doses (>150 mg/day) inhibit prostacyclin synthesis and increase GI bleeding risk (>2/1000 patients/year) and should be avoided. Enteric-coated aspirin reduces GI side effects by delivering the drug to the intestine rather than to the stomach, but at the cost of reduced bioavailability (suboptimal response). Dyspepsia occurs in nearly 20%. Aspirin reduces renal excretion of uric acid and creatinine and raises the level of these parameters, especially in the elderly (caution). There is a marginal increase in intracranial haemorrhage.

3. What is the role of aspirin in primary and secondary prevention?

While in secondary prevention indications, aspirin is clearly the winner –46% reduction of unstable angina, 25% reduction of myocardial infarction (MI), 22% reduction of stroke and 23% reduction of peripheral arterial disease (PAD) compared with placebo – in primary prevention, the role of aspirin is controversial: the reduction of stroke in women and MI in men is almost counterbalanced by the increase in bleeding so the net benefit is minimal.

4. What is aspirin resistance?

Aspirin resistance (5%–20% of aspirin users) due to glycoprotein polymorphism and/or activation of non-COX pathways of platelet aggregation is a cause of recurrent vascular thrombosis even on a therapeutic dose of aspirin, especially in diabetics.

5. What is the mechanism of action of ticagrelor?

Ticagrelor is a reversible P2Y12 receptor inhibitor binding to the non-adenosine triphosphate (ADP)-binding site of the receptor.

DOI: 10.1201/9781003027584-16

6. What are the pharmacokinetics of ticagrelor?

The drug and its hepatic CYP3A4-generated metabolite are *both* active and undergo *faecal excretion*. It has a plasma half-life of 8–12 hr and achieves steady state in 2–3 days. The onset of action is rapid (40% platelet inhibition by 30 min) with a peak effect in 2 hr and quick offset. Being a substrate of CYP3A4, concomitant use with enzyme inducers (phenytoin, rifampicin and dexamethasone) or inhibitors (ketoconazole, clarithromycin and ritonavir) should be avoided. In that case, clopidogrel/prasugrel should be used. There is no dose modification required in renal failure or the elderly or lower body weight. This is an advantage over prasugrel.

7. What are the adverse effects of ticagrelor?

Adverse effects of ticagrelor include dyspnoea, ventricular pauses and increased level of creatinine – this could be due to the adenosine-like effect on the equilibrative nucleoside transducer (ENT1). In the PLATO trial, dyspnoea was more common in the ticagrelor group than the clopidogrel group (13.8% versus 7.8%), but this led to discontinuation of the drug in only 0.9% of patients.

8. What is the role of ticagrelor?

Ticagrelor is the drug of choice in both in medically and interventionally managed acute coronary syndrome (ACS) as a part of dual antiplatelet therapy (DAPT) for up to a year. It can also be used after 1 year at a dose of 60 mg twice daily in those with MI for 3 years. The landmark PLATO trial showed that in ACS, ticagrelor reduced all-cause mortality by 16% compared to clopidogrel. The role of aspirin overlapping with that of ticagrelor for 3 months after stenting followed by ticagrelor monotherapy up to a year is being actively investigated. The TWILIGHT trial showed there was decrease in bleeding without an increase in ischaemic events when DAPT was abbreviated to 3 months.

9. What is the usual dosage of ticagrelor?

The loading dose is 180 mg followed by a maintenance dose 90 mg twice daily.

10. What is the pharmacology of irreversible P2Y12 antagonists?

Clopidogrel and Prasugrel: They are irreversible P2Y12 receptor blockers. Both are prodrugs activated in the liver. Fifteen per cent of clopidogrel and 85% of prasugrel are converted into the active metabolite predominantly by the CYP 2C19 and CYP 3A4 enzyme systems, respectively. Prasugrel (½–4 hr) has a faster onset of action than clopidogrel (2–8 hr). Both have a long duration (7–10 days) of action. The increased effect of prasugrel compared to clopidogrel is due to better absorption of the drug (95%) and increased availability of its active metabolite – the potency of active metabolites of both drugs is the same.

11. What are the contraindications for prasugrel?

Prasugrel is contraindicated in previous stroke/transient ischaemic attack (TIA), age >75 years and weight <60 kg. It is not used if ACS is managed medically.

12. What is clopidogrel resistance?

Clopidogrel has a reduced effect in the following subsets (clopidogrel resistance): Diabetes, smoking, renal failure, ACS, faster platelet turnover, genetic polymorphism (CYP 2C19*2 loss-of-function allele – increased thrombosis). Interestingly the variant CYP 2C19* 17 causes more active metabolites, resulting in increased bleed. Thus, prasugrel is preferred in diabetics and those with the CYP 2C19 *2 allele.

13. What is the role of clopidogrel and prasugrel?

In the TRITON TIMI 58 trial, prasugrel compared to clopidogrel reduced major acute cardiovascular events (MACEs) by 19% in ACS patients undergoing percutaneous coronary intervention (PCI).

Dose

Clopidogrel: Loading dose 300 mg for medically managed and 600 mg prior to primary PCI followed by 75 mg once daily.

Prasugrel: Loading dose 60 mg then maintenance 10 mg once daily.

14. What are the newer antiplatelet agents?

Vorapaxar: The human platelet aggregatory response to thrombin is primarily mediated through two G-protein-coupled protease-activated receptors (PARs): PAR1 and PAR4. The PAR 1 antagonist vorapaxar has been shown to decrease ischaemic events in patients with previous MI or peripheral vascular disease. The addition of vorapaxar to antiplatelet agents causes increased bleeding risk, especially intracranial bleed (TRACER trial). The drug is contraindicated in patients with a history of stroke (increased risk of intracranial bleed), TIA or intracranial haemorrhage and has limited use.

Cangrelor: A direct-acting reversible platelet P2Y12 antagonist with a very short half-life (3–6 min). It is a useful intravenous drug in those ACS patients who are vomiting/drowsy while being taken to catheterization lab but are yet to be given a P2Y12 loading dose. Another use may be where the anatomy is unknown and cardiac surgery may be required.

15. What are the causes of ACS in the perioperative period?

Reasons for perioperative ACS (**Table 16.1**) are (1) plaque rupture, (2) increased platelet aggregability, (3) sympathetic activation and (4) inflammation. The perioperative risk of stent thrombosis is increased by certain patient and procedural characteristics enumerated in **Table 16.2**.

Table 16.1: Pathophysiology of Perioperative ACS

Absence of Antiplatelet Cover	Perioperative Prothrombotic State
Unendothelized stent struts	Increased platelet reactivity
Incompletely revascularized or non-revascularized vessels	Increased cytokines and sympathetic activation
Vulnerable plaque	Increased procoagulants
	Decreased fibrinolysis

Table 16.2: High-Risk Features that Predispose to Stent Thrombosis in the Perioperative Period

Patient Characteristics	Lesion Characteristics
ACS at the time of index procedure	>3 stents/overlapping stents
Past history of stent thrombosis	>3 lesions treated
Multiple previous MI	>60 mm stent length
LVEF <35%	Chronic total occlusion
Kidney disease	Incomplete revascularisation
Diabetes	Bifurcation with two stents
	Small stent (2.5 mm)

16. What is the protocol for withholding antiplatelets (Figure 16.2)?

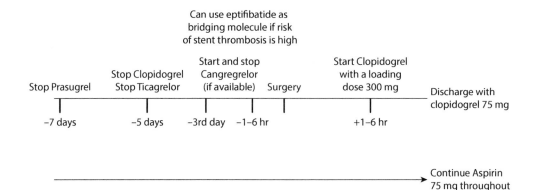

Figure 16.2 Timeline of antiplatelet withdrawal.

Aspirin should be stopped 7 days before surgery and restarted after a week in routine cases. Stopping and restarting aspirin in established or those at risk of atherosclerotic disease for a minimum 3 days before (median 7 days) and 8 days after does not increase adverse cardiac events (POISE 2 trial, 2014). For some spinal/neurosurgical operations, discontinuation may extend to 10 days before surgery.

The exceptions where aspirin should be continued are stenting by drug-eluting stent (DES) within one year (especially if the indication was ACS) or by bare metal stent (BMS) in the past 6 weeks or carotid endarterectomy was recently performed or is currently considered.

17. What is the timing of DAPT discontinuation in non-cardiac surgery?

DAPT discontinuation prior to non-cardiac surgery can be considered in:

- *Post-BMS implantation*: After 4–6 weeks

- *Post-DES implantation*: After 6 months (non-ACS, new-generation DES), 12 months (ACS indication)

If surgery is unavoidable/emergent, in the setting of newly (1–3 months) implanted new-generation DES, the operation should be carried out in a centre with a catheterization laboratory so that in the eventuality of stent thrombosis, immediate thrombus aspiration is possible.

Clopidogrel and ticagrelor should be withheld for 5 days and prasugrel for 7 days. The DAPT should be restarted within 48 hr, if possible, especially in post-stent cases.

In cases of very high risk of stent thrombosis (**Table 16.2**), bridging with eptifibatide and, recently, with the reversible intravenous P2Y12 inhibitor cangrelor has been tried in some cases.

18. What is the antithrombotic discontinuation protocol related to surgery in non-vitamin K antagonist (VKA) use?

See the Chapter 14 on non-VKAs.

19. What is the perioperative protocol in the case of VKA use?

Patients on VKA are at increased risk of periprocedural bleeding. In cases of low thrombotic risk, surgery is safe once the international normalization ratio (INR) drops to 1.5. Heparin/low-molecular-weight (LMWH) bridging is not necessary.

20. When is bridging with heparin required during VKA discontinuation?

In patients with a high risk of thromboembolism bridging with unfractionated heparin (UFH)/LMWH is necessary:

a. Atrial fibrillation (AF) with high CHADVAS score

b. Mechanical prosthetic heart valves

c. Newly inserted bioprosthetic valve

d. Venous thromboembolism <3 months

e. Thrombophilia

21. What is the protocol of bridging with heparin?

VKA should be discontinued 3–5 days prior to surgery. UFH/LMWH should be started once the INR <2 or 1 day after discontinuation of the VKA. The last dose of LMWH should be given >12 hr before the procedure. Once the INR <1.5 one can proceed to surgery. The bridging molecule is often LMWH (more data), but in mechanical valves UFH can be used. In the case of UFH, the last dose should be > 4 hr before surgery. If the INR is still >1.5, postpone surgery until it is at that level. After surgery, UFH/LMWH is resumed at the preprocedural dose after 1–2 days depending on the bleeding risk but usually >12 hr post-procedure. VKA is started after 1–2 days at the preoperative dose plus an extra 50% booster dose for 2 days. Then UFH/LMWH should be continued until the INR reaches therapeutic levels.

FURTHER READING

1. Fox K A A, White H D, Gersh B, Opie L J. Antithrombotic Agents: Platelet Inhibitors, Acute Anticoagulants, Fibrinolytics, and Chronic Anticoagulants, in Opie L, Gersh B J (Ed). Drugs for the Heart. 8th Edition. (2013), pp 332–397. Elsevier.
2. McFadyen J D, Schaff M, Peter K. Current and Future Antiplatelet Therapies: Emphasis on Preserving Haemostasis. Nat Rev Cardiol 2018 Mar;15(3):181–191.
3. Rossini R, Tarantini G, Musumeci G, et al. A Multidisciplinary Approach on the Perioperative Antithrombotic Management of Patients with Coronary Stents Undergoing Surgery. J Am Coll Cardiol Intv 2018;11:417–434.

17 Non-Vitamin K Oral Anticoagulants

Sunandan Sikdar

1. What are the non-vitamin K antagonist (VKA) oral anticoagulants or newer oral anticoagulants (NOACs)?

The list of NOACs is given below (landmark trials of the drugs in atrial fibrillation (AF) are given in parentheses). Their mechanism of action has been depicted in **Figure 17.1**.

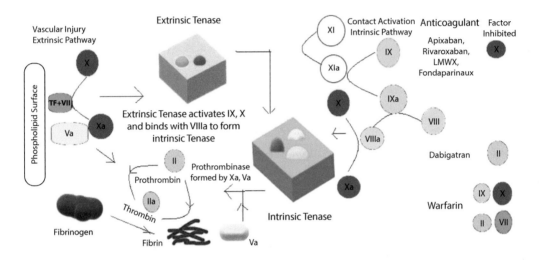

Figure 17.1 Clotting mechanism and site of action of anticoagulant drugs.

a. Direct factor Xa inhibitors

- Rivaroxaban (ROCKET AF)
- Apixaban (ARISTOTLE)
- Edoxaban (ENGAGE AF-TIMI 48)

b. Direct thrombin inhibitors

- Dabigatran (RE-LY)

2. What are the advantages of NOACs over VKAs?

They have (1) more efficacy, (2) more safety, (3) no need for regular international normalization ratio (INR) monitoring and (4) fewer drug interactions.

3. How do you adjust the VKA dose as per the INR?

The dosage adjustment of VKA as per INR is given in **Table 17.1**.

Table 17.1: Adjusting the Dose of VKA (e.g. Warfarin) by Using INR	
INR	**Dose Adjustment per Week**
≤1.5	Increase by 15%/week
1.6–1.9	Increase by 10%/week
2–2.9	Unchanged
3–3.9	Decrease by 10%/week
4–4.9	Hold one dose, then restart with dose decreased by 10%/week
≥5	Hold until INR is 2–3, then restart with dose decreased by 15%/week

DOI: 10.1201/9781003027584-17

4. What are the current indications of VKA?

There are only a few conditions where VKA has no alternative: (1) *Mechanical valve prosthesis* (with or without AF) (in the REALIGN trial dabigatran caused both more bleeding and increased thrombotic events compared to VKA when used in patients with mechanical valves). (2) *Moderate to severe mitral stenosis with AF.* INVICTUS trial showed that in patients with rheumatic heart disease–associated AF, VKA therapy led to a lower rate of a composite of cardiovascular events or death than rivaroxaban therapy, without a higher rate of bleeding. (3) Use of VKAs in *AF patients in advanced renal failure or in those undergoing dialysis* is standard of care, but the evidence base of the practice is limited. Apixaban has some evidence in its favour. Warfarin accelerates medial arterial calcification and this effect is markedly accentuated in advanced kidney disease.

5. What are the indication for NOACs?

a. All types of AF except moderate to severe mitral stenosis

b. Prophylaxis for venous thromboembolism

c. Treatment of pulmonary embolism

d. Left ventricular (LV) thrombus (off-label indication)

6. What are relative pharmacokinetics of different NOACs?

Table 17.2: Pharmacokinetics of NOACs

Parameter	Dabigatran	Rivaroxaban	Apixaban	Edoxaban
Bioavailability	3%–7%	• 60% without food • 100% with food	60%	60%
Prodrug	Yes	No	No	No
Half-life	12–17 hr	• 5–10 hr in young • 11–14 hr in elderly	12 hr	10 hr
Food	No effect	Increased absorption	No	Minimal
Protein binding	35%	95%	87%	55%
Renal clearance	80%	35%	27%	50%
Hepatic elimination (CYP3A4)	No	18%	25%	Minimal

7. What is the dose modification for apixaban?

The dose modification for Apixaban from 5 mg twice daily to 2.5 mg twice daily is required if any of the two are present:

1. Age > 80 years

2. Body weight < 60 kg

3. Serum creatinine > 1.5 mg/dL

Renal dose modifications for NOACs are provided in **Table 17.3**. Creatinine Clearance is given in mL/min/1.73m²

Table 17.3: Renal Dose Modification for NOACs

Creatinine Clearance	Dabigatran	Rivaroxaban	Apixaban
> 50	150 mg BD	20 mg OD	5 mg BD
30–50	110 mg BD	15 mg OD	2.5 mg BD
15–30	×	15 mg OD	2.5 mg BD
<15	×	×	Limited evidence in favour, continue in selected cases

8. Which NOACs have been proven superior to warfarin in preventing strokes?

Dabigatran 150 mg twice daily and apixaban 5 mg twice daily have been proven superior to warfarin in preventing strokes. However, head-to-head comparison among different NOACs has not been prospectively studied in large populations.

9. What is the preoperative regimen of NOACs in non-cardiac surgery?

The procedures are divided into three groups:

1. *Minor bleeding risk*: Dental procedure, ophthalmologic (cataract and glaucoma) procedure, endoscopy without biopsy, superficial surgery like abscess drainage.

2. *Low bleeding risk*: Endoscopy with biopsy, prostate biopsy, pacemaker and automatic implantable cardioverter defibrillator (AICD) implantation, peripheral angiography.

3. *High bleeding risk*: Abdominal and thoracic surgeries, spinal and epidural anaesthesia, transurethral prostate resection, orthopaedic surgery.

4. *For minor bleeding risk*: Stoppage is required only on the day of surgery. It can be restarted after >6 hr.

5. *For low bleeding risk*: Stoppage is required on the day of surgery, and it can be restarted after 24 hr (on the day after surgery).

6. *For high bleeding risk*: Stoppage is required 48 hr prior to surgery and should be restarted after 48 hr.

10. How do you switch from warfarin to a NOAC?

When INR <2, we can start a NOAC immediately. If the INR 2–2.5, then start the NOAC the next day. If the INR >3, recheck in 3 days until the INR drops to <2.

11. How do you switch from a NOAC to warfarin?

Continue the NOAC and start warfarin until three consecutive INR readings are 2–3. If the INR <2, then repeat it in 3 days, taking a sample before the NOAC intake. If the INR >2, then repeat it the next day after stopping warfarin.

12. What is the renal dose modification for NOACs?

Dose reduction is needed for creatinine clearance (CrCl): 50–30 mL/min – dabigatran 110 mg twice daily, rivaroxaban 15 mg once daily, edoxaban 30 mg twice daily and apixaban 2.5 mg twice daily (**Table 17.3**). For CrCl 15–30 mL/min, dabigatran is contraindicated, while the other drugs continue at previously mentioned doses. Below CrCl 15 mL/min, all NOACs are contraindicated and VKA use is the usual convention, though apixaban now has limited evidence from small studies in advanced renal failure, even in those on dialysis.

13. What is the status of NOACs with liver disease?

Avoid rivaroxaban in liver disease. All NOACs are contraindicated in liver disease Child-Pugh category C.

14. What regimen is used in cases of patients requiring antiplatelets after stenting but who are on NOACs due to chronic AF?

For elective percutaneous cardiac intervention (PCI) (stent thrombosis risk lower): Triple therapy (NOAC + aspirin + clopidogrel) for the hospital stay (1–7 days), then dual therapy (NOAC + clopidogrel) for 6 months, then only the NOAC is continued.

For acute coronary syndrome (ACS)-related PCI (stent thrombosis risk higher) with current drug-eluting stent (DES): Triple therapy (NOAC + aspirin + clopidogrel) for 1 month (in exceptional cases, 3 months), then dual therapy for 1 year (NOAC + clopidogrel), then only NOAC is continued (dual therapy can be extended beyond 1 year at the discretion of the physician). It is important to use an approved NOAC for stroke prevention.

In contrast to the European guidelines summarized earlier, the AUGUSTUS trial showed that apixaban (dose 5 mg twice daily), when added to clopidogrel monotherapy from 1 week after PCI for ACS in an AF cohort, significantly reduces the risk of bleeding at a non-significantly increased risk of ischaemic events. The avoidance of aspirin after a week of triple drug therapy post-PCI in ACS with AF may thus be justified. It also supports the already established fact that NOAC causes less bleeding than VKAs, and the deadly trio aspirin + clopidogrel + VKA must no longer be used post-PCI for prolonged periods. The PIONEER AF (rivaroxaban) and REDUAL PCI (dabigatran) trials also had similar results.

15. How do you manage ischaemic stroke when a patient is on a NOAC?

For a patient already on a NOAC, the following subgroups can proceed for stroke thrombolysis: (1) NOAC intake >48 hr with normal renal function; (2) if NOAC plasma level is available, the value below the lower limit of detection; (3) NOAC intake 24–48 hr with normal renal function, in selected cases, use of thrombolytics is an option that has insufficient data; and (4) if <24 hr, give antidote and proceed for thrombolysis or use endovascular thrombectomy (lack of quality evidence) – this is valid for dabigatran where a specific antidote is available.

16. Post-ischaemic stroke, how do you initiate a NOAC?

There are four scenarios

a. *For transient ischaemic attack*: Start NOAC >1 day after stroke onset

b. *For acute ischaemic stroke with mild neurological deficit*: NOAC >**3 days** after stroke onset

c. *For acute ischaemic stroke with moderate neurological deficit (CT/MRI 24 hr before starting NOAC shows no haemorrhagic transformation)*: NOAC >**6–8 days** from stroke onset

d. *For acute ischemic stroke with severe neurological deficit (CT/MRI 24 hr before starting NOAC shows no haemorrhagic transformation)*: NOAC >**12–14 days** from stroke onset

This can be summarized as the "1-3-6-12 Rule."

17. What is the NOAC regimen in post-intracranial haemorrhage with AF (who were on anticoagulation)?

An assessment has to be made whether to restart anticoagulation at all. The factors to be taken into account before re-anticoagulation include large bleed, severity and location, multiple microbleeds, bleeding on underdosage of NOACs, elderly, alcoholic and dual antiplatelet therapy.

18. What is the definition of a major bleed in a patient on a NOAC?

Across various NOAC trials, approximately 4% of patients had major bleeds and 0.4% had intracranial haemorrhage. A bleed is called major if it is:

1. Associated with haemodynamic compromise

2. Occurring in an anatomically critical site (e.g. intracranial)

3. Associated with a decrease of haemoglobin >2 g/dL (when the baseline is known)

4. Requires transfusion of >2 unit of packed red blood cells (RBCs)

19. How do you monitor a NOAC-related bleed?

Blood levels of a NOAC, if available, can be measured. Reversal agents are required if:

a. NOAC level >50 ng/mL + major bleed

b. NOAC level >30 ng/mL + emergency invasive procedure

NOAC levels are often not available. Ideal tests are thrombin time and ecarin clotting time for dabigatran and anti-Xa levels for others, but these are also not available in most centres. However, activated partial thromboplastin time (aPTT) and prothrombin time (PT) can give an idea if the results are used in perspective.

In the case of dabigatran, measure aPTT. A prolonged aPTT suggests significant drug levels in the blood.

In the case of rivaroxaban, apixaban or edoxaban, measure PT. Elevated PT suggests an increased drug level.

20. How do you treat NOAC-induced bleeding?

A reasonable strategy is as follows (**Figure 17.2**):

Step 1. Assess the severity of the bleed. If non-major and non- significant, then continue the NOAC. If a major bleed or if the bleed is non-major but significant (hospitalization required), then stop the NOAC.

Step 2. Control the bleed in all cases by local measures. If bleeding is at a critical site (e.g. intracranial) or is still uncontrolled, then reversal agents are required.

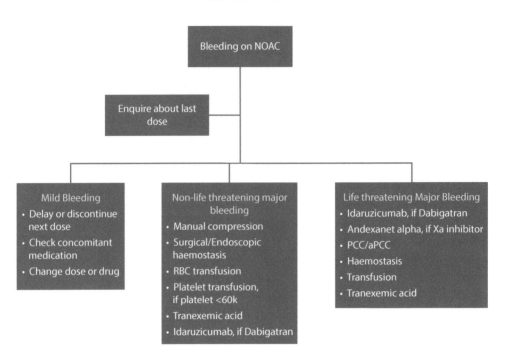

Figure 17.2 Management of bleeding on NOACs.

Step 3. Determine if the NOAC needs to be restarted. If there is no persisting indication for the NOAC, there is no need to restart. If indications are still there for the NOAC, then check if contraindications to starting are there: Critical site of the bleed, high risk of rebleed, death/disability if rebleed occurs, unknown site, plan for operation and lack of consent from the patient. If no contraindications are there, the NOAC can be restarted. If one or more contraindications are there, do not restart.

21. How do you control a bleed?

a. Repletion and fluid resuscitation strategies

b. Prothrombin complex concentrates (PCCs)

c. Fresh-frozen plasma

d. Specific reversal agents for DOACs (**Table 17.4**):

   i.   Idarucizumab for dabigatran

   ii. Andexanet alfa for rivaroxaban and apixaban

   iii. Citaparantag for apixaban (no recommendation)

22. How do you use the antidote for dabigatran?

a. The Fab fragment idarucizumab is a humanized monoclonal antibody fragment which is directed specifically at dabigatran. The affinity of idarucizumab for dabigatran is approximately 350 times that of dabigatran for thrombin.

b. In the RE-VERSE AD (Reversal of Dabigatran Anticoagulant Effect with idarucizumab) study, patients were given 5 g idarucizumab as a fixed-dose intravenous infusion of two 2.5 g aliquots.

c. Among patients with bleeding, cessation was achieved within a median time of 3.5–4.5 hr, depending on the location of the bleed.

d. Idarucizumab was safe.

e. The rate of thrombotic complications was 6%, with approximately two-thirds of those events occurring in patients not receiving anticoagulation post-reversal.

Table 17.4: Reversal Agents for NOACs

Parameters	Idarucizumab	Andexanet alpha	Citaparantag
Structure	Humanized monoclonal antibody fragment	Recombinant truncated factor Xa variant (decoy)	Synthetic water-soluble cation consisting of two L-arginine molecules with a piperazine linker
Binding	Non-competitive binding >350 times affinity to factor IIa compared to dabigatran	Competitive binding Combines with factor Xa inhibitors with similar affinity	Covalent hydrogen binding
Onset	<5 min	2 min	5–10 min
Duration t 1/2	Initial – 47 min Terminal – 10 hr	6 hr	Duration 24 hr
Storage	Refrigerated	Refrigerated	Room temperature
Agents reversed	Dabigatran	Apixaban, rivaroxaban	Argatroban, fondaparinux, apixaban, rivaroxaban
Dose	2.5 g IV two doses 15 min apart	400–800 mg loading then 4–8 mg/hr	100–300 mg IV

23. How do you reverse rivaroxaban and apixaban?

a. Andexanet alfa (andexanet) is a specific reversal agent for factor Xa (FXa) inhibitors.

b. There is a similar structure to endogenous FXa that binds FXa inhibitors, but it is not enzymatically active.

c. A bolus and 2-hr infusion of andexanet alfa rapidly reversed the anticoagulant effects of apixaban and rivaroxaban in older healthy volunteers in the ANNEXA-4 (Andexanet Alfa in Patients Receiving a FXa Inhibitor Who Have Acute Major Bleeding) trial.

d. Due to the short half-life of andexanet alfa, some anticoagulant effects of the direct FXa inhibitor return within 1 to 3 hr of stopping the infusion.

e. Eighteen percent of patients experienced thrombotic events within 30 days of andexanet infusion, the majority of whom (92%) had not restarted anticoagulant therapy.

The regimen used was as follows

Patients on apixaban or >7 hr from last rivaroxaban dose: Bolus 400 mg + infusion 480 mg @ 4 mg/min

Patients on enoxaparin, edoxaban or ≤7 hr from last rivaroxaban dose: Bolus 800 mg + infusion 960 mg @ 8 mg/min

24. How do you use the four-factor (4F) PCC?

It is purified, heat-treated, nanofiltered and lyophilized plasma. It contains the vitamin K-dependent coagulation factors II, VII, IX and X and the anti-thrombotic proteins C and S. Factor IX is the lead factor for the potency of the preparation. The excipients are human anti-thrombin III, heparin, human albumin, sodium chloride and sodium citrate. It overcomes the problems with delay and volume related to plasma. PCC reduced all-cause mortality in comparison with plasma.

4F-PCC is the most extensively studied nonspecific reversal strategy for FXa inhibitors. A dose of 25–50 U/kg can be used for emergency reversal such as severe or life-threatening bleeding in patients anticoagulated with oral direct FXa inhibitors. Contraindications to therapy include allergy to any factor, heparin-induced thrombocytopenia and disseminated intravascular coagulation. Adverse effects include thromboembolism, transmission of infection (virus, Creutzfeldt-Jakob disease [CJD] variants – but rare), hypersensitivity and fluid overload.

25. What is the safest NOAC in cases of gastrointestinal (GI) ulcer disease or those with a history of melena?

The results from various NOAC trials indicate that

1. Overall bleeding risk is low (about 1.5%).

2. Among the different NOACS, dabigatran (odds ratio 1.58) and rivaroxaban (odds ratio 1.48) have a higher bleeding risk than apixaban.

It must be remembered that NOACs do not precipitate bleeding per se, but may magnify the extent of a bleed.

Risk factors of GI bleed include age >75 years, concomitant use of antiplatelets, HAS-BLED score >3, previous disease (peptic ulcer, angiodysplasia, diverticulosis) and renal impairment.

26. What is the NOAC dosage for pulmonary embolism (PE)?

Rivaroxaban: 15 mg twice daily × 3 weeks then 10 mg once-daily maintenance

Apixaban: 10 mg twice daily for a week then 5 mg twice-daily maintenance

Dabigatran: Heparin/low-molecular-weight heparin (LMWH) for a week then 150 mg twice-daily maintenance

27. What is the dose for long-term prevention of recurrent deep vein thrombosis (DVT)/PE (i.e., after 6 months)?

Rivaroxaban 10 mg once daily

Apixaban 2.5 mg twice daily

Dabigatran 150 mg twice daily

28. What is the dose for thromboembolism prophylaxis post-orthopaedic surgery?

Recommendations in major orthopaedic surgery (e.g. hip or knee replacement, duration 35 days for hip, 12 days for knee) include

Apixaban 2.5 mg twice daily

Rivaroxaban 10 mg once daily

Dabigatran 110 mg first dose then 220 mg once daily

29. Is there any beneficial effect of NOACs in atherosclerotic disease?

Rivaroxaban 2.5 mg twice daily showed encouraging results in atherothrombotic states when added to antiplatelets in the COMPASS trial, particularly for patients with peripheral arterial disease (PAD).

ACKNOWLEDGEMENTS

Professor Renato D. Lopes had gone through the manuscript in 2020, and his suggestions were incorporated. I thank him for his kindness.

FURTHER READING

1. Lopes RD, Heizer G, Aronson R, Vora AN, et al. Anti-thrombotic Therapy after Acute Coronary Syndrome or PCI in Atrial Fibrillation (AUGUSTUS Trial). N Engl J Med (2019);380(16):1509–1524.
2. Steffel J, Verhamm P, Potpara T S, et al. The 2018 European Heart Rhythm Association Practical Guide on the Use of Non-vitamin K Antagonist Oral Anticoagulants in Patients with Atrial Fibrillation. Eur Heart J (2018);39:1330–1393.

18 Acute Aortic Syndromes

Sunandan Sikdar and Arunansu Dhole

1. What are the functions of the aorta?

The aorta (1) functions as a conduit; (2) maintains pulsatility, generating blood flow in both systolic and diastolic phases (the Windkessel effect) due to elastin in the tunica media of vessel wall; and (3) provides early diastolic reversed flow in the ascending aorta, which generates coronary perfusion.

2. What is the clinical measure of aortic stiffness?

The pulse wave velocity (PWV) between the carotid and femoral artery is a measure of aortic stiffness. The stiffer the aorta, higher the velocity. In the young it is 4–5 m/sec, while in an 80 year old, it is 8–15 m/sec.

3. What is an aortic aneurysm?

An abnormal dilation more than 50% for the age, sex and particular aortic segment of the reference population.

The aortic aneurysm is divided into the following types.

Thoracic aorta aneurysm (TAA): Ascending aorta aneurysm (60%), arch of aorta aneurysm (<10%), descending thoracic aorta aneurysm (35%)

Abdominal aorta aneurysm (AAA): Suprarenal aorta/thoracoabdominal aorta aneurysm (10%) involving the renal arteries, infrarenal aorta aneurysm (>80%)

4. What are acute aortic syndromes (AASs)?

There are three conditions under this heading:

a. Acute aortic dissection (AAD)

b. Intramural haematoma (IMH)

c. Penetrating atherosclerotic ulcer (PAU)

5. What are the risk factors of AAS?

Genetic factors (connective tissue disease): Marfan syndrome, Turner syndrome, Ehlers-Danlos syndrome, bicuspid aortic valve

Acquired factors: Systemic hypertension, aortic aneurysm, atherosclerotic heart disease, history of cardiac surgery

6. What is aortic dissection?

AAD is defined as the disruption of the medial layer due to intramural bleeding leading to a separation of the aortic wall layers, leading to formation of true and false lumen (**Figure 18.1**).

7. What are the types of AAD?

*Stanford Type A (**Figure 18.2a**)*: Ascending aorta involved (usually two-thirds of all AADs)

*Stanford Type B (**Figure 18.2b**)*: Ascending aorta not affected (usually one-third of all AADs)

8. What are the clinical features of AAD?

a. Abrupt, severe, sharp, "tearing" pain in the anterior chest (common for Type A) and back (more common for Type B).

b. Dyspnoea (due to pleural/pericardial effusion, acute aortic regurgitation).

c. Syncope (due to hypotension).

d. Stroke (due to dissection flap involving the carotid artery).

e. Myocardial infarct (10%) due to flap covering the coronary ostia or dissection involving the coronary ostia. The right coronary artery is more commonly involved.

DOI: 10.1201/9781003027584-18

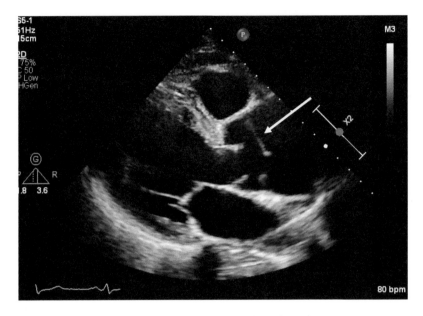

Figure 18.1 Aortic dissection: Note the flap in the ascending aorta *(arrow)*.

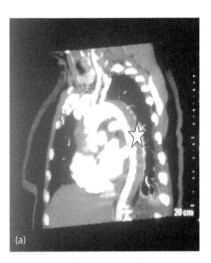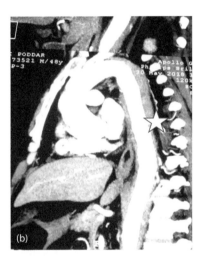

Figure 18.2 Aortic dissection Type A (a) and Type B (b). Note involvement of the ascending aorta from the coronary cusp to the arch in A but not in B. The true lumen appears white on contrast, and the thrombosed lumen (*) appears black.

 f. Limb ischaemia (mostly in the dissection flap involving aortic bifurcation).

 g. In 5% of patients the classical signs may be absent.

9. What are the diagnostic modalities to confirm the diagnoses?

Chest X-ray (CXR): The most common investigation may be CXR, which often shows a widened mediastinum.

Echocardiography: Transthoracic imaging shows ascending aorta quite well from the parasternal views and the arch from the suprasternal view. A flap can be demonstrated (**Figure 18.1**) with colour flow seen in the true lumen. Differentiating a flap from an artefact is of utmost importance.

Transechocardiography, with its clearer images, is invaluable in evaluation of the descending thoracic aorta.

D-dimer: This test has a negative predictive value; a D-dimer <0.5 mg/L rules out the diagnosis in most cases. The exceptions in AAS where D-dimer is not raised are IMH, PAU and AAD with a thrombosed true lumen (rare).

Troponin: Mostly done as a routine test in acute chest pain; in the context of AAD, it rules out myocardial ischaemia.

Contrast-enhanced CT (CECT): This is the confirmatory test of AAS, and given the rapidity required to reach a diagnosis, it should be done early if the suspicion is high. It confirms the true lumen, the extent of the flap, the entry points to the false lumen and any organ compromise. If multislice (16–64) CT is available, often a 3D reconstruction can be done. These views are helpful in surgical or endovascular repair.

10. What is the plan of management?

Guidelines suggest that any patient with chest/abdominal pain/syncope/perfusion deficit be assessed for (1) high-risk predisposing factors (e.g. Marfan syndrome), (2) high-risk pain feature (e.g. abrupt ripping pain) and (c) high-risk exam (e.g. pulse deficit, hypotension). If more than two risk features are present, then urgent aortic imaging is required. Once AAD is confirmed, the next step is to evaluate haemodynamics.

If hypotensive, start fluids (and, if required, vasopressors) and then refer to surgery (if Type A, then emergent surgery).

If the patient is hypertensive/normotensive, the goal is to maintain systolic BP (SBP) at 100–120 mmHg and a heart rate about 60–80/min.

Control of SBP

a. Beta-blockers are the drugs of choice to reduce aortic wall stress until the patient reaches urgent surgery. Labetalol, which unlike esmolol, is widely available, is given at an initial IV bolus of 20 mg over 2 min and then started at an infusion of 2–10 mg/min.

b. Sodium nitroprusside increases wall stress, and it should only be used in conjunction with beta-blockers, at a dose of 0.5 mcg/kg/min.

c. Intravenous nitroglycerin may also be used.

Whenever an AAD patient is hypertensive, three possibilities are present: That hypertensive crisis may have been a causal factor of AAD, or the AAD flap is involving the renal artery, or this hypertension is due to severe pain.

For the first two possibilities (always check with the radiologist about the status of the renal artery), anti-hypertensive therapy is beneficial. For the third possibility, reduction of pain may lead to sudden hypotension.

After medical therapy the patient is wheeled for open surgical repair for Type A AAD. For Type B AAD, medical therapy is the first option. Thoracic endovascular repair by stent graft may be indicated in selected cases of Type B AAD.

11. What are the surgical options in Type A AAD?

Definitive surgery. For Type A AAD, the surgical options (to treat/avoid tamponade, aortic regurgitation [AR], aortic rupture, stroke, visceral ischaemia) include:

a. *Type A AAD with dilated aortic sinus*: Modified Bentall (composite valve + root replacement + graft)

b. *Type A AAD with AR*: AVR + ascending aorta replacement or repair with valve resuspension

c. *Type A AAD with head-neck vessel involvement*: Total arch replacement with anastomosis to all head vessels

d. *Type A AAD*: Ascending aorta graft

12. What are the indications for repair in Type B AAD?

Type B AAD often has a variable course. Though medical management usually suffices for the majority with acceptable mortality (about 60% of cases, with a mortality rate of 8%), some cases may progress to require endovascular repair (about 20%, with a mortality of about 12%). Open surgical repair entails a high mortality (17%–30%) and is usually considered if endovascular repair (thoracic endovascular aortic repair [TEVAR]) is not feasible. The indications for proceeding for repair in Type B AAD are:

a. Rupture/impending rupture

b. Hypoperfusion of organs

c. Aneurysmal dilation >55 mm/rapid dilation

d. Refractory pain/hypertension

e. Haemorrhagic pleural effusion

13. What are the features of IMH?

The intramural haematoma is a special group of AASs, characterized by accumulation of blood in the aortic wall in the absence of an entrance tear. Since communication from the true to false lumen is absent, it is picked up by CT and transoesophageal echocardiography (TEE) but not by aortography. On CT, there is crescentic or circular wall thickening without tear, which shows high attenuation prior to contrast. There is no enhancement on contrast. The possible aetiology is believed to be a microtear in the wall that sealed by itself. More prevalent in elderly Asians, it has a favourable natural history, with many patients with IMH showing spontaneous resorption of the haematoma and only a few progressing to AAD.

14. What is the differential diagnosis of IMH?

Aneurysm with a mural thrombus mimics IMH, both of which show apparent thickening of the aortic wall without contrast enhancement. However, high attenuation prior to contrast is a characteristic feature of IMH.

15. What is a PAU?

A PAU is defined as an ulceration of aortic atherosclerotic plaque penetrating through the internal elastic lamina into the media. PAU is a disease of the intima, while AAD and IMH are diseases of the media. PAU usually involves the middle and distal parts of the descending thoracic aorta, especially in elderly males and often with comorbidities like coronary artery disease or hypertension. Though they commonly occur in the dilated aorta they can occur in aorta of normal calibre. The PAU can be detected only if it is big enough to protrude outside the contour of the aortic lumen. CT, MRI and TEE are the modalities for diagnosis. PAU may remain quiescent for years, but a few may progress to rupture, and some others lay the groundwork for saccular or fusiform aneurysms in later years. The adverse risk markers for PAU are growth rate >5 mm/year, initial depth >10 mm and diameter >20 mm. For a quiescent PAU, initially 3-monthly and later 6-monthly assessment by CT angiography and medical treatment with a beta-blocker and antihypertensive drugs suffices. For those with persistent pain, IMH, periaortic haemorrhage or AAS, endovascular repair with TEVAR is the treatment of choice.

16. What is the differential diagnosis of PAU?

Non-penetrating atheromatous ulcers and ulcer-like projections with concomitant IMH are difficult to distinguish from PAU even on CT.

17. What is the indication for surgery in TAA?

Ascending aorta diameter: Non-syndromic patients: 55 mm; syndromic (connective tissue disease) patients: 50 mm

Descending thoracic/thoracoabdominal diameter: 60 mm

A lower threshold (55 mm) may be indicated in case of small body surface area, certain risk factors and in cases where endovascular repair (TEVAR) is being considered.

The operative options are:

- Valve-sparing aortic root replacement (young)

- Composite (valve + graft)

- Ascending aorta graft (elderly)

- Frozen elephant trunk technique (arch + descending aorta)

18. What are the diagnostic modalities of an AAA?

AAA is diagnosed when infrarenal aorta diameter >30 mm. Risk factors include elderly male (>65 years), hypertension, smoking and family history. Diabetes is not a risk factor. There is a long asymptomatic period from onset to rupture (growth 1–6 mm/year). Though men are more prone to aneurysm, women are more prone to rupture. Palpation of the abdomen (pulsatile swelling in the midline for larger aneurysms) during first contact, ultrasound/echocardiography-based screening and confirmation by multidetector CT angiography are the methods of diagnosis.

19. What are the options in AAA?

Surgery: Ruptured/symptomatic abdominal aneurysm: Urgent open repair/EVAR

Asymptomatic aneurysm: 55 mm or more (open repair/EVAR)

- EVAR is especially suitable for an infrarenal aneurysm with a proximal (infrarenal) neck and distal landing zone (proximal to bifurcation).

Medical: Diameter 40–54 mm requires aggressive risk factor modification, as the 10-year risk of mortality from ischaemic heart disease (38%) is higher than the risk of death from rupture (2%).

Frequency of imaging surveillance:

- 30–40 mm: 3-yearly
- 40–50 mm: 1-yearly
- 50–55 mm: 6-monthly

FURTHER READING

1. Erbel R, Eboyans V, Boileau C et al. 2014 ESC Guidelines on the diagnosis and treatment of aortic diseases. European Heart Journal (2014) 35, 2873–2926.
2. Goria R, Bossone E, Erbel R. 2019 Acute Aortic Syndrome: Diagnostic Strategy and Clinical Features in Camm A J, Luscher T F, Maurer G, Serruys P W (Ed). ESC textbook of Cardiovascular Medicine third edition. Oxford University Press. pp. 2589–2591.

19 Refractory Hypertension in Critical Care

Sunandan Sikdar and Rathindra Nath Karmakar

1. What is a hypertensive emergency?

A hypertensive emergency is defined as a major and often sudden elevation of blood pressure (BP) leading to acute and progressive organ dysfunction. Though in previously stable and well-controlled patients a BP level of >180/120 mmHg may qualify for this definition, in pre-eclampsia a BP of >140/95 mmHg or in aortic dissection a BP of >160/110 mmHg may also be taken with the same urgency. Thus, it is the context and the presence of organ damage that may be more important than the numbers recorded.

The organs involved are the heart, retina, brain, kidneys and large arteries resulting in acute heart failure, myocardial infarction, retinopathy, stroke, acute kidney injury and aortic dissection. It is estimated that 0.5%–1% of emergency/healthcare encounters are due to this condition.

2. What is hypertensive urgency?

Hypertensive urgency is major elevation of BP without acute or progressive target organ dysfunction (grade II retinopathy, left ventricular hypertrophy and stable proteinuria are acceptable).

Both hypertensive emergency and urgency come under the heading of hypertensive crisis.

3. How do you measure BP in the cardiac care unit (CCU)?

Though the manual auscultatory method was commonly used, increasingly it is being replaced by oscillometric methods. However, in the case of arrhythmia, the manual method is the recommended one. The cuff must be at the heart level. If arm circumference >32 cm, the standard (12 cm × 35 cm) cuff will not suffice and a larger cuff is required. Invasive BP measurement is also available in the CCU. It is useful for those on vasopressors.

4. How do you classify hypertension?

The European Society for Cardiology (ESC) 2018 classification, with the level of cardiovascular (CV) risk is as follows (**Table 19.1**).

Table 19.1: Classification of Hypertension

Hypertension Disease Staging	Risk Factors	High-Normal SBP 130–139 DBP 85–89	Grade 1 Hypertension SBP 140–159 DBP 90–99	Grade 2 Hypertension SBP 160–179 DBP 100–109	Grade 3 Hypertension SBP ≥180 DBP ≥110
Stage 1 (uncomplicated)	No risk factors	Low risk	Low risk	Moderate risk	High risk
	One to two risk factors	Low risk	Moderate risk	Moderate to high risk	High risk
	Three or more risk factors	Low to moderate risk	Moderate to high risk	High risk	High risk
Stage 2 (asymptomatic disease)	HMOD, CKD grade 3, diabetes without organ damage	Moderate to high risk	High risk	High risk	High to very high risk
Stage 3 (established disease)	ASCVD, CKD 4, diabetes with organ damage	Very high risk	Very high risk	Very high risk	Very high risk

DOI: 10.1201/9781003027584-19

See **Table 19.2** for general principles of drug therapy.

Table 19.2: Hypertension Classification and Treatment (Based on ESC)

Classification	High-Normal BP	Grade 1	Grade 2	Grade 3
Definition	130–139/85–89	140–159/90–99	160–179/100–109	>180/110
Treatment initiation guideline Target SBP • *<65 yr*: <130 mmHg • *>65 yr*: 130–139 mmHg • *DBP*: 70–79 mmHg	Drug therapy in high risk, especially in those with CAD	Drug treatment in those with high/very high risk or those with CAD, renal disease	Immediate drug treatment, control BP in 3 months	Immediate drug treatment, control BP in 3 months
Associated condition	HTN (uncomplicated)	HTN + CAD	HTN + HFrEF	HTN + CKD
Particular therapy Step 1	ACEI/ARB + CCB/ diuretic	ACEI/ARB + BB Or CCB + BB	ACEI/ARB + BB + diuretic (ARNI may replace ACEI)	ACE/ARB + CCB + loop diuretic
Additional therapy if Step 1 fails to achieve target	Beta-blocker	Diuretic/ Spironolactone	Spironolactone	Alpha-blockers, alpha-2 agonist, spironolactone, beta-blocker

5. What is thrombotic microangiopathy?

Sometimes an acute BP rise may precipitate Coombs test–negative haemolytic anaemia and thrombocytopenia without any other obvious cause that resolves with control of BP.

6. What is hypertensive encephalopathy (HE)?

HE occurs in 10%–15% of malignant hypertension. It is characterized by severe hypertension and seizures, lethargy, cortical blindness and coma with no other explanation. Retinopathy is commonly present. MRI demonstrates cerebral oedema, microscopic haemorrhages and infarctions.

7. What is posterior reversible encephalopathy syndrome (PRES)?

PRES is a disorder of reversible subcortical vasogenic oedema (disruption of the blood-brain barrier with fluid transudation), which is a part of HE. The posterior circulation is more prone to lack of autoregulation due to a paucity of sympathetic innervations of this area. Encephalopathy, seizures, headache and visual disturbances may occur. Children with autoimmune disorders or those receiving cytotoxic therapy are more prone. MRI with T2-weighted fluid-attenuated inversion recovery (FLAIR) shows parieto-occipital or posterior frontal oedema bilaterally with haemorrhage. SBP reduction by 10% in the first hour and 25% in the next few hours and a target below 160 mmHg is recommended. Clevidipine is the drug of choice, though labetalol or fenoldopam may also be used.

8. What is the natural history of hypertensive emergency?

The natural history available from c. 1939 showed a mortality of 17% in a year, the majority due to renal failure (40%), followed by stroke (24%), myocardial infarct (11%) and heart failure (10%). Early studies c. 1970 had a documented mortality rate of ~79%, with a mean survival of 10 months. Though the initial prognosis was equivalent to some malignancies (hence the term malignant hypertension), after the development of effective therapies, the prognosis has improved. Now, mortality is ~5% in Western populations and ~15% in developing countries.

9. What are the conditions associated with hypertensive crisis?

The most common presentation of hypertensive emergency is neurological deficit, followed by chest pain. While doing a history and physical exam, the following needs to be kept in mind:

1. History of missing anti-hypertensive drugs, e.g. clonidine (rebound hypertension) or taking drugs like erythropoietin or cyclosporine

2. History of taking recreational drugs (cocaine, LSD, phencyclidine)

3. History suggestive of pheochromocytoma.

4. History of kidney disease (glomerulonephritis, vasculitis, polycystic kidney)

5. History of taking monoamine oxidase inhibitors (MAOIs) (tyramine-MAOI interactions)

6. Rule out eclampsia

7. Look for papilledema, retinal haemorrhages

8. Check whether BP is different between left and right arm (aortic dissection)

9. Look for signs of heart failure

10. Look for abdominal bruit (renal artery stenosis)

11. Look for neurological signs (HE/stroke), check autonomic function (e.g. Gullian-Barre syndrome)

12. Look for signs of scleroderma (renal crisis) and any connective tissue disorder

Clues for secondary hypertension are given in **Table 19.3**.

Table 19.3: Clues for Suspicion of Secondary Hypertension

- Childhood hypertension or onset of Grade II hypertension at <40 years of age
- Acute worsening of stable hypertension
- Grade III hypertension or hypertensive crises
- Resistant hypertension
- Organ involvement extensive
- *Identified*: Endocrine (hyperthyroidism, hyperparathyroidism, Cushing, primary hyperaldosteronism), sleep apnea, CKD, renovascular hypertension, pheochromocytoma, coarctation, aortoarteritis
- *Drugs*: NSAIDs, erythropoietin, cyclosporin, steroids, OCP, VEGF inhibitors (bevacizumab), tyrosine kinase inhibitors (sunitinib), cocaine, amphetamine, nasal decongestants

---

10. What are the complications of hypertensive emergency?

The prevalence of complications in hypertensive emergency are as follows: Cerebral infarction (20%–25%), pulmonary oedema (14%–31%), HE (0%–16%), acute coronary syndrome (12%–25%), intracerebral or subarachnoid haemorrhage (4%–15%), eclampsia (0%–4%) and aortic dissection (0%–2%).

11. How do you assess hypertension-mediated target organ damage?

The following investigations may be considered (**Table 19.4**).

Table 19.4: Assessment of Hypertension-Mediated Organ Damage

Test	Interpretation/Significance
ECG	LVH (SV1 + RV5 >35 mm, R aVL >11 mm)
Echocardiography	LVH/structural changes LV (mass/BSA) (gm/m^2) >115 (male) >95 (female)
CXR	Mediastinal widening, fluid overload
Urine albumin creatinine ratio, toxicology	Albuminuria/renal dysfunction Check for amphetamines
Fundoscopy	Retinal haemorrhage in Grade II and III hypertension
Pulse wave velocity	>10 m/sec – stiff aorta
USG abdomen	Look for renal parenchymal disease, pheochromocytoma, abdominal aneurysm Doppler for renal artery stenosis
Carotid Doppler (Intima media thickness)	Carotid plaques (IMT >1.5 mm) Carotid disease (IMT >0.9 mm)
Ankle Brachial Index	<0.9 – peripheral arterial disease
Electrolytes, creatinine, eGFR	Hyperaldosteronism, renal injury
Troponin	Cardiac injury
Brain imaging	Ischaemic brain injury

---

a. 12-Lead ECG

b. Fundoscopy

c. Urine albumin/creatinine ratio, urine microscopy for red cells, cast

d. Creatinine and estimated glomerular filtration rate (eGFR)

e. Troponin, lactate dehydrogenase (LDH), NT-pro-BNP

f. Electrolytes

g. Haemogram, platelet count, fibrinogen

h. *Ultrasound sonography (USG) of abdomen with Doppler*: Renal size and echotexture, abdominal aorta size, adrenal gland

i. Echocardiography, including suprasternal views, to exclude coarctation

j. Chest X-ray to exclude aortic pathology, fluid overload

k. Peripheral arterial imaging

l. Brain imaging

Rise of creatinine >30% after starting an angiotensin receptor blocker (ARB) may be a subtle hint of underlying renal disease. eGFR <45 mL/min/m^2 must prompt stoppage of spironolactone.

12. What is resistant hypertension?

Resistant/refractory hypertension is defined as the inability to achieve a BP goal of <140/90 mmHg even after using three antihypertensive drugs of which one is a diuretic (others being an ARB + calcium channel blocker [CCB]), provided that patient is compliant with drugs.

13. What is pseudo-resistant hypertension?

The caveats to the resistant hypertension definition constitute pseudo-resistant hypertension. They are:

a. Non-compliance

b. White coat effect

c. Poor BP measurement technique

d. Brachial artery calcification

e. Inadequate doses

14. What are the drugs used in hypertensive emergencies and their dosages?

Table 19.5: Intravenous Antihypertensives in Use in Hypertensive Crisis

Drug	Dosage	Onset of Action	Duration of Action	Contraindication	Adverse Effects
Nitroglycerin	5–200 µg/min IV infusion, 5 µg/min increase every 5 min	1–3 min	3–5 min	*Relative contra*: Inferior wall MI	Headache, reflex tachycardia
Nitroprusside	0.3–10 µg/kg/min IV infusion, increase by 0.5 µg/kg/min every 5 min until goal BP	Immediate	1–2 min	Liver/Renal failure	Cyanide toxicity
Labetalol	• 0.25–0.5 mg/kg IV bolus • 2–4 mg/min infusion until goal BP is reached, thereafter 5–20 mg/hr	5–10 min	3-6 hr	Heart block, bradycardia, asthma, heart failure	Broncho-constriction, bradycardia
Nicardipine	5–15 mg/hr (IV) starting dose 5 mg/hr, increase every 15–30 min with 2.5 mg until goal BP, thereafter decrease to 3 mg/hr	5–15 min	30–40 min	Liver failure	Headache, reflex tachycardia

(Continued)

Table 19.5 (*Continued*): Intravenous Antihypertensives in Use in Hypertensive Crisis

Drug	Dosage	Onset of Action	Duration of Action	Contraindication	Adverse Effects
Esmolol	0.5–1 mg/kg as IV bolus, 50–300 µg/kg/min as IV infusion	1–2 min	10–30 min	Heart block, bradycardia, asthma, heart failure	Bradycardia
Clevidipine	2 mg/h IV infusion, increase every 2 min with 2 mg/hr until goal BP	2–3 min	5–15 min		Headache, reflex tachycardia
Fenoldopam	0.1 mg/kg/min IV infusion, increase every 15 min with 0.05–0.1 mg/kg/min increments until goal BP is reached	5–15 min	30–60 min	Caution in glaucoma	

15. What are the hypertensive emergencies requiring immediate BP lowering with intravenous agents?

The different clinical presentations of hypertensive emergencies and their therapy are shown in **Table 19.6**.

Table 19.6: Clinical Presentation of Hypertensive Emergencies and Their Treatment

Clinical Presentation	Target BP	Drug Preferred
Hypertensive emergency with or without renal failure	Reduce MAP by 25% early	Labetalol Nicardipine
Hypertensive encephalopathy	Reduce MAP by 25% immediately	Labetalol Nicardipine
Acute coronary syndrome with hypertension	Reduce SBP <140 mmHg, but reduce gradually	Nitroglycerin Labetalol
Acute cardiogenic pulmonary oedema	Reduce SBP <140 mmHg	Nitroglycerin Nitroprusside
Acute aortic dissection	Reduce SBP <120 mmHg and heart rate >60 /min	Labetalol/esmolol/nitroglycerin
Eclampsia/Pre-eclampsia	Reduce SBP <160 mmHg and DBP <105 mmHg	Labetalol/nicardipine/ magnesium sulphate

16. What are the principles of management of hypertensive emergencies?

Several principles should be kept in mind:

a. Normotensives have vascular beds that autoregulate between 60 mmHg and 180 mmHg, but chronic hypertensives have this autoregulation curve shifted to the right. Hence lowering BP to normal levels may cause hypoperfusion in these beds. Thus, BP needs to be lowered by 25% in the first 2 hours. After 160/100 mmHg is achieved, maintain it for 6 hours; further reduction should take place over next 24 hours. Once the patient is stable, taper intravenous drugs and switch to oral drugs.

b. Exceptions to the above rule:

- Aortic dissection where BP lowering is to be done rapidly to 120 mmHg by 20 min.

- Ischaemic stroke where the BP threshold is higher (discussed later).

c. If the patient has clinical evidence of volume overload or is in pulmonary oedema, only then give intravenous diuretics at admission. Use oral diuretics only if there is lack of control of BP after the use of vasodilators because there is sodium and water retention with these agents (tachyphylaxis).

d. Rapid reduction of BP >50% may be associated with ischaemic strokes and fatality.

e. In coronary artery disease with hypertension, when left ventricular hypertrophy is present, it may be prudent to gradually reduce the BP, as coronary perfusion occurs in diastole and ischaemia may be exacerbated by sudden reduction of diastolic BP (DBP). Beta-blockers should be used with caution and as an additive agent over nitroglycerin.

f. Angiotensin-converting enzyme (ACE) inhibitors and ARBs may have unpredictable responses due to variable activation of the renin-angiotensin-aldosterone system (RAAS).

g. In HE, labetalol may be safer than nitroprusside, as the later has a negative impact on cerebral autoregulation.

h. Nitroprusside causes coronary steal and hence should be avoided in hypertensive emergencies with acute coronary syndrome (ACS). Here the drug of choice is nitroglycerin followed by labetalol. Urapidil is an alternative.

i. In acute pulmonary oedema caused by hypertensive crisis, the drug of choice is nitroprusside owing to its after and preload lowering efficiency (balanced vasodilator). Nitroglycerin is an alternative but only reduces preload. Urapidil has been shown to have better BP-lowering efficacy than nitroglycerin without reflex tachycardia but may not be available.

j. Often secondary hypertension, especially renovascular cause may be the culprit. In such cases we must be cautious about using RAAS blockers, as there may be a precipitous fall in renal perfusion.

17. How do you manage hypertensive emergency due to sympathetic overactivity?

Recreational drugs (cocaine), autonomic instability and pheochromocytoma are causes of this rare condition, which requires a different approach. Benzodiazepines are the initial drugs for recreational overdose. A selective beta-blocker (without alpha blockade) should not be used, as coronary and peripheral vasoconstriction may occur, and paradoxical hypertension may occur due to unbalanced alpha activity.

Anti-hypertensives useful in sympathetic overactivity include phentolamine, nicardipine and clonidine.

Autonomic dysfunction may occur in spinal cord lesions (above T6) and intracerebral haemorrhage. Noxious stimuli below the lesion leads to sympathetic hyperactivity, vasoconstriction and hypertension. Parasympathetic overactivity occurs on stimulus above the lesion. Below T6 due to compensatory splanchnic vasodilation, this hypertensive crisis does not occur. Treatment involves placing the patient in as much of an upright position as possible, reducing the noxious stimuli and using nitroglycerin, labetalol and nicardipine. Dexmedetomidine, a central-acting α2 agonist, may be helpful in autonomic dysfunction with dystonia.

Pheochromocytoma presents with paroxysmal hypertensive crisis with palpitation especially during stress. The drug of choice in pheochromocytoma is intravenous phentolamine. A beta-blocker may be added to treat reflex tachycardia. Labetalol and nitroprusside have also been used.

Phentolamine: Onset of action 1-2 min, duration 30 min

Infusion dose: 0.5–1 mg/kg bolus (usually 5–15 mg IV)

                    Then 50–300 mcg/kg/min

Side effect: Reflex tachycardia

18. What is the protocol of BP lowering in stroke with hypertensive crisis?

Up to 80% of strokes present with hypertension. The Cushing reflex is responsible for hypertension only in large strokes with raised intracranial pressure. Often the raised BP resolves by a week.

Lowering of BP in ischaemic stroke is tricky. If the patient is a thrombolysis candidate, the antihypertensive threshold is 180/110 mmHg. BP should be kept below 180/105 mmHg at least for 24 hours. Those who are not candidates for thrombolysis should be initiated on antihypertensive treatment if BP >220/120 mmHg. Cautious lowering of BP 15%–20% should be tried with intravenous drugs.

Lowering of BP in intracranial haemorrhage is to be started if SBP is >140 mmHg, as it reduces haematoma progression. The ICH-ADAPT study showed that cerebral perfusion is not reduced by the protocol described earlier.

Nitroprusside and esmolol are preferred by some physicians for this indication and nicardipine and labetalol by others. There is a risk of a rise in intracranial pressure with CCBs, though nimodipine has been used in subarachnoid haemorrhage.

Subarachnoid haemorrhage, presenting as a thunderclap headache within an hour of onset, has a high mortality of 67%. Non-contrast CT is the test of choice with a high negative predictive value in the initial 6 hours. Though guidelines do not specify a protocol, nimodipine has traditionally been used to reduce BP and reduce vasospasm, a feared complication that occurs after a week of aneurysm rupture.

19. What is the BP management protocol of acute renal insufficiency?

BP management in renal hypertensive emergency patients includes fenoldopam, nicardipine and clevidipine, as they reduce systemic vascular resistance while preserving renal blood flow. In scleroderma renal crisis and Takayasu arteritis, the ACE inhibitor enalaprilat and an ARB are first-line agents.

20. What is the management protocol for pre-eclampsia?

Preeclampsia is characterized by severe hypertension (typically $\geq$160/110 mmHg) in patients who have progressed beyond the 20th week of gestation (it can occur up to 8 weeks postpartum). Magnesium sulphate, alpha methyl dopa, hydralazine, labetalol and nifedipine are all useful. ACE inhibitors, ARBs and nitroprusside are contraindicated.

21. What is the non-pharmacologic treatment of resistant hypertension?

Renal denervation therapy, where catheter-based radiofrequency or catheter-based ultrasound ablation of the sympathetic plexus is done, has shown conflicting results in multiple trials. Hence, it is yet to establish itself as a definitive therapy. Stimulation of the carotid sinus baroreceptor has shown no benefit.

FURTHER READING

1. Williams B, Mancia G, Spiering E, et al. ESC/ESH Guideline for Management of Arterial Hypertension. European Heart Journal (2018);39:3021–3014.
2. Bobrie G, Amar L,Faucon A, et al. Resistant Hypertension, in Bakris G L, Sorrentino M J (eds). Hypertension: A Companion to Braunwald's Heart Disease, 3rd Edition (2018), pp 398–408.

20 Pulmonary Embolism

Sunandan Sikdar, Arindam Pande, and Gautam Das

1. What are the risk factors for pulmonary embolism (PE)?

The risk factors of pulmonary embolism can be divided into strong , moderate and weak risk factors and are discussed below in Table 20.1.

Table 20.1: Risk Factors for Pulmonary Embolism

Strong Risk Factors (Odds Ratio >10)	Moderate Risk Factors (Odds Ratio 2–9)	Weak Risk Factors (Odds Ratio <2)
Fracture of lower limb	• Arthroscopic knee surgery	Bed rest >3 days
Hospitalization for heart failure or atrial fibrillation/flutter (within previous 3 months)	• Central venous lines • Catheters • Leads	Diabetes mellitus
Hip or knee replacement	• Oral contraceptive therapy, chemotherapy	Immobility due to sitting (e.g. prolonged car or air travel)
Myocardial infarction (within previous 3 months)	• Infection (specifically pneumonia, urinary tract • infection and HIV) • Inflammatory bowel disease • Autoimmune diseases • Cancer (highest risk in metastatic disease) • Paralytic stroke	Pregnancy
Previous VTE	• Congestive heart failure or respiratory failure	Obesity
Spinal cord injury	• Hormone replacement therapy (depends on formulation) • In vitro fertilization • Postpartum period	Arterial hypertension
Major trauma	• Blood transfusion	Laparoscopic surgery (e.g. cholecystectomy)

2. What are the presentations of a PE?

a. *Massive PE* (systolic blood pressure [SBP] <90 mmHg + organ hypoperfusion + saddle/main pulmonary artery/right pulmonary artery/left pulmonary artery [RPA/LPA] thrombus) – divided into three types: (1) Cardiac arrest, (2) obstructive shock and (3) persistent hypotension (SBP <90 mmHg, BP drop >40 mmHg for >15 min in absence of arrhythmia, hypovolemia, sepsis)

b. *Submassive PE, high risk* (SBP >90 mmHg + right ventricular [RV] dysfunction + biomarker rise)

c. *Submassive PE, low risk* (SBP >90 mmHg + RV dysfunction/biomarker rise)

d. *Small to moderate PE* (normal SBP, normal RV function)

3. What is the role of common ancillary tests in PE?

The most common ECG finding (**Figure 20.1**) may be sinus tachycardia and occurs in mild to the most severe cases. Features of RV strain like a qR in V1, T inversion in V1–V4 and S1Q3T3 are more specific but rare and are indicative of severe disease.

Arterial blood gas may show hypoxemia but may be normal or may have an increased alveolar-arterial gradient in the majority (due to increased dead space) but not all cases.

Chest X-ray may be frequently normal, and it rules out other pathologies. Hampton hump (peripheral wedge-shaped density above the diaphragm), Palla's sign (enlargement of the right descending pulmonary artery) and Westermarck sign (focal oligemia) may be present but are very rare. In fact, a near-normal chest X-ray in the presence of falling saturation in a hyperventilating and hypotensive patient suggests this diagnosis.

DOI: 10.1201/9781003027584-20

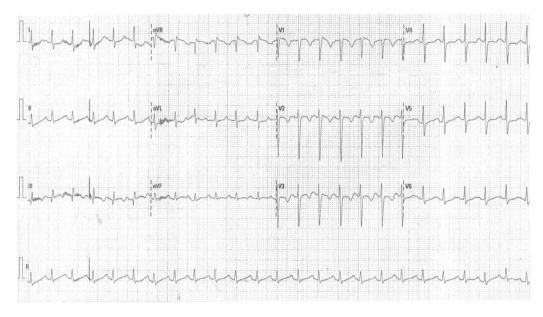

Figure 20.1 Acute massive pulmonary embolism: Note sinus tachycardia, T-wave inversion in precordial leads and S1Q3T3.

4. What are the echocardiographic signs of PE?

Acute pressure overload of the RV is the cause of echocardiographic changes. The negative predictive value is only 30%–40%, but being a convenient and widely available test, it must be used routinely. The most common finding may be RV dilatation. The myriad of findings include:

a. Enlarged RV in parasternal long axis (PLAX) view

b. *McConnell's sign*: Hypokinesia of RV with sparing of apex

c. Basal RV diameter/basal left ventricle (LV) diameter ratio >1 in apical four-chamber view

d. *60/60 Rule*: Coexistence of acceleration time of pulmonary ejection <60 ms and mid-systolic "notch" with mildly elevated (<60 mmHg) peak systolic gradient at the tricuspid valve

e. Decreased tricuspid annular plane systolic excursion (TAPSE) measured with M-mode (<16 mm)

f. Decreased peak systolic (S') velocity of tricuspid annulus (<9.5 cm/sec)

g. *Visualization of mobile thrombus*: A specific sign

h. *Sign of RV overload*: Flattening of interventricular septum

i. *Sign of raised RV pressure*: Dilated and non-collapsing inferior vena cava (IVC)

5. What is the role of the D-dimer test?

D-dimer, a marker of thrombosis, is primarily a rule-out test in a hospitalized patient. The D-dimer test is usually an enzyme-linked immunosorbent assay (ELISA)–based test (see biomarker section). A negative test rules out both deep vein thrombosis (DVT) and PE. A positive test, on the other hand, may occur in infection, pregnancy, malignancy and hospitalized patients. The cut-off is usually taken to be 500 μg/L (taking 1000 μg/L will increase specificity). But in the elderly, especially 80 years and older, in such cases the formula age × 10 μg/L as the cut-off limit may be more appropriate. D-dimer measurement is not useful in patients with high clinical probability, as a normal result does not safely exclude PE.

6. What is the role of CT pulmonary angiography (CTPA)?

CTPA is the imaging test of choice to diagnose PE (**Figure 20.2**), having the capacity to image subsegmental pulmonary vessels. A segmental or more proximal filling defect can be recognized in

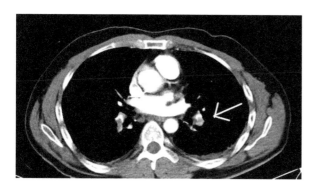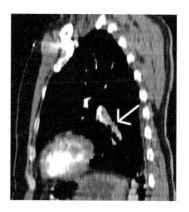

Figure 20.2 An elderly man post-gastrectomy for stomach cancer collapsed on the first postoperative day. CECT showing massive pulmonary embolus (*arrow*).

positive cases. A positive CTPA is suggestive of the diagnosis, while a negative CTPA virtually rules out the diagnosis if the clinical probability is low or intermediate. A negative CTPA with high clinical probability requires further tests – but this situation is rare. The strength of this test lies in its accuracy, ability to provide an alternative diagnosis if there is one and the rarity of inconclusive results (3%–5%). The limitations include contraindications in advanced renal failure, pregnancy and in cases of contrast allergy, apart from radiation exposure.

7. What is the role of lower limb Doppler (compression) ultrasound in diagnosis of PE?

The cardinal sign of DVT on ultrasound is loss of vein collapsibility on compression of the skin overlying it (**Figure 20.3**). If there is clinical suspicion of PE, a diagnosis of proximal DVT by compression ultrasound confirms it. However, if there is distal (below the knee) DVT, further tests are required to confirm the diagnosis.

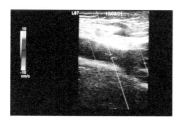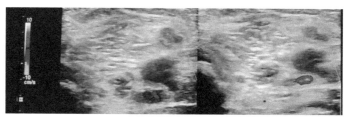

Figure 20.3 Lack of compressibility and colour flow in the common femoral vein.

8. What is the simplified Pulmonary Embolism Severity Index (sPESI) criteria?

If any one or more of the following factors are present: age >80 years, history of cancer, history of heart failure/lung disease, SBP <100 mmHg, heart rate (HR) >110/min, SpO_2 <90%, then it is high-risk PE by sPESI criteria. sPESI is used to triage haemodynamically stable patients into intermediate- and low-risk groups.

9. What is the management protocol for PE?

The following protocol is adapted from the European Society for Cardiology (ESC) guideline in a simplified form (**Table 20.2**).

10. What is the anticoagulation regimen in PE?

The mainstay of anticoagulation in haemodynamically unstable patients/high-risk PE, those with renal failure or acute kidney injury (common) or pregnancy is unfractionated heparin (UFH).

For intermediate- or low-risk patients, anticoagulation by parenteral (low-molecular-weight heparin [LMWH] or fondaparinux) or oral (newer oral anticoagulants [NOACs]) methods can be used. NOAC is contraindicated in renal failure, pregnancy and antiphospholipid antibody syndrome.

Table 20.2: Management Protocol of Pulmonary Embolism

Presentation	Risk Category	Anticoagulation	Thrombolysis	Hospital Monitoring
Shock	High	Yes	Yes	Yes
RV dysfunction/sPESI 1 or more plus troponin +ve	High intermediate	Yes	Individualize if worsening	Yes
RV dysfunction/sPESI 1 or more but troponin –ve	Low intermediate	Yes	No	Yes
No RVD, sPESI 0	Low	Yes	No	Yes, if comorbidity, individualize if no comorbidity

Dosage of UFH
For patients with average bleeding risk, UFH should be started with an intravenous bolus of 80 units/kg, followed by a continuous infusion at 18 units/kg/hr (activated partial thromboplastin time [aPTT] 1.5–2.5 times control, range 60–80 sec).

LMWH-based regimen
Since LMWH has better bioavailability, more predictable response and longer duration of action, it is preferred over UFH in all cases except in renal failure. The usual dosage is 1 mg/kg SC q12hr OR 1.5 mg/kg SC once daily (administer at the same time each day). Warfarin should be started within 3 days of the start of LMWH. LMWH should be continued until the international normalization ratio (INR) reaches 2–3 and then it can be discontinued.

Fondaparinux-based regimen

- *<50 kg*: 5 mg SC once daily

- *50–100 kg*: 7.5 mg SC once daily

- *>100 kg*: 10 mg SC once daily

Administer for 5–9 days

Dosages for NOAC

- *Rivaroxaban*: 15 mg twice daily × 3 weeks then 10 mg once-daily maintenance

- *Apixaban*: 10 mg twice daily for a week then 5 mg twice-daily maintenance

- *Dabigatran*: Heparin/LMWH for the initial week then 150 mg twice-daily maintenance

11. How is thrombolysis given?

Systemic thrombolysis is the cornerstone of treatment of haemodynamically unstable PE. By causing dissolution of the thrombus, it causes relief of physical obstruction and reduces the release of serotonin and other neurohormonal mediators that cause pulmonary hypertension. The drug of choice is a tissue plasminogen activator (tPA), though other agents (streptokinase, reteplase and tenecteplase) can be used. The tPA is usually given as 100-mg infusion over 2 hr. It can be used for up to 2 weeks after symptom onset. The mortality is reduced by half, and recurrent embolism is reduced by two-thirds. However, this comes at the cost of three times increase in major bleeding (including intracranial haemorrhage).

12. What are the alternatives to systemic thrombolysis?

In order to reduce bleeding complications (2% intracranial haemorrhage), pharmacoinvasive therapy (**Figure 20.4**) may be used with reduced-dose thrombolysis (even one-quarter of the systemic dose may suffice). The following techniques have been tried:

a. Pigtail catheter rotational embolectomy

b. Clot pulverization

c. Rheolytic thrombectomy

d. Low-intensity ultrasound-facilitated fibrinolysis

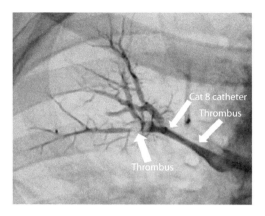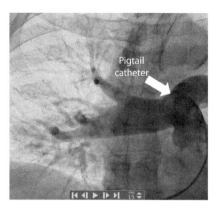

Figure 20.4 Thrombus lodged near a pulmonary artery bifurcation in the same patient as in Figure 20.2. An aspiration device (Penumbra System) was used to aspirate the thrombus.

13. How is warfarin used in DVT and PE?

Warfarin should be initiated with LMWH overlap (for 5 days), as it not only inhibits factors II, VII, IX and X but also proteins C and S, thus causing paradoxical thrombogenic milieu in the initial few days. Start at 5 mg and titrate the dose to reach an INR 2–3 (the algorithm is given in the chapter on NOACs). All antibiotics used in intensive care (except rifampicin), and paracetamol tend to accentuate the bleeding risk. There are numerous drug interactions, especially those related to, more commonly, CYP 2C9 and, rarely, VKORC1 genes.

In patients without a recognized precipitating factor or those having cancer as the precipitating factor, there must be an extended duration of DVT prophylaxis compared to those with a reversible or transient trigger (e.g. surgery). Male gender episodes of PE and raised D-dimer predict an increased risk of venous thromboembolism (VTE).

However, numerous clinical trials have proven that use of NOACs is noninferior to warfarin with regard to efficacy but is safer. Hence, current guidelines emphasize that NOACs should be the default choice in short- and long-duration DVT/PE anticoagulation rather than warfarin.

14. What is the anticoagulation regimen?

Duration

a. DVT/PE with known reversible risk factors (surgery/fracture) – 3 months

b. DVT/PE without known risk factor – preferable to continue indefinitely

c. DVT/PE with persistent risk factor – indefinite anticoagulation

d. DVT/PE with cancer – continue until cancer is cured

e. DVT/PE with antiphospholipid antibody syndrome (APLAS) – indefinite

Regimen

a. *For cancer*: LMWH for 6 months (or rivaroxaban); post 6 months, indefinite anticoagulation can be continued with rivaroxaban

b. *For APLAS*: A vitamin K antagonist (VKA)

c. *For routine anticoagulation up to 3 months*: Dabigatran 150 mg twice daily/rivaroxaban 10 mg once daily/apixaban 5 mg twice daily

d. *For extended-duration (>3 months) anticoagulation*: Apixaban 2.5 mg twice daily/rivaroxaban 10 mg once daily

15. How should PE be managed in pregnancy?

PE is a leading and catastrophic cause of postpartum mortality and morbidity, and its diagnosis is challenging and difficult to predict. The problem is compounded by the fact that D-dimer levels progressively increase until the third trimester, increasing the chance of a false-positive result. If clinical suspicion is high or if the D-dimer is positive, a chest X-ray (CXR) and Doppler ultrasound of the lower limb is performed. If a proximal DVT is present, then LMWH should be started. If DVT is not confirmed, the next test of choice is CTPA (if the CXR is abnormal) or ventilation and perfusion scan (if available, especially if the CXR is normal). Thrombolysis or surgical embolectomy is the treatment of choice in pregnancy-related PE with shock. The time of withholding of anticoagulation by LMWH prior to giving spinal/epidural anaesthesia during delivery is usually 24 hr. It should not be restarted until at least 4 hr after delivery.

FURTHER READING

1. Konstantinides S V, Meyer G, Becattini C, et al. 2019 ESC Guidelines for the Diagnosis and Management of Acute Pulmonary Embolism Developed in Collaboration with the European Respiratory Society (ERS). European Heart Journal (2019);00:1–61.

21 Pulmonary Hypertension

Sunandan Sikdar and Auriom Kar

1. What is pulmonary hypertension (PH)?

PH is defined by a mean pulmonary artery pressure (mPAP) >20 mmHg at rest measured by right heart catheterization (RHC) (6th World Symposium on Pulmonary Hypertension 2018). It is also recommended that the cut-off for pulmonary vascular resistance (PVR) of >3 Wood units (WU) be used to detect patients with idiopathic pulmonary arterial hypertension (iPAH) and other forms of PH, who have a significant component of pre-capillary disease. In the ESC 2022 guideline, PVR > 2 WU has been taken as threshold for diagnosis of PH.

2. How do you classify PH?

Haemodynamic Classification

PH can be classified as pre- or post-capillary PH. Pre-capillary PH is due to a primary elevation of pressure in the pulmonary arterial system alone (e.g. PAH), while post-capillary PH is that due to elevations of pressure in the pulmonary venous and pulmonary capillary systems.

Pre-capillary pulmonary hypertension (primary PH): Pulmonary artery wedge pressure (PAWP) <15 mmHg

Post-capillary PH (left-sided heart disease): PAWP >15 mmHg

Aetiological Classification (Table 21.1)

I. Pulmonary Arterial Hypertension (PAH)

II. PH due to left heart disease

III. PH due to lung disease or hypoxia

IV. Chronic thromboembolic PH (CTEPH) and other pulmonary artery obstruction

V. PH due to unknown/multifactorial mechanism

Table 21.1: Classification of PH

Type	Description	Example
I	Pulmonary arterial hypertension	• Idiopathic PAH • Inherited • Drugs and toxins • Schistosomiasis • Connective tissue disease • Portopulmonary hypertension • HIV • Sickle cell anaemia
II	Pulmonary hypertension due to left heart disease	• Systolic LV dysfunction • Diastolic LV dysfunction • Valvular heart disease
III	Pulmonary hypertension due to lung disease or hypoxia	COPD, ILD, sleep apnoea, high altitude
IV	Chronic thromboembolic pulmonary hypertension and other pulmonary artery obstruction	
V	Pulmonary hypertension due to unknown/multifactorial mechanism	Myeloproliferative disease, glycogen storage disease, sarcoidosis, renal failure on dialysis

---

3. What is the normal value of mPAP?

The normal value of mPAP is 14 ± 3 with a maximum upper limit of 20 mmHg. Borderline PAH is thus 20–25 mmHg. Resting mPAP <25 mmHg and post-exercise mPAP >30 mmHg can be said to be exercise-related PAH.

DOI: 10.1201/9781003027584-21

4. How do you classify the haemodynamic parameters related to PH?

- All PH have mPAP > 20 mmHg.
- PVR = (mPAP-PAWP) / Cardiac Output Precapillary PH(iPAH): PAWP<15 mmHg, PVR > 2WU.
- *Combined Pre and Post Capillary PH:* PAWP > 15mmHg, PVR > 2WU.
- *Isolated Post Capillary PH:* PAWP > 15 mmHg, PVR < 2WU.
- *Exercise PH:* mPAP/ Cardiac output, slope between rest and exercise > 3mmHg/L/min.

5. What is the pathophysiologic basis of PAH?

In iPAH, three pathologic changes occur: *Intimal fibrosis, muscularization* of small arteries (<200 microns) and *plexiform lesions* – capillary-like formations of the small pulmonary arteries.

Three major pathways are involved in pathogenesis: Endothelin, nitric oxide and prostacyclin pathways.

6. What are the symptoms of idiopathic PAH?

The typical patient with iPAH is a young adult woman. The patient with CTEPH is older, and both sexes are equally affected. Elderly patients may also have left ventricular pathology as a cause of PAH.

Breathlessness (initially at exertion, then at rest), fatigue, weakness, angina and syncope are the symptoms that appear after a long asymptomatic period of subclinical PH (often the diagnosis is delayed by 2 years). Dyspnoea is caused by hyperventilation induced by hypoxemia and low cardiac output. Syncope is due to lack of increase of cardiac output with exercise/stress and reduced venous return on bending forward. Syncope is more common in iPAH. Angina is due to ischaemia of a pressure-overloaded right ventricle (RV) and coronary compression by a dilated pulmonary artery, particularly in patients with a pulmonary artery trunk at least 40 mm in diameter. Oedema and hae-moptysis are more common in CTEPH. Symptoms of PH has been graded in WHO Functional Class from I to IV. It is like NYHA classification except that syncope is considered instead of palpitation.

On examination, a left parasternal heave, narrowly split S2, loud P2, RVS3, systolic murmur of tricuspid regurgitation (TR) or diastolic murmur of pulmonary regurgitation (PR) may occur. Clubbing suggests pulmonary veno-occlusive disease and congenital heart disease. Increased jugular venous pressure (JVP), hepatomegaly and pitting oedema indicate the onset of RV failure. Signs of scleroderma like sclerodactyly and signs of liver disease like telangiectasia must be sought. A history of drugs/medications is helpful in determining aetiology (**Table 21.2**).

Table 21.2: Drug-Induced Pulmonary Hypertension

Evidence	Agents
Definite	• Fenfluramine • Dexfenfluramine • Toxic rapeseed oil
Likely	• Amphetamine • L-Tryptophan • Dasatinib
Possible	• Cocaine • Chemotherapeutic agents • Selective serotonin reuptake inhibitors
Unlikely	• Oral contraceptive • Oestrogen • Smoking

7. What are the chest X-ray (CXR) findings of PH?

Chest radiograph (CXR) may be normal but may show enlarged central pulmonary arteries with attenuation of the peripheral vessels, resulting in oligemic lung fields. RV enlargement (diminished retrosternal space), right atrial dilatation (prominent right heart border) and pleural effusions may also be seen as PH progresses. Lung disease may be evident on CXR.

8. What are the echocardiographic findings of PH?

In general an estimated pulmonary artery systolic pressure (ePASP) of 35 mmHg in the young and 40 mmHg in the elderly qualifies as possible PH in day-to-day practice. However, it is a fact that ePASP corelates poorly with RHC values. ePASP >50 mmHg makes the diagnosis probable PH (**Figure 21.1**). Echocardiographic findings of PH are summarized in **Table 21.3**.

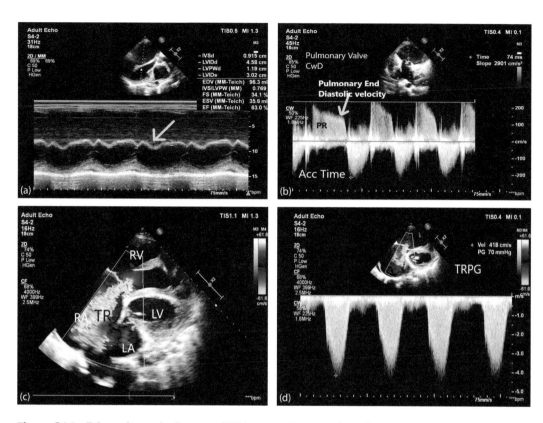

Figure 21.1 Echocardiography features of PH in a case of untreated atrial septal defect (ASD). (a) Paradoxical movement of septum. (b) Increased PR end-diastolic velocity and shortened acceleration time. (c) and (d) RA and RV dilation with TR velocity >4 m/sec.

Table 21.3: Echocardiography Findings in PH

Ventricle	Pulmonary Artery	IVC/RA
RV/LV basal diameter ratio >1	RVOT acceleration time <105 ms	IVC >21 mm with <50% collapse on inspiration
• Flattening of ventricular septum. • *LV eccentricity index*: bigger diameter/smaller diameter of LV short axis cross-section >1.1	Mid-systolic closure of pulmonary valve on 2D echocardiogram and corresponding notching of pulmonary artery Doppler flow	RA area >18 cm^2

• Peak velocity of TR
  • 3.4 m/s, high probability of PAH
  • 2.9–3.4m/s, intermediate probability of PAH
  • <2.8 m/s, low probability of PAH
	Early diastolic pulmonary regurgitation velocity >2.2 m/s	Presence of pericardial effusion

TAPSE for RV function	PA diameter >25 mm	

9. What is the role of the CT scan in PH?

CT scan may play a supportive role as enumerated below:

a. A pulmonary artery diameter larger than 2.9 cm, pulmonary artery:ascending aorta (ratio) >1 and segmental artery:bronchus (ratio) >1 in three or more lobes are suggestive of PH.

b. Lung disease can be evaluated. Pulmonary capillary haemangiomatosis can be recognized from small nodular opacities with bilateral thickened interlobular septa.

c. CTEPH can be diagnosed by contrast CT angiography.

10. What are the lab tests for PH workup?

Before labelling it as iPAH, secondary causes should be ruled out by the following lab tests:

a. *Connective disease profile*: Antinuclear antibody, rheumatoid factor, anti CCP, anti-centromere, anti–RNA polymerase III, anti-Ro, anti-La and U1RNP antibodies

b. *Infectious profile*: HIV, stool and urine for parasites (schistosomiasis)

c. *Haematologic profile*: Peripheral smear for sickle cell

11. What is the role of RHC?

RHC, the gold standard for PH diagnosis, is valuable in:

a. Confirming the diagnosis (mPAP >25 mmHg) in doubtful cases.

b. Differentiating pre- and post-capillary PH (pulmonary artery occlusion pressure <15 mmHg in pre- versus >15 mmHg in post-).

c. Performing oximetry run in suspected left-to-right shunt.

d. Measuring cardiac output (thermodilution or the Fick principle) pulmonary resistance (>3 WU in PH).

e. Performing vasoreactive tests.

f. Pulmonary angiography is the final test for candidate selection in CTEPH prior to surgery.

g. Coronary angiogram may be performed in the case of definite angina to rule out coronary obstruction and left main compression by an enlarged pulmonary artery.

However, RHC may not be required in definite cases of left ventricular failure (LVF), obstructive sleep apnoea and severe lung disease with a total lung capacity (TLC) <65%.

12. What are the complications of PAH?

PAH has a 1-year mortality of over 10%. Among the causes of mortality, sudden death constitutes 25%. Right-sided heart failure (HF), atrial flutter/fibrillation, haemoptysis, pulmonary artery dissection and rupture, pulmonary artery compression by the left main artery and pericardial effusion are other causes.

13. What is a positive vasoreactivity test?

A positive vasoreactivity test means a >10 mmHg reduction of mean pulmonary pressure or a reduction to <40 mmHg mean pressure without a reduction (or an increase) in cardiac output on application of the drug. Inhaled nitric oxide (10–20 ppm) or intravenous epoprostenol is used for this test. Adenosine is no more recommended.

14. What are the indications of the vasoreactivity test?

It is indicated in iPAH, inheritable causes of PH and drug-induced PAH to determine the possible response to a calcium channel blocker (CCB).

15. What are the contraindications to the vasoreactivity test?

Contraindications to the vasoreactivity test include low systemic blood pressure (e.g. SBP <90 mmHg), low cardiac index (cardiac index <2 L/min/m²) or the presence of severe (functional class IV) symptoms, since hypotension and occasionally cardiovascular collapse can occur with the administration of the vasodilator.

16. How do you predict the prognosis in the case of iPAH?

See **Table 21.4** for determining the prognosis in iPAH.

17. What is the role of anticoagulation in PH?

Oral anticoagulation is generally not indicated in PH though exceptions can be made..
    It is not beneficial in PH due to associated diseases and in portopulmonary hypertension.

Table 21.4: Risk Stratification of PH

Parameter	Low Risk <5%	Intermediate Risk 5%–10%	High Risk >10%
Signs of HF	Absent	Absent	Present
Symptom progression	No	Slow	Rapid
Syncope	No	Occasional	Recurrent
WHO Class	I, II	III	IV
6MWD (meters)	>440	440–165	<165
NT-pro-BNP	<300	300–1400	>1400
RA area on echocardiogram cm^2	<18	18–26	>26
RAP	<8	8–14	>14
SvO$_2$	>65%	60–65	<60%
CI	>2.5	2.5–2.0	<2.0

Note: Percentages in risk stratification pertains to estimated 1 year mortality

18. What is the role of oxygen?

In PH, a pO_2 <60 mmHg warrants O_2 therapy to improve exercise performance. This is also indication of in-flight oxygen therapy.

19. What is basic medical therapy in PH?

Diuretics may reduce congestion and are widely used. Spironolactone may improve the prognosis. However, angiotensin-converting enzyme inhibitors (ACEIs), angiotensin receptor blockers (ARBs), beta-blockers and ivabradine have no data favouring their use. Digoxin may be used for rate control. Beta-blockers must be avoided in portopulmonary hypertension, as they may adversely affect haemodynamics. Pneumococcal, influenza and COVID vaccination must be considered. Anemia should be corrected.

20. What are the targeted therapies in PH?

Targeted therapies are the mainstays of PH treatment, singly or in combination, and each of them is directed towards a particular signalling pathway involved in PH (**Table 21.5**). However, in those with response to vasoreactivity test and WHO class I - II (mPAP < 30 mmHg, PVR < 4 WU), high dose CCBs (Amlodipine 15–30 mg) should be used. Approved therapies target three main pathways important in endothelial function: The prostacyclin and nitric oxide (NO) pathways, which are underexpressed in PAH patients, and the endothelin pathway, which is overexpressed. For World Health Organization (WHO) functional classes II–III, for PAH with intermediate- low risk of death an endothelin receptor A (ERA), a phosphodiesterase 5 inhibitor (PDE5I) and selexipag are recommended. 2022 ESC guideline recommends that in non vasoreactive high-risk patients with idiopathic, heritable or drug induced hypertension but no cardiopulmonary comorbidity an ERA, PDE5I and s.c / i.v prostaglandins should be considered:

A. Ambrisentan (10 mg/day) plus tadalafil (40 mg/day) (AMBITION trial). This is the best initial combination.

B. Macitentan (3 mg or 10 mg/day) plus sildenafil (SERAPHIN trial). ESC recommended Macicentan + Tadalafil.

Table 21.5: Treatment Pathways in PH

Endothelin Pathway	NO-cGMP Pathway	Prostacyclin Pathway
Endothelin receptor antagonists (ERAs)	*Phosphodiesterase 5 inhibitors (PDE5Is)*	*Prostacyclin analogues*
• Bosentan • Ambrisentan • Macitentan	• Sildenafil • Tadalafil • Vardenafil	• Beraprost • Epoprostenol • Iloprost • Treprostinil
	Soluble guanylate cyclase stimulator Riociguat	*IP receptor agonist* Selexipag

ERA: *Ambrisentan* is specific ERA antagonist improving symptoms, exercise capacity, haemodynamics and natural history at a dosage of 5 mg/day. Abnormal liver function occurs rarely (0.8%–3%). There is increased peripheral oedema.

Bosentan is a dual endothelin receptor A and B antagonist. It has data in iPAH, PH with connective tissue disease and Eisenmenger syndrome. However, it causes dose-dependent reversible liver dysfunction (10%). Bosentan and sildenafil should not be combined.

Macitentan is also a dual antagonist which has shown mortality and morbidity reduction. The dose is 3 mg or 10 mg/day. Its specific side effect may be anaemia. It causes fetal harm.

NO-cGMP Pathway

NO plays an anti-proliferative and vasodilatory role in the pulmonary circulation. The PDE5Is sildenafil, tadalafil and vardenafil inhibit PDE5, which is responsible for the breakdown of cyclic guanosine monophosphate (cGMP) and thereby promotes the NO-cGMP pathway. Riociguat, on the other hand, is a guanylate cyclase stimulator enhancing cGMP production.

Sildenafil: It is an orally active potent inhibitor of PDE5 and improves exercise capacity, symptoms and haemodynamics in PAH at a dose of 20 mg thrice daily. Headache, flushing and epistaxis are the side effects caused by vasodilation.

Tadalafil: It is similar to sildenafil except that it is given *once* daily at a dose of 20 or 40 mg.

Vardenafil: It is similar to sildenafil except that it is given at a dose of 5 mg twice daily.

Riociguat: A guanylate cyclase stimulator, given at a dose of 2.5 mg thrice daily, it causes improvement in exercise capacity, symptoms and haemodynamics. A specific side effect is syncope. Riociguat cannot be co-administered with PDE5I.

Prostacyclin Pathway

Prostacyclin is a prominent vasodilator, platelet aggregation inhibitor, antiproliferative and cytoprotective agent.

Beraprost: This is an orally active prostacyclin analogue with improvement in exercise capacity but no improvement in haemodynamics or outcomes. Side effects include headache, flushing, jaw pain and diarrhoea.

Epoprostenol: It is a synthetic prostacyclin with a short half-life and is administered by continuous infusion by a permanent catheter. It improves symptoms, exercise capacity and haemodynamics and is the only drug shown to reduce mortality. It can be used in a dosage of 2–4 ng/kg/min in iPAH, scleroderma-related PAH and non-operable CTEPH. Side effects are as before for prostacyclin analogues.

Selexipag: It is an orally available selective prostacyclin IP receptor agonist. Selexipag has been shown to reduce pulmonary vascular resistance after a few months of use in combination with ERA or PDE5I and also to reduce composite mortality and morbidity end points.

21. When should therapy be escalated or changed?

Those on monotherapy must change to combination therapy if not responding in 3 months. For high risk cases without cardio pulmonary comorbidities, combination therapy (ERA+ PDE5I + Prosacyclin Analogue), must be initial strategy. For intermediate risk, no cardio pulomonary comorbidities initial therapy is with ERA + PDE5I. For those with cardiopulmonary comorbidities, either ERA or PDE5I is the initial drug. For patients not responding to combination therapy, lung transplant may be considered.

22. What is the treatment modality in PH due to chronic lung disease?

Targeted therapies have no clear benefit in lung disease–related PH. Non-invasive ventilation and long-term oxygen therapy are indicated in hypercapnic and hypoxemic patients, respectively, and improve pulmonary haemodynamics.

23. What are the specific management principles in PH due to associated diseases?

Portopulmonary hypertension: Anticoagulation and beta-blockers are contraindicated. Ambrisentan can be used with caution.

Pulmonary veno-occlusive disease: Lung transplant may the only option. Standard target-based therapy is associated with life-threatening pulmonary oedema due to pulmonary vasodilation with post-capillary venous obstruction.

Eisenmenger syndrome: An ERA (Bosentan) has class I indications. Anticoagulation can be used in right HF and pulmonary artery (PA) thrombosis in the absence of haemoptysis. Tadalafil has also been used with good results. Calcium channel blockers should not be used. It is of paramount importance to maintain hydration, avoid iron deficiency and use air filters during intravenous fluid administration. Pregnancy is contraindicated, and a progesterone-based contraceptive should be used (oestrogen based may increase thrombotic risk). An intrauterine device may be used. Hyperviscosity syndrome may require venesection if haematocrit >65%.

PAH in HIV: Antiretroviral therapy (especially protease inhibitors) has been associated with a reduction in PH. Bosentan, tadalafil and prostanoids have been shown to be useful.

PAH in connective tissue disease: Standard targeted therapy is applicable.

24. What is CTEPH?

It is a rare progressive pulmonary vascular disease due to persistent obstruction of *large and medium-sized pulmonary arteries* by organized thrombi, usually as a consequence of prior pulmonary embolism. The clinical presentation is often only subtle signs of right-sided HF.

The diagnosis of CTEPH requires 3 months of anticoagulation, V/Q scan showing mismatched perfusion defects followed by RHC (mPAP >25 mmHg, PAWP <15 mmHg) and pulmonary angiography (ring-like stenosis, webs, slits, pouch lesions/tapered lesions). Multidetector CT pulmonary angiography can also confirm the diagnosis, though haemodynamic information is not available.

Therapy consists of pulmonary endarterectomy (PEA) in operable cases (**Figure 21.2**) and a possible role of interventional balloon angioplasty in surgery-ineligible ones. Medical therapy with anticoagulation (vitamin K antagonist [VKA]) is recommended in all cases. Riociguat, bosentan and macitentan have all been used in inoperable cases with a reduction in PVR but no reduction in mortality.

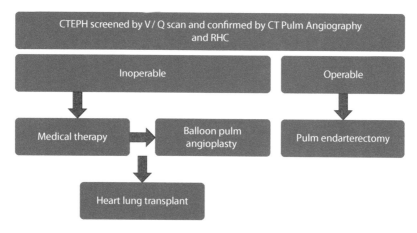

Figure 21.2 Treatment of CTEPH simplified.

25. What are the newer therapies in PH?

Experimental therapies in PH include the following:

a. Pulmonary artery denervation by radiofrequency ablation

b. Ultrasound-based denervation

c. Stenting of the left main coronary stenosis caused by compression from a dilated pulmonary trunk

BOX 21.1 COVID-19 AND PULMONARY HYPERTENSION

COVID-19 increases the mortality in PH, which approaches nearly 12%. During COVID-19, echocardiography-based follow-up of PH has decreased and V/Q scans have shifted to perfusion-only scans. COVID-19 itself has emerged as a cause of PH.

CASE STUDY 21.1: ANECDOTAL CASE

A 25-year-old young woman presented with class III dyspnoea with restriction of her daily activities. ECG showed atrial fibrillation. Echocardiography suggested a mitral valve area of 0.8 cm^2 with a mean pressure gradient of 16 mmHg and moderate TR with a peak gradient of 60 mmHg. So, this was a case of PH Type 2 (left-sided heart disease). Balloon mitral valvuloplasty was performed, and the mean gradient dropped to 5 mmHg and the valve area increased to 1.2 cm^2. The ePASP dropped to 30 mmHg. This case highlights the fact that PH Type 2 is quite common in the cardiac care unit (CCU) and effective treatment is often available.

FURTHER READING

1. Humbert M, Kovacs G, Hoeper M, et al. 2022 ESC/ERS Guidelines for the Diagnosis and Treatment of Pulmonary Hypertension. Eur Heart J (2022)43:3618–3731.
2. Frost A, Badesch D, Gibbs JSR, et al. Diagnosis of Pulmonary Hypertension. Eur Respir J 2019;53:1801904. https://doi.org/10.1183/13993003.01904-2018.

22 Narrow QRS Tachycardia

Sunandan Sikdar and Debabrata Bera

1. What is a narrow QRS tachycardia (NQRST)?

An NQRST is a tachycardia with a QRS duration of <120 msec. Usually due to supraventricular tachycardia (**Figures 22.1–22.5**), they include:

a. **Source from the atrium**

Sinus tachycardia (ST)

Inappropriate sinus tachycardia (IST)

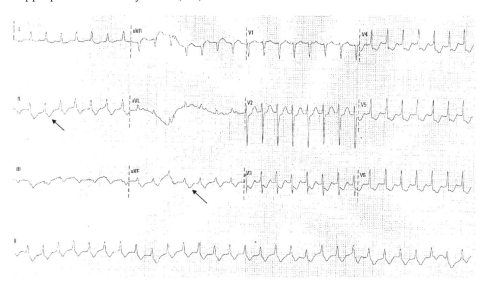

Figure 22.1 Regular narrow QRS tachycardia with short RP with secondary ST depression. Inverted P wave seen in inferior leads *(arrow).*

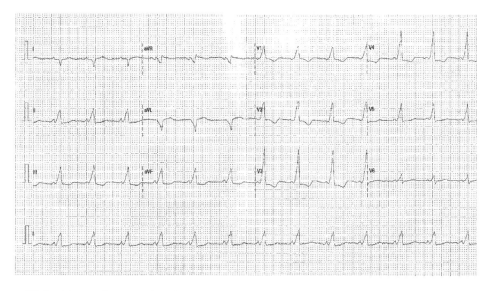

Figure 22.2 After cardioversion by adenosine: Baseline pre-excitation with positive delta in V1–V6 and negative in I and aVL, suggesting a left lateral AP.

DOI: 10.1201/9781003027584-22

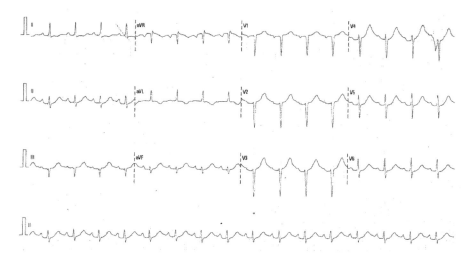

Figure 22.3 Radiofrequency Ablation (RFA) done. Absence of delta wave after ablation of the left lateral pathway.

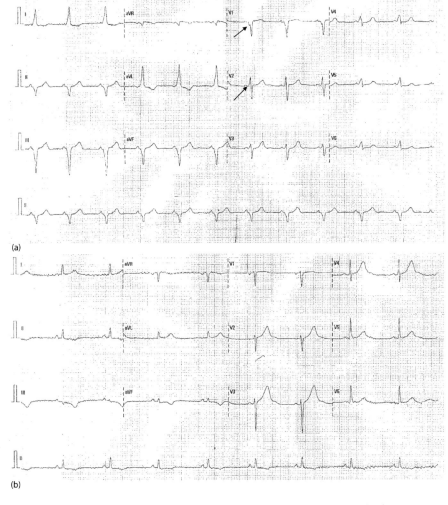

Figure 22.4 (a) WPW due to posteroseptal AP. Note the negative delta in inferior leads suggesting a posterior location. The transition from negative delta in V1 to positive delta in V2 suggests a septal location (arrow). (b) Same patient after RFA of posteroseptal pathway.

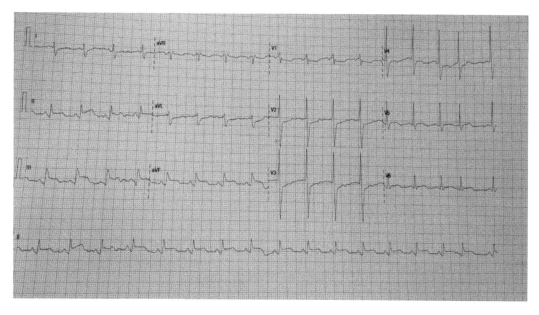

Figure 22.5 WPW: Right-sided AP mimicking inferior wall myocardial infarction (MI) (pseudoinfarct pattern): Delta negative in 2, 3 and F and positive in V1.

Sinoatrial nodal re-entrant tachycardia (SANRT)

Focal atrial tachycardia (AT)

Multifocal AT (MAT)

Atrial fibrillation (AF)

Atrial flutter (AFL)

b. **Obligatorily involving the AV node**

Junctional tachycardia (JT)

Atrioventricular nodal re-entrant tachycardia (AVNRT)

Atrioventricular re-entrant tachycardia (AVRT)

A "supraventricular" origin of a tachycardia implies the obligatory involvement of one or more cardiac structures above the bifurcation of the His bundle.

Wolff-Parkinson-White (WPW) syndrome occurs when at baseline, ventricular activation is caused by impulses coming down from the atrium both by the accessory pathway (AP) and the atrioventricular (AV) node (hence, it is a fusion complex). Because of the faster conduction by the AP, there is eccentric activation of the ventricles (especially for APs inserting into the free wall of the ventricles). This leads to a triad of a short PR (as the AV node is bypassed), slurred up (or down) stroke of the QRS (due to eccentric activation) and a wide QRS complex (due to activation of the ventricles sequentially rather than simultaneously).

2. What is paroxysmal supraventricular tachycardia (SVT)?

Paroxysmal SVT usually denotes an intermittent SVT other than AF, AFL and MAT and describes a clinical syndrome characterized by the presence of a regular and rapid tachycardia of abrupt onset and termination. The major causes are AVNRT (50%–60% of cases), AVRT (30%) and focal AT (10%).

3. How do you analyse NQRST on ECG?

Step 1. *NQRST: Is it regular?*

If it is irregular, then it is likely to be any of AF, atrial tachycardia/flutter with variable AV conduction or MAT. If it is regular, then go to Step 2.

Step 2. *Are P waves visible?*

If P waves not visible, then AVNRT is more likely.

If P waves are visible, then go to Step 3.

Step 3. *Are the P waves more than the QRS?*

If there are multiple P waves for each QRS, then it is likely to be AFL or AT.

If P = QRS, then go to Step 4.

Step 4. *What is the RP interval?*

If RP > PR: AT, PJRT, atypical AVNRT

If RP < PR, then go to Step 5.

Step 5. *What is the RP?*

RP <90 msec – AVNRT

RP >90 msec – AVRT

4. What are the exceptions to the rule that NQRSTs are SVTs?

Fascicular ventricular tachycardias (VTs) may have a relatively narrow QRS, but they may show AV dissociation. Sometimes due to retrograde conduction of ventricular impulses to the atrium, veno-atrial (VA) association, rather than dissociation, may be present.

5. How do you terminate SVT?

All manoeuvres target and block the AV node (**Figure 22.6**), as it is the weakest link in the loop.

a. *Try vagal manoeuvres*: They have a 30% success rate, especially near the onset of tachycardia, when sympathetic response to the tachycardia is yet to be established. The Valsalva is the most effective technique. In modified Valsalva, while the patient is doing a standard Valsalva, the leg is lifted to reduce sympathetic overdrive. Carotid sinus massage is also effective. Facial immersion in cold water is the method of choice for infants.

b. *Adenosine*: Its success rate for SVT termination nears 90%. Adenosine binds to G-coupled adenosine receptors, activating the acetylcholine-induced potassium channel and antagonizing the sympathetic drive–induced rising cyclic adenosine monophosphate (AMP) and calcium currents. Its actions on the atrium, sinus and AV nodes cause shortening of the action potential, hyperpolarization and reduced automaticity. It thus slows down the sinus node, terminates the SVT by blocking the AV node and can terminate VT induced by delayed afterdepolarization. Rarely, it may precipitate AF. A bolus of adenosine can paradoxically produce transient sympathetic activation by interacting with carotid baroreceptors, while a continuous infusion can cause hypotension.

   It has a rapid onset of action (10 sec) and a short half-life (10 sec) and is transported into endothelial cells and metabolized by adenosine deaminase. The usual dose for the peripheral vein is 6 mg or 12 mg (if the first one fails) in 1–2 sec with a vigorous flush of saline. Inadequate flush may lead to longer transport times and its elimination even before it reaches its site of action. For the central vein, the dose is 3 mg at the most and can often do with 1 mg. A second dose, often 12 mg, can be given after 60 sec. Due to the short half-life, reinitiation of SVT can occur soon after. In such a case verapamil, diltiazem or a beta-blocker should be started. Patients on theophylline or its cogeners require higher doses of adenosine, as they block adenosine receptors. In post–cardiac transplant patients, denervation hypersensitivity causes potentiation of adenosine effects and are better avoided.

   There is occasional asystole <5 sec, but this is rarely of consequence, and there may be a sensation of chest tightness.

c. *Verapamil*: Dosage 5 mg IV over 2 min followed after 5–10 min by 5–7.5 mg.

d. *Diltiazem*: 20 mg IV bolus then a second bolus of 25–35 mg if the first dose is ineffective. Infusion of diltiazem is given at 5–15 mg/hr if necessary.

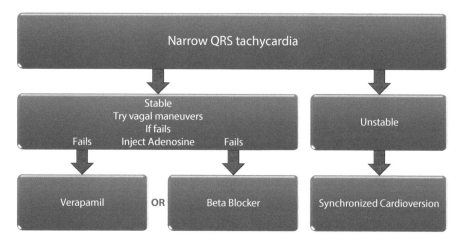

Figure 22.6 Management of narrow QRS tachycardia.

e. *Metoprolol*: 5 mg IV bolus every 5 min to a maximum of 15 mg. Verapamil/diltiazem should not be given intravenously in close succession after or before intravenous beta-blockers, as fatal AV block may occur.

6. Can adenosine cause haemodynamic collapse?

This is a rare event but can occur in patients with accessory pathway (AVRT). That is the reason an SVT patient being given adenosine must be admitted and a crash trolley and monitor must be ready. By shortening the effective refractory period of atrial tissue, Adenosine can precipitate AF. Those with an accessory pathway with robust antegrade conduction (and an AV node blocked by adenosine) can conduct the atrial impulses unchecked to the ventricle, triggering ventricular fibrillation (VF) and collapse.

7. What are the different types of AT?

The different types of AT are:

a. *Focal AT*: Originates from a small focus and I usually caused by automaticity. The initiating P wave has the same morphology on ECG as the tachycardia P waves. The tachycardia gradually speeds up at initiation and slows down at termination. Adenosine does not usually terminate the tachycardia. Focal AT caused by triggered activity can, however, be terminated by adenosine.

b. *Macro–re-entrant AT (MRAT)*: Tachycardia circuit around a large obstacle (valve/scar).

MRAT can be of three types:

a. *Cavotricuspid isthmus (CTI)*: Dependent right AT – These are actually AFL

b. *CTI-independent right AT*: These are the actual MRATs

c. Left ATs

8. What is the site of origin of AT?

The most common site of origin of AT is the right atrium (RA), around the crista terminalis due to anisotropic conduction in the region. In the left atrium (LA), the most common site of origin is around the pulmonary veins. Atrial appendage, coronary sinus os and either vena cava are other sources of AT.

9. How do you determine the site of AT focus by ECG?

RA vs LA: Lead V1 negative and aVL predominantly showing positive P waves implies an RA focus as the activation wave travels posteriorly (away from V1) and leftward (toward aVL) from the crista. The converse is true for an LA focus.

Cristal AT: If the P wave is negative in aVR, cristal AT is strongly suggested.

Superior versus inferior focus for RA-related AT: If the RA focus is confirmed, look at the inferior leads (II, III, aVF). Positive P in these leads suggests a superior focus (high RA) as the activation front is travelling towards them; a negative P suggests the focus in an inferior part of the RA.

10. What is MAT?

MAT has the following characteristics:

a. Discrete P waves with a rate >100/min

b. P waves with three different morphologies in the same lead

c. P waves separated by isoelectric intervals

d. No dominant driving foci – This differentiates it from sinus rhythm with multiple premature atrial contractions (PACs)

MAT occurs with chronic obstructive pulmonary disease (COPD) treated with theophylline, heart failure treated with digoxin, post-surgery or in those with electrolyte abnormalities. Treatment of the underlying condition, IV magnesium for rhythm control and a beta-blocker/calcium channel blocker (CCB) for rate control if symptomatic due to fast the ventricular rate are the treatment options. Amiodarone may be used in refractory cases.

11. How do you treat focal AT in the acute setting?

A patient who is haemodynamically stable can be converted by intravenous beta-blockers, verapamil and diltiazem. If a satisfactory result is not obtained, amiodarone or ibutilide may be used.

If the patient is unstable, IV adenosine is the drug of choice; electrical cardioversion may be required if it fails.

For chronic therapy, catheter ablation is the first choice. If medical management is preferred, then for rate control, a beta blocker/CCB, and for rhythm control, flecainide for a structurally normal heart and amiodarone for structural heart disease are the options.

12. How do you recognize AFL?

AFL circuit: The re-entrant circuit, which provides the path for perpetuation of classic flutter, is bounded anteriorly by the tricuspid annulus and posteriorly by undefined barriers. The flutter waveform rotates counterclockwise or clockwise (based on the left anterior oblique [LAO] view) around this pathway (**Figure 22.7**). The CTI is a protected zone of slow conduction bounded by the tricuspid annulus anteriorly and the inferior vena cava (IVC) and eustachian ridge posteriorly, running from the low anterolateral RA to the low septal RA. It forms clinically the most important part of the flutter circuit and is the target of flutter ablation.

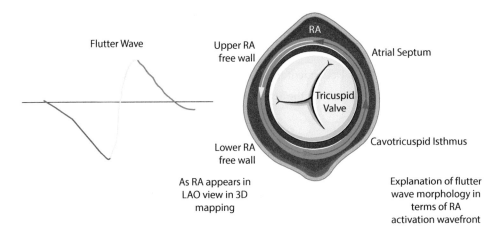

Figure 22.7 Flutter wave morphology on ECG explained.

ECG: AFL consists of atrial complexes of constant morphology, polarity and cycle length (average atrial rate 240–340/min) without an isoelectric interval, prominent in the inferior leads and lead V1.

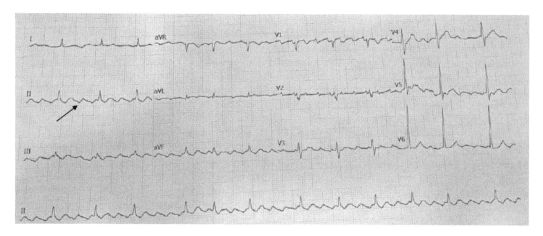

Figure 22.8 Counterclockwise atrial flutter with variable conduction: Note negative flutter waves in inferior leads *(arrow).*

In the case of counterclockwise AFL, the inferior leads record a predominantly negative deflection (**Figure 22.8**), with an initial slow downslope coinciding with the CTI slow conduction, followed by a rapid downslope due to the activation waveform moving up caudocranially (away from the inferior leads) along the RA side of the septum rapidly. This is followed by a sharp upstroke due to the craniocaudal direction of the wavefront travelling down the RA free wall (toward the inferior leads and, hence, positive). In clockwise flutter, the direction of the wavefront is opposite to the previous direction and records a predominant positivity in the inferior leads and negativity in lead V1.

The classical ECG of typical CTI-dependent flutter (counterclockwise/clockwise) may be altered by previous ablation or the presence of a scar. In atypical flutter, which may involve sites other than CTI, the P-wave morphology is different.

The ventricular rate (150/min) is often half the atrial rate (2:1 conduction), and in such cases one of the P waves is buried in the QRS complexes and may be missed by the untrained eye. Thus, such a rhythm may appear like sinus tachycardia. It can be confirmed by carotid sinus massage or adenosine, which can increase the degree of AV block and uncover the P waves. Sometimes spontaneously or due to use of antiarrhythmic drugs, 4:1 or 6:1 AV block occurs, often due to blocks at multiple levels (AV node, bundle of His and below).

13. How do you treat AFL?

These are the steps to manage AFL in the acute setting:

a. Decide whether rate control or rhythm control is best: Most patients benefit from rhythm control with respect to three issues: Symptoms, avoidance of tachycardiomyopathy and reduced risk of thromboembolism. However, elderly/frail patients with multiple comorbidities, a very large atrium, a history of multiple recurrence even on rhythm control drugs/ablation, intra-atrial thrombi or those with contraindications to anticoagulation may be candidates for rate control.

b. Decide whether the patient is haemodynamically stable or not.

All rhythm control scenarios in the acute setting involve full anticoagulation with intravenous unfractionated heparin (100 units/kg) immediately.

Scenario 1: *Haemodynamically unstable, rhythm control*: Electrical cardioversion with 50 joules. Success rate 95%. Contraindications: Digitalis toxicity and hypokalaemia.

Scenario 2: *Haemodynamically unstable, rate control*: Intravenous amiodarone is the best option in intensive care, especially those with associated heart failure or comorbidities. This drug may also inadvertently convert AFL to sinus rhythm and hence anticoagulation is necessary.

Scenario 3: *Haemodynamically stable, rhythm control*: Electrical cardioversion is again the safest method.

However, in those who cannot be sedated, two other methods can be tried: Atrial overdrive pacing if a pacemaker or dual-chamber automatic implantable cardioverter defibrillator (AICD) is in place and pharmacological cardioversion.

Overdrive pacing may be done by increasing the atrial rate 10% higher than the atrial rate of the flutter for 15 sec or more. The rate is increased incrementally until the flutter terminates or AF develops. The success rate is about 82% and is even better in those taking antiarrhythmics. A temporary pacing wire-based overdrive may be considered in a situation like a patient with digitalis toxicity.

Pharmacological cardioversion may be considered in those cases where sedation is contraindicated. Ibutilide is an effective drug which can terminate flutter in half an hour in one-half to three-fourths of subjects regardless of the duration of arrhythmia. Amiodarone can terminate flutter in only one-third of subjects. The serious side effect of ibutilide is polymorphic VT in about 2%, especially in those with left ventricular (LV) dysfunction. The patient given ibutilide must be monitored for at least 8 hr post-administration for this complication.

Scenario 4: *Haemodynamically stable, rate control*: Rate control is best done by beta-blockers/non-dihydropyridine CCBs (verapamil/diltiazem), provided the patient is not in heart failure. Beta-blockers are preferred in cardiomyopathy, ischaemic heart disease and post-surgery. Verapamil is preferred in the case of an obstructive airway. In patients with flutter in the setting of heart failure, amiodarone may be the best option for rate control. Digoxin may be used in refractory cases, but in those with heart failure, this drug may be proarrhythmic. Further, because efficacy of this drug is based on increasing the vagal tone, this drug may not be very effective in ambulatory patients.

Scenario 5: *Flutter with an accessory pathway*: Flutter in the presence of an accessory pathway can lead to very high ventricular rates and haemodynamic collapse. Prompt electrical cardioversion should be done. Those who are stable can be treated by ibutilide or procainamide. However, drugs that predominantly block the AV node (like beta-blockers, CCBs, adenosine and IV amiodarone) should not be used, as they may facilitate antegrade conduction via the accessory pathway and precipitate ventricular fibrillation. Peculiarly, oral amiodarone acts on both the AV node and AP equally and does not have the disadvantage of IV amiodarone. Thus it can be used in chronic therapy in AFL with AP.

14. What is the management of AFL in the chronic setting?

Once AFL is cardioverted, determine whether a reversible cause is present. Flutter in the setting of acute myocardial infarction, pulmonary embolism, cardiac surgery and hyperthyroidism does not require chronic therapy. In other cases, catheter ablation is the treatment of choice, as all antiarrhythmic drugs used (flecainide, amiodarone, sotalol, dofetilide) have a limited efficacy. Risk of stroke in AFL is similar to AF, and CHADVAS-based anticoagulation should be done.

15. How do you treat pregnancy with SVT?

Verapamil is the treatment of choice in the acute setting. If there is no pre-excitation, selective beta-blockers or verapamil may be used as maintenance therapy during discharge. If there is baseline pre-excitation, flecainide is used. In general, antiarrhythmics are avoided in pregnancy.

16. There is baseline pre-excitation in the ECG, but symptoms causing cardiac care unit (CCU) admission are not due to the ECG finding. When is catheter ablation required?

An electrophysiology (EP) study may be considered for risk stratification once the index admission is over. The indications for catheter ablation of the accessory pathway are:

a. EP testing with the use of isoprenaline identifies high-risk properties: Shortest pre-excited RR interval during AF (SPERRI) <250 ms, AP ERP ≤250 ms, multiple APs and an inducible AP-mediated tachycardia.

b. LV dysfunction due to electrical dyssynchrony induced by the AP.

FURTHER READING

1. Issa Z, Miller J M, Zipes D P. Paroxysmal Supraventricular Tachycardia, in Cardiac Arrhythmology and Electrophysiology, Third Edition, pp 697–729 Elsevier.
2. Brugada J, Katritis D G, Arbelo E, et al. 2019 ESC Guidelines for the Management of Patients with Supraventricular Tachycardia. European Heart Journal 2020;41(5):655–720.
3. Bera D, Mukherjee S, Narasimhan C, Lokhandwala Y, Halder A, Reddy P, Majumder S, Sikdar S. Precordial reverse pattern break: A predictor of posteroseptal accessory pathways ablatable from the proximal coronary sinus. Heart Rhythm. 2022 Aug;19(8):1386–1388.

23 Atrial Fibrillation

The CCU Perspective

Anunay Gupta and Sunandan Sikdar

1. What are the types of atrial fibrillation (AF)?

AF is the most common tachyarrhythmia encountered in critical care. AF can be classified in the following ways:

a. *Paroxysmal*: AF episodes that terminate spontaneously or with intervention within 7 days of onset

b. *Persistent*: Lasts longer than 7 days and often requires termination by cardioversion (pharmacological/electrical)

c. *Long-standing persistent*: Continuous AF lasting for ≥1 year.

d. *Permanent*: Persistent AF when the clinician and patient has decided not to pursue a rhythm control strategy

e. *Lone AF*: AF without any structural heart disease and risk factors for stroke. Less commonly used term these days.

f. *Subclinical AF (SCAF)*: SCAF is defined as episodes of AF detected by intracardiac, implantable or wearable monitors and confirmed by intracardiac electrogram or review of the recorded rhythm on the ECG.

g. *Valvular AF*: Patients with mitral stenosis or artificial heart valves and post–mitral valve repair should be treated with vitamin K antagonists only instead of novel oral anticoagulants (NOACs).

2. What is new-onset AF?

This term encompasses new symptoms attributable to AF, asymptomatic patients with a newly discovered irregularly irregular pulse with suggestive ECG or AF detected by a device for the first time.

3. What is the mechanism of AF?

For AF to be initiated and maintained, the following are important (**Figure 23.1**):

Initiation – Triggers: In 90% of cases of paroxysmal AF, the initiating trigger is pulmonary vein ectopy. In these cases, the sleeves of atrial myocytes entering the pulmonary veins are electrically active (focal driver) and have decreased refractoriness, delayed afterdepolarization and show an

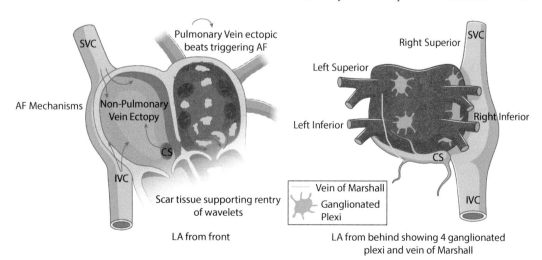

Figure 23.1 Mechanisms of AF simplified.

DOI: 10.1201/9781003027584-23

anisotropic condition, especially in response to catecholamines and atrial stretch. The superior vena cava, ligament of Marshall and coronary sinus also show such activity. Atrial tachycardia, atrial flutter and other supraventricular tachycardias can also initiate AF in predisposed patients. Atrial flutter and AF commonly coexist, and elimination of atrial flutter will diminish and/or eliminate episodes of AF.

Maintenance – Substrate: Persistent AF occurs due to atrial substrate changes that allow perpetuation of the arrhythmia. Long-standing AF includes loss of myofibrils with an increase in interstitial fibrosis, disruption of cell-to-cell gap junctions and enlargement of the atria. These anatomic and electrophysiologic alterations of conduction and refractoriness may lead to re-entry, possibly rotors or spiral wave re-entry. It is known that "AF begets AF," and the longer a patient is in AF, the less likely that sinus rhythm can be restored and maintained.

4. What are vagal and adrenergic AF?

1. Vagal AF occurs in young males with a structurally normal heart during sleep or in the postprandial state.

2. Adrenergic AF occurs in the elderly with heart disease and occurs predominantly in the daytime during episodes of emotional stress.

3. In patients with paroxysmal AF, vagal and adrenergic types occur in 15% and 10%, respectively.

5. What are the risk factors for AF?

1. Genes – 20% have family history in those with AF with a normal heart

2. Age >60 yr

3. Hypertension (most common modifiable risk factor)

4. Heart failure

5. Ischaemic heart disease

6. Valvular heart disease

7. Obesity

8. Sleep apnoea (reversible)

9. Thyroid disease (reversible cause)

10. Diabetes

11. Chronic obstructive pulmonary disease

12. Chronic kidney disease

13. Alcohol (>7 drinks/week or binge drinking of >5 drinks in a day) (holiday heart)

14. Smoking

15. Surgery (reversible cause)

6. What are the causes of drug-induced AF?

The following drugs/substances have been implicated in AF:

1. Adenosine

2. Noradrenaline/dopamine

3. Milrinone

4. Digitalis

5. Bisphosphonates

6. Aminophylline

7. Ivabradine

8. Cannabis

7. What is the epidemiology of postoperative AF?

Around one-third of patients develop AF after open-heart surgery. AF even without drug therapy usually resolves within 4–6 weeks in such patients. One study compared rate vs rhythm control strategies for postoperative AF and demonstrated no difference in the absence of AF at 2 months. Therefore, adequate anticoagulation and rate control are required in these patients and rhythm control can be avoided, and patients reassessed later after discharge.

8. What is silent AF?

AF without symptoms occurs in one-third of the total AF population. This is called silent AF. The actual prevalence of AF is likely much more than reported in large epidemiological studies because many patients have "silent" AF and are not included in such studies

9. What is device-detected AF?

AF detected by a cardiac implantable electronic device (often on the basis of cut-off atrial episodes with a rate ranging between >175 and >220/min and lasting >6 min) while patients are usually asymptomatic. For a device-detected AF with duration >24 hr, anticoagulation may be considered depending on the risk of stroke. Whether patients with an AF duration between 5.5 hr and <24 hr need anticoagulation is currently being assessed in randomized controlled trials.

10. What is the CHA2DS2-VASc score?

Table 23.1: CHADVASc Score Calculation

Letter	Parameter	Points
C	CHF or LV dysfunction	1
H	Hypertension	1
A2	Age >75	2
D	Diabetes	1
S2	Stroke, TIA, emboli	2
V	Vascular disease	1
A	Age 65–74	1
S	*Sex*: Female	1

Maximum points are 9. Low risk – score 0, intermediate risk – score 1, high-risk – score 2 or more.
Anticoagulation is required if the CHADVAS is 2 or more in males and 3 or more in females. In nonvalvular AF, it is reasonable to omit anticoagulation with a score of 0 in men and 1 in women (class IIa indication); for a score of 1 in men and 2 in women, oral anticoagulation may be considered (class IIb).

11. Which anticoagulation method should be used?

NOACs should be preferred over vitamin K antagonists in non-valvular AF. Currently, only severe mitral stenosis and metallic valves are considered absolute contraindications for NOACs.

Table 23.2: Oral Anticoagulants and Their Dosages

Drug	Mechanism of Action	Dosage
Warfarin/Acitrom	Vitamin K antagonist	2–10 mg/day, target INR 2–3
Direct Acting (NOACs)		
Dabigatran	Thrombin inhibitor	150 mg BD/110 mg BD
Apixaban	Factor Xa Inhibitor	5 mg BD/2.5 mg BD (if more than two out of three criteria are met: Age >80, creatinine >1.5 and weight <60 kg)
Rivaroxaban	Factor Xa Inhibitor	20 mg OD/15 mg OD if CrCl 15–50 mL/min
Edoxaban	Factor Xa Inhibitor	30 mg OD/15 mg OD

12. How is bleeding risk stratification for anticoagulation in AF done?

Their can be done by using the HAS-BLED score.

Table 23.3: HAS BLED Score and Bleeding Risk Stratification

Letter	Parameter	Points
H	Hypertension (systolic BP >160 mmHg)	1
A	Abnormal liver/renal function	1 or 2
S	Stroke	1
B	Bleeding	1
L	Labile INR (high INR/time in therapeutic range <60%)	1
E	Elderly (age >65 yr)	1
D	Drugs (antiplatelet or NSAID)/alcohol	1 or 2

Risk of bleeding: Low-risk score 0–1, intermediate-risk score 2, high-risk score 3.

It is important to understand that a high bleeding risk score is not a reason to withhold NOAC. However, a high score should prompt careful review and follow-up, as well as aggressive efforts at amelioration of potentially reversible bleeding risk factors (e.g., uncontrolled hypertension, labile international normalized ratios [INRs] and renal or hepatic insufficiency).

13. What are the symptoms of AF?

The symptoms are many and variable and may relate to the arrhythmia itself or some of its severe consequences, for example, stroke and heart failure.

Four major presentations of AF are:

a. Palpitation (the most common symptom, especially in paroxysmal AF)

b. Chest pain (demand ischaemia)

c. Syncope (due to a long ventricular pause following AF termination or loss of cardiac output at AF initiation in hypertrophic cardiomyopathy [HCM], aortic stenosis, bypass tract with antegrade conduction)

d. Embolic manifestation

Due to loss of an atrial kick at end diastole, there is underfilling of the ventricles and loss of a quarter of cardiac output compared to those without AF at the same heart rate; this may lead to fatigue.

14. How do you measure blood pressure in AF?

In AF, the blood pressure is determined as an average value of multiple cycles, usually five.

15. What is the diagnostic workup for AF?

ECG, echocardiogram, electrolytes (especially hypokalaemia), thyroid-stimulating hormone (TSH), live function test (LFT) and creatinine are the basic investigations in AF. Holter monitoring is often necessary to look for rate control. CT angiography or invasive angiography may be considered if clinical findings are suggestive of ischaemia.

16. What is the characteristic ECG of AF?

AF is characterized by rapid, typically more than 400/min, disorganized atrial activation, which appears as an undulating baseline without any distinct P waves (**Figure 23.2**) or as a tracing that at times gives the appearance of a flutter-like rhythm. However, true AF has an atrial rate with a clocklike regularity, and careful measurement of the flutter-like appearance in the AF tracing shows the atrial rate is irregular. The ventricular rate is usually irregularly irregular unless the patient has heart block. A standard 12-lead ECG recording or a single-lead ECG tracing of ≥30 sec shows a heart rhythm with no discernible repeating P waves and irregular RR intervals.

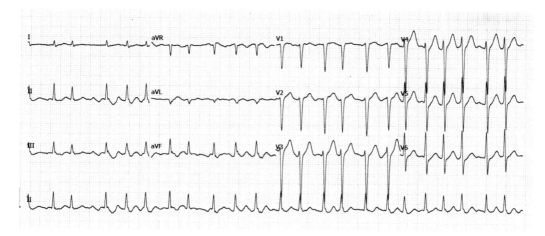

Figure 23.2 ECG of atrial fibrillation.

17. What are the indications for admission in AF and urgent rhythm control?

a. Presence of antegrade conducting accessory pathway

b. Haemodynamic instability

c. Ischaemia

d. Heart failure

e. Comorbidities like acute coronary syndrome, pneumonia, hyperthyroidism and pericarditis

18. What is the ABC pathway in the management of AF?

2020 AF Guidelines suggest ABC care:

a. Anticoagulation/Avoid stroke

b. Better symptom management – Better rate and rhythm control

c. Comorbidities and Cardiovascular risk factor management – Treating comorbidities like hypertension along with smoking cessation, reduction of weight, treatment of sleep apnoea, avoiding excess alcohol and moderate-intensity exercise

19. What are the indications for rate versus rhythm control therapy?

The two principal treatment strategies for patients with AF are controlling the ventricular rate when AF occurs but making no attempt to restore and maintain sinus rhythm (rate control) or, as a main goal, to keep the patient in sinus rhythm (rhythm control). Newer studies have shown benefits of rhythm control therapy with ablation if attempted in the initial course of the illness. Most of the trials involved relatively young patients with normal left ventricular (LV) function. Nothing can be generalized, however, and the decision should be individualized (**Figure 23.3**).

The rhythm control strategy is indicated in patients who are symptomatic on rate control drugs or have heart failure where AF is a contributing factor.

The rate control strategy is indicated in elderly patients with mild symptoms or infrequent symptoms in a younger population.

In new-onset AF, where recurrence is low, antiarrhythmic drugs for maintenance of rhythm control may not be necessary.

20. How do you control the rhythm with drugs?

Amiodarone is the most effective drug but with a significant side effect profile. Therefore, it should not be used as a first-line drug in most instances except in patients with heart failure, coronary

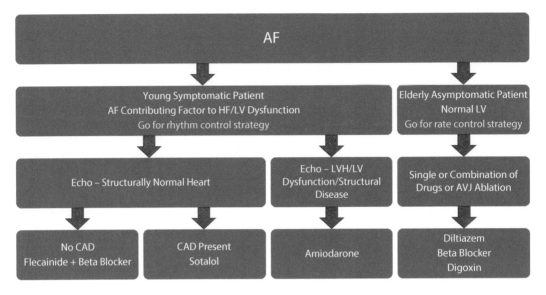

Figure 23.3 AF – Choice of drug therapy.

heart disease or substantial left ventricular hypertrophy (LVH) >15 mm on echocardiogram and if used should be at the lowest possible maintenance dose of 100–200 mg/day to avoid side effects.

Table 23.4: Drugs Available in India for Maintenance of Sinus Rhythm

Name of Drug	Dosing	Precautions
Flecainide	50–200 mg BD	• Needs AV nodal blocker concomitantly • QRS widening can occur • QRS Should not exceed 150% of baseline
Amiodarone	• *Loading*: 400–600 mg/day for a month • *Maintenance dose*: 100–300 mg/day	• Lung, liver or thyroid toxicity • Prolonged QT interval (torsade de pointes, ventricular tachycardia rare)
Sotalol	40–60 mg OD	• Prolonged QT interval with torsade de pointes, ventricular tachycardia • QTc should not exceed 520 msec • SA or AV nodal dysfunction

Flecainide is the drug of choice for AF with a structurally normal heart.

Sotalol is useful in coronary artery disease (but not in heart failure).

Amiodarone is used in those with LV hypertrophy, LV dysfunction or heart failure.

Disopyramide may be used to convert vagally mediated AF due to its anticholinergic action, provided prostatism and glaucoma are ruled out.

Beta-blockers may be used in adrenergic-mediated AF.

To avoid proarrhythmic side effects, an ECG should be done at 7 days and a Holter at 14 days to check for bradyarrhythmia, QRS duration and QT interval.

21. How do you control rate?

Controlling the rate is critical in AF both during the acute state to provide symptomatic relief and in the long term to develop tachycardiomyopathy. Optimum rate control is debatable but usually 60–80 beats per minute at rest and 90–115 beats per minute with exercise is considered. When large doses of a drug are needed to control rate, it can cause significant side effects. Therefore, it may be better to use two different agents at moderate doses to achieve rate control with minimal side effects, for example, a beta-blocker and calcium channel blocker.

Table 23.5: Drugs Used for Rate Control

Beta-Blockers	Dosage	Remarks
Metoprolol succinate	50–100 BD	Not preferred in the young and active
Bisoprolol	2.5–10 mg BD	
Propranolol	10–40 mg TDS	
Calcium channel blockers	Dosage	Avoided in heart failure and LV dysfunction
Verapamil (Calaptin)	120–480 mg/day	Preferred in asthma and COPD
Diltiazem	120–360 mg/day	
Digoxin	0.25–0.5 mg/day 5 days a week	Cautious use in kidney failure and hypokalaemia
Acute rate control		
Esmolol	500 mcg/kg bolus over 1 min, then 50–300 µg/kg/mL	Avoided in decompensated heart failure
Diltiazem	0.25 mg/kg bolus over 2 min, then 5–15 mg/hr	
Digoxin	0.25 mg stat	Additional dosing allowed, but max 1.5 mg in 24 hr

22. What are the contraindications for pharmacological cardioversion?

In patients with (1) sick sinus syndrome, (2) long QT (>500 msec) or (3) atrioventricular conduction disturbance, pharmacological cardioversion should not be used. If a pacemaker is present already, patients in items (1) and (2) can undergo drug therapy.

23. How is cardioversion performed?

It can be either electrical direct current cardioversion (DCCV) through a defibrillator or pharmacological through drugs. DCCV requires a shock synchronized to the QRS complex to be given through electrode pads on the chest timed to the QRS complex. The patient should be adequately sedated to avoid pain. A fasting state is preferable (the 6-hr standard may not be achievable in an emergency). Anticoagulation by heparin is essential (**Figure 23.4**). Most authors consider using a 200-joule biphasic shock as standard for cardioversion of AF due to its higher efficacy and also higher energy is unlikely to cause ventricular fibrillation (VF) if it falls on the T wave. The side

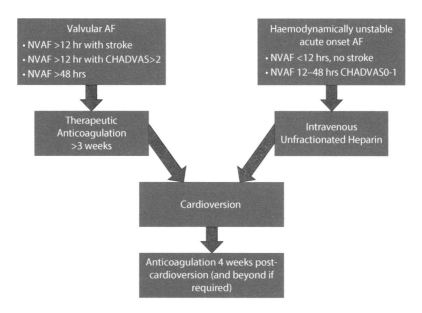

Figure 23.4 Protocol for cardioversion in AF.

effects of electrical cardioversion are thromboembolism, bradyarrhythmia and pulmonary oedema due to ventricular stunning (rare).

Pharmacologic cardioversion is less effective than DCCV. It is considered only in haemodynamically stable patients.

Oral drugs include a single dose of 300 mg flecainide or 600 mg propafenone, which can be used if no contraindications are present. An atrioventricular (AV) nodal blocking agent should be administered concomitantly to minimize the chance of 1:1 ventricular conduction if drug conversion of AF to atrial flutter occurs.

The recommended dose of ibutilide varies with patient weight. For patients weighing less than 60 kg, the dose is 0.01 mg/kg infused over 10 min. If the arrhythmia does not terminate within 10 min after the end of the infusion, a second bolus (same dose over 10 min) may be given. For patients weighing more than 60 kg, the dose is 1 mg over 10 min. Again, if the arrhythmia does not terminate within 10 min after the end of the infusion, a second bolus of 1 mg over 10 min may be given. The QTc interval needs to be monitored; therefore, it should be given in intensive care unit (ICU) settings. Intravenous magnesium sulphate enhances the ability of ibutilide to successfully convert AF or flutter, and it can attenuate the QT interval prolongation associated with ibutilide therapy.

Amiodarone is also used for pharmacological cardioversion. The dosing is 150 mg IV bolus over 10 min followed by 60 mg/hr for 6 hr and then 30 mg/hr for a total dose of 900 mg.

24. How do you anticoagulate pre- and post-cardioversion?

During cardioversion, if there is a thrombus, the risk of clot dislodgement is real. Hence, the requirement of anticoagulation except in an emergency, where intravenous heparin is the drug of choice (**Figure 23.4**).

25. What are the indications for catheter ablation in AF?

AF catheter ablation may be considered as first-line rhythm control therapy to improve symptoms in patients with symptomatic paroxysmal AF episodes or in persistent AF without major risk factors for AF recurrence as an alternative to antiarrhythmic drug class I or III, considering patient choice, benefit and risk. It is also indicated as a second-line treatment in symptomatic paroxysmal/persistent AF with beta-blocker failure or intolerance where the risks of the procedure are acceptable and the patient is motivated. Another indication based on recent trials is symptomatic AF with heart failure with reduced ejection fraction (HFrEF), especially if tachycardiomyopathy is suspected.

26. With post-catheter ablation of AF, what is the role of antiarrhythmics and anticoagulation?

Anticoagulation will be according to CHA2DS2VASc, and ablation doesn't eliminate the need for anticoagulation. If antiarrhythmics are decided on (may reduce recurrence), they can be continued for 3 months (at least 2 months) and stopped thereafter. The efficacy of antiarrhythmics increases post-ablation.

27. What is the indication for AF cardioversion in pregnancy?

In pregnancy with HCM, persistent AF requires cardioversion.

28. What drugs can be used for long-term management of AF during pregnancy?

For rhythm control: Sotalol, flecainide

For rate control: Digoxin, verapamil

29. When is anticoagulation for AF re-introduced after intracranial haemorrhage (ICH)?

Provided bleeding and the risk factors of bleeding are controlled, a 4- to 6-week waiting period is recommended.

30. What is the role for left atrial (LA) appendage occlusion?

Since the LA appendage is the source of the embolus in nearly 90% of cases, occlusion of the LA appendage may be a useful alternative to anticoagulation and free of its systemic side effects.

LA appendage closure through percutaneous closure is indicated in non-valvular AF if the subject has contraindications to anticoagulation or has bleeding on NOACs. It is comparable to warfarin in efficacy; however, direct comparison to NOACs is lacking.

Patients undergoing cardiac surgery can undergo surgical occlusion of the LA appendage.

FURTHER READING

1. Hindricks G, Potpara T, Dagres N, et al. 2020 ESC Guidelines for the Diagnosis and Management of Atrial Fibrillation Developed in Collaboration with the European Association for Cardio-Thoracic Surgery (EACTS). European Heart Journal (2020);42:373–498.
2. Andrande J G, Aguilar M, Atzema C, et al. The 2020 Canadian Cardiovascular Society/Canadian Heart Rhythm Society Comprehensive Guidelines for the Management of Atrial Fibrillation. Canadian Journal of Cardiology 36;(2020):1847–1948.

24 Wide QRS Tachycardia

Sunandan Sikdar and Subramanian Anandaraja

1. What is a wide QRS tachycardia (WQT)?

Tachycardia (ventricular rate >100/min) with QRS duration >120 msec is referred to as WQT.

2. What are the causes of WQT?

The causes of WQT and their corresponding prevalence figures are:

1. Ventricular tachycardia (VT) – 80%

2. Supraventricular tachycardia (SVT) with aberrancy/baseline wide QRS – 15%

3. Pre-excited tachycardia, drug (class 1A, 1C or III)– or hyperkalaemia-induced widened QRS, paced complexes – 5%

3. How do you differentiate VT from SVT with wide QRS?

Differentiating VT from SVT with wide QRS is often difficult and in a few cases may require invasive electrophysiologic study for confirmation. Numerous difficult-to-remember algorithms are available (**Figures 24.1** and **24.2** for the Brugada algorithm), but the basic principle is based on few simple facts.

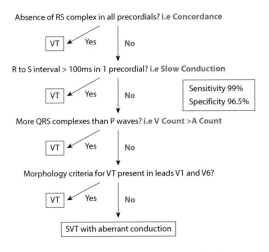

Figure 24.1 Brugada criteria for differentiating VT from SVT with aberrant intraventricular conduction (3C + 1M). (From Brugada P, Brugada J, Mont L, et al. A new approach to the differential diagnosis of a regular tachycardia with a wide QRS complex. Circulation.1991. 83, 1649–1659.)

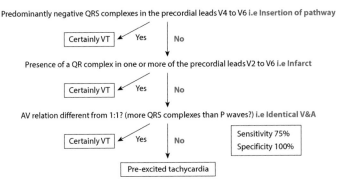

Figure 24.2 Brugada criteria for differentiating VT from antidromic tachycardia over an accessory pathway. (From Brugada P, Brugada J, Mont L, et al. A new approach to the differential diagnosis of a regular tachycardia with a wide QRS complex. Circulation.1991. 83, 1649–1659.)

 DOI: 10.1201/9781003027584-24

Morphology: **VT** (especially those arising from the free wall) results from slow, muscle-to-muscle conduction and sequential (instead of simultaneous) activation of the ventricles. Hence, the His-Purkinje conduction system is engaged much later in the QRS timeline in VT. This causes both the upstroke and downstroke of the QRS to be gradual (broad and notched QRS). VTs arising from the ventricular septum are an exception because they engage the conduction system much earlier and cause simultaneous activation of both ventricles, leading to a comparatively narrower QRS. On the other hand, SVT engages the conduction system early. Though a bundle branch block (aberrancy) also causes sequential ventricular activation, the initial upstroke/downstroke of the QRS is sharper. Further, in all SVTs, the activation is from the base of the ventricle towards the apex (V5–V6 should be positive), so any activation travelling from the apex of the left ventricle (LV) to the base (V5–V6 should be negative) cannot be an SVT and hence is a VT. All these are reflected in the following criteria (**Figures 24.3–24.6**):

WQT with right bundle branch block (RBBB) morphology (V1, initial part positive): QRS duration >140 msec – VT

Morphology favouring VT in RBBB morphology: Monomorphic R or R > r in V1, S > R in V6

WQT with left bundle branch block (LBBB) morphology (V1, initial part negative): QRS duration >160 msec – VT

Morphology favouring VT in LBBB morphology: Initial r duration >30 msec, S >60 msec, notch in S downslope in V1 (slow downslope), qR in V1, Q in V6

Lead aVR in the diagnosis (Vereckei algorithm) (**Figure 24.7**): V1 and aVR are the two most important leads. If monomorphic R is present in aVR (activation from apex to base), the diagnosis is VT. Other clues exclusively for aVR which favours VT are initial r >40 msec, notch on the initial downstroke and Vi/Vt <1.

Vi/Vt concept (**Figure 24.8**): The Vi/Vt criterion is based on the estimation of initial (Vi) and terminal (Vt) ventricular activation velocity. Higher velocity (distance/time) translates to larger myocardial activation in a shorter time (larger vertical distance). The ratio (Vi/Vt) is determined by measuring the vertical excursion (in millivolts) recorded on the ECG during the initial (Vi) and terminal (Vt) 40 msec of the QRS complex.

SVT captures His early with rapid conduction, so Vi (initial vertical excursion) is more, and VT captures myocardium early with slow conduction, hence Vi is less.

Thus, SVT – Vi/Vt >1, VT – Vi/Vt <1.

Advantage: Not affected by antiarrhythmic drugs, as they reduce conduction in the His and myocardium equally.

Disadvantage: Extensive myocardial scar, fascicular VT (VT close to septum) can cause an erroneous result.

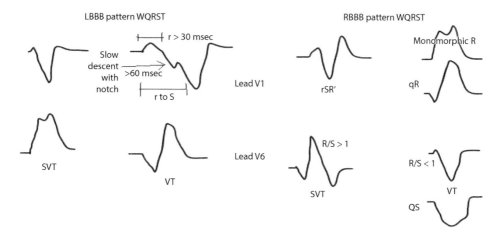

Figure 24.3   Morphology criteria for SVT versus VT.

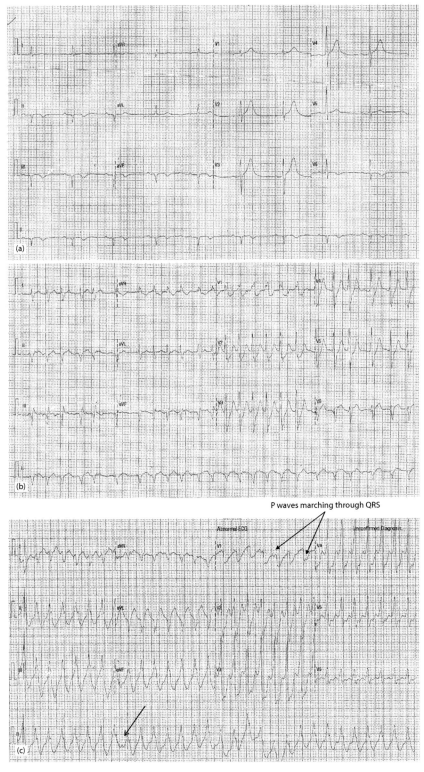

Figure 24.4 (a) An 80-year-old man with ACS – ECG after successful percutaneous coronary intervention (PCI) of occluded left circumflex artery (LCX). (b) Palpitation next day – WQT with RBBB morphology and varying RR interval with initial sharp deflection in QRS. No P wave is discernible. Rhythm is AF with RBBB aberrancy. (c) Same patient on day 3. WQT with LBBB right axis morphology with regular RR interval, QRS >160 msec in V1 with AV dissociation. Rhythm is VT.

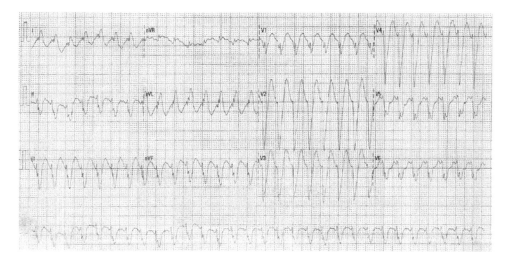

Figure 24.5 WQT LBBB left axis morphology with regular RR interval: QRSd >160 msec in V1, all precordial leads negative (negative concordance), slow notched descent in V1 (r to s >60 msec) and qR in aVR, all suggest VT with an apical exit.

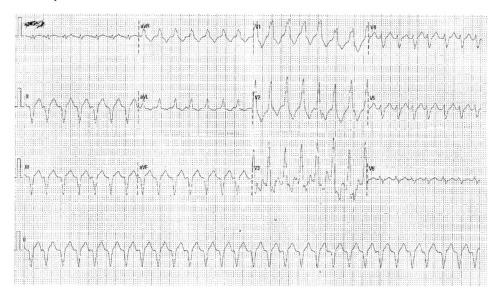

Figure 24.6 WQT, RBBB superior axis morphology with regular RR interval. QRSd >140 msec V1, monophasic R V1 and aVR suggest VT with exit inferior wall of LV. Echocardiography revealed an inferior wall scar.

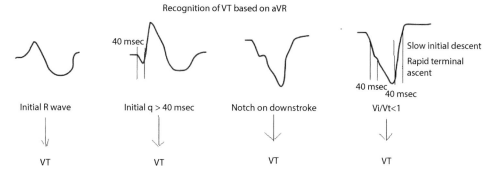

Figure 24.7 aVR-based Vereckei algorithm.

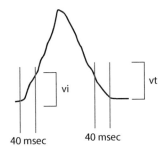

40 msec   40 msec

- The vi/vt criterion based on the estimation of initial (vi) and terminal (vt) ventricular activation velocity ratio (vi/vt) by measuring the vertical excursion (in millivolts) recorded on the ECG during the initial (vi) and terminal 40 msec (vt) of the QRS complex.
- SVT captures His early so Vi more, VT captures Myocardium early Vi less
- SVT – Vi/Vt >1, VT Vi/Vt <1
- Adv: Not Affected by Anti Arrhythmic Drugs
- Disadv: Myocardial Scar, Fascicular VT may affect

Figure 24.8 Concept of the velocity ratio.

QRS axis (**Table 24.1**): A frontal axis between **–90 and +180 degrees** (northwest axis) cannot be achieved by any combination of bundle branch block and therefore suggests VT. Negative QRS complexes in leads I, II and III make VT likely. LBBB with a right axis is usually VT.

Table 24.1: The Significance of Determining the Axis

- A frontal axis between *–90 and +180 degrees* (NW) cannot be achieved by any combination of bundle branch block and therefore suggests VT.
- Negative QRS complexes in leads I, II and III suggest VT.
- LBBB with right axis is usually VT.
- *LBBB-like morphology in V1*: An exit in the right ventricle or the interventricular septum.
- *QRS axis that is directed **superiorly** generally indicates an exit in the inferior wall; an axis directed *inferiorly* indicates an exit in the anterior (superior) wall.
- *In V2–V4, dominant R waves* usually indicate an exit near the base of the ventricle.

Concordance: Negative concordance (all precordial complexes are initially negative – the foci of VT is near the apex) is more likely to be VT than positive concordance (all precordial complexes are positive – the foci are likely at the base and posteriorly). The latter may also occur with posteriorly inserted bypass tracts.

Timing (**Table 24.2**): The majority of VTs will have atrioventricular (AV) dissociation (V more than A and unrelated), as the AV node is rendered refractory by concealed retrograde conduction, but in about 30% of cases retrograde P waves may occur. Thus, retrograde P waves may regularly follow QRS even in VT. Further, in atrioventricular nodal re-entry tachycardia (AVNRT) with aberrancy, Ventriculo-atrial (VA) dissociation may occur. In slow VTs (due to antiarrhythmic use), despite AV dissociation, the sinus beat may get an opportunity to capture the ventricle, leading to capture (morphology like sinus beat) and fusion (partly sinus and partly like premature ventricular contraction [PVC]) beats. Capture and fusion beats are the hallmarks of a VT.

Table 24.2: Importance of AV Dissociation

- This is one of the most useful criteria for distinguishing VT from SVT – but SVT *can have* AV dissociation (AVNRT, JT).
- Occurs in *20%–50%* of VT cases and *almost* never in SVT.
- *30% of VTs have 1:1 retrograde conduction.*
- Capture beats (more specific).
- Fusion beats (can occur in SVT with VPC).

4. What is the management protocol for WQT?

There are two diagnoses (SVT vs VT) and two presentations (haemodynamically stable vs unstable) to consider (**Table 24.3** and **Figure 24.9**).

Table 24.3: Differential Diagnosis of WQT

RBBB Morphology	LBBB Morphology
SVT with RBBB	SVT with LBBB
Pre-excited tachycardia with left-sided AP	SVT with bystander right-sided AP (also Mahaim-like pathway)
Antidromic tachycardia with left AP conducting in antegrade direction	Antidromic tachycardia with right-sided AP
Ischaemic VT with LV exit	RV – VT
Fascicular VT with posterior fascicle exit	LV – VT (aortic cusp, mitral isthmus)
LVOT VT	

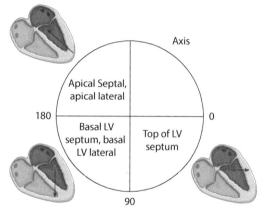

- LBBB – VT – LV septum, RV
- RBBB VT – LV anterolateral wall
- Positive concordance – LV base
- Negative Concordance – LV apex
- QS complex
  - –aVF – inferior
  - V2–4 – Ant lat wall
  - V3–5 – Apex
  - V5–6 – Lat wall

Figure 24.9 Determination of VT exit sites.

In unstable haemodynamics, synchronized direct current (DC) cardioversion by 50–100 J shock by biphasic external defibrillator is given after ensuring conscious sedation. Amiodarone may be considered in a bolus (150 mg) diluted in 5% dextrose in water given via filter to reduce recurrent episodes of VT. Lidocaine, with limited efficacy, may be administered while the sedation is underway.

If haemodynamics are stable and SVT is almost certain, adenosine is reasonable. It can terminate the SVT and expose atrial tachycardia (AT) or atrial flutter by nodal block. If it is an outflow tract VT, it also may respond to adenosine. In the case of VT, it can make the AV dissociation obvious. However, verapamil/diltiazem is contraindicated because profound hypotension may occur in case of VT.

If the patient is stable and VT is more likely, amiodarone is the drug of choice, especially if there is structural heart disease/LV dysfunction. The rate of VT termination is about 38%. After the 150-mg bolus dose (may be given over half an hour to reduce hypotension), 1 mg/min infusion over 6 hr (360 mg) and 0.5 mg/min over the next 18 hr (540 mg) is given. Procainamide is an alternative, though it is not readily available. Intravenous amiodarone may cause hypotension, especially if administered rapidly. Lidocaine can be used if amiodarone is ineffective or if ischaemia is the probable cause (50-mg loading dose, followed by a second loading dose of the same amount after 5–10 min then 2 mg/min IV infusion).

Correction of potassium and magnesium is paramount. After cardioversion, actively search for any reversible causes like ischaemia or granuloma (e.g. in sarcoidosis, cardiac MRI or positron emission tomography [PET] may give a clue) which may respond to revascularization or immunosuppression, respectively.

5. What is non-sustained ventricular tachycardia (NSVT)?

NSVT is defined as three or more consecutive ventricular complexes with a mean rate >100/min and a duration <30 sec.

6. What is the significance of NSVT?

NSVT can be found incidentally in the cardiac care unit (CCU) monitor, in the Holter or in the routine ECG. It occurs in 0%–3% of normal hearts and is mostly without significance. The importance is based the presence or absence of structural heart disease.

In the absence of heart disease (or channelopathies), NSVT may induce symptoms like palpitation but does not increase mortality. However, the only exception is if the ectopic burden is >20% on Holter, the patient requires follow-up by Echo, as there is a possibility of LV dysfunction later. NSVT with normal hearts often is caused by outflow tract in the right or left ventricle (RVOT/LVOT) ectopics either during exercise and rarely, in salvos during rest. If the patient is symptomatic, verapamil or a beta-blocker may be used.

In the presence of heart disease, in nonischaemic cardiomyopathy (NICM), nearly half of the patients may have NSVT on the Holter monitor, with the percentage increasing as heart failure progresses. NICM patients with NSVT have a higher mortality than those without. One-third of patients with HCM may have NSVT on the Holter monitor. Repetitive NSVT may confer increased risk of mortality in hypertrophic cardiomyopathy (HCM), especially in symptomatic patients and is an indication for an automatic implantable cardioverter defibrillator (AICD). While in stable coronary artery disease, NSVT may occur only in 5%, the situation changes after infarction, where in the first 24 hr 30% of patients may have this transient arrhythmia. The prevalence comes down in the next 2–4 weeks to 15%. When NSVT occurs 10–30 days after myocardial infarction (MI), it confers increased mortality risk. An electrophysiologic study of patients with coronary artery disease and LV systolic dysfunction may help identify those who would benefit from AICD based on VT inducibility.

7. How do you manage patients with monomorphic VT with structural heart disease?

In monomorphic VT with structural heart disease, etiological causes are ischaemic heart disease (IHD) (35%), NICM (18%), arrhythmogenic right ventricular cardiomyopathy (ARVC) (5%), valvular heart disease (4%), idiopathic and channelopathies (15%).

Lead V1 classifies VT into an LBBB- or RBBB-type morphology. The LBBB type originates from the LV septum in IHD or from the right ventricle (RV) in the case of NICM. The RBBB type usually originates from the LV (often its free wall). The morphology is dictated by the exit site of the VT circuit (where the depolarizing wave emerges from the protected channel to depolarize the large ventricular mass).

Pharmacological management in acute situations is discussed earlier. For long-term therapy amiodarone is a useful agent (200 mg twice daily), especially when used with a beta-blocker – both in preventing recurrent VT and avoiding AICD shocks. However, non-cardiac side effects are a cause of concern and are discussed in the section on cardiac drugs. Sotalol may be used in patients who already have an AICD because it reduces the defibrillation threshold and does not have the side effects of amiodarone.

However, in VT with structural heart disease, pharmacological treatment is inadequate and AICD is the therapy of choice. Patients with LV dysfunction and wide QRS may benefit from cardiac resynchronization therapy with a defibrillator (CRT-D), especially if left ventricular ejection fraction (LVEF) <35% and there are concomitant antiarrhythmic drugs (which may increase the pacing requirement). Patients on AICD who receive recurrent electrical therapies may require catheter ablation to reduce episodes of VT.

8. How do you manage bundle branch re-entry tachycardia (BBR-VT)?

It is a monomorphic VT with re-entry circuit involving the right and left bundle branches and the ventricular septum with rates >200/min and haemodynamic instability (syncope/arrest). The substrates are NICM, valvular heart disease, IHD, ARVC and even with those with His-Purkinje system disease and, rarely, in an apparently normal heart.

The ECG shows an LBBB (type A BBR-VT) or RBBB (type C BBR-VT) pattern VT and sometimes both. When the wavefront travels antegrade down the RBB and retrograde up the LBB towards the AV node (counterclockwise sequence), the more common (98%) type A BBR VT is manifested. The reverse (clockwise) sequence creates type C BBR VT. In the rare type B BBR VT (also called interfascicular re-entry), the left anterior and posterior fascicle form two limbs of the circuit.

Antiarrhythmics are less effective, and catheter ablation of the RBB is the treatment of choice for type A and C BBR-VT. Acute success rate approaches 100%. For those who have LBBB at a baseline sinus rhythm, LBB ablation may be safer, as ablation of the RBB may lead to complete AV block. Those with type B require fascicular ablation. After ablation, the merits of AICD/CRT-D implantation should be considered, as other VTs are not uncommon in NICM.

9. How do you manage outflow tract VT?

Commonly associated with a normal heart, outflow tachycardias (80% from RVOT, a few from LVOT) are arrhythmias caused by triggered activity due to delayed afterdepolarizations (DADs).

The ECG is important to localize the VT site and look for subtle signs of structural heart disease (QRS fragmentation, QRS prolongation, T-wave inversion). The ECG with RVOT VT shows an inferior QRS axis with a tall R in the inferior leads with a transition at V3 or V4 and an LBBB pattern in V1. A positive R in lead I implies a posterior (rightward) focus. In contrast, LVOT/coronary cusp VT has a precordial R-wave transition in V1 or V2 (small r present in V1). VT arising from an aorto-mitral continuity has a qR in V1.

It is important to recognize that ARVC may present with a VT resembling RVOT VT of a structurally normal heart. The baseline ECG showing a T-wave inversion in V1–V3 and QRS fragmentation, a VT ECG showing an R-wave voltage in inferior leads equalling the R wave in lead I and VT with multiple morphologies are suggestive of underlying cardiomyopathy. Echocardiography is essential, and cardiac MRI may be considered while planning therapy.

Outflow VTs usually have a good prognosis and if symptomatic (palpitation, syncope, chest pain) respond to beta-blockers and to verapamil. Symptomatic patients, especially those who are symptomatic despite medications, can be considered for catheter ablation, as the efficacy and safety of RVOT VT ablation are favourable.

10. How do you manage fascicular VT?

Classified under idiopathic LV VT, the most common site of origin of fascicular VT is the posterior fascicle (90% of cases) of the LV in a structurally normal heart in young individuals. The ECG of posterior fascicular VT shows RBBB V1 VT morphology with an rSR' pattern, S wave in V5–V6, left superior QRS axis and relatively narrow QRS morphology. Anterior fascicular VT shows the same V1 morphology with the right axis. These VTs are sensitive to verapamil (intravenous/oral). Catheter ablation has high success rates.

FURTHER READING

1. Cha Y M, Asirvatham S J. Approach to Wide QRS Tachycardia, in Asirvatham S J (Ed). Mayo Clinic Electrophysiology Manual. (2014), pp 137–169.
2. Vereckei A. Current Algorithms for the Diagnosis of Wide QRS Complex Tachycardias. Curr Cardiol Rev. (2014 Aug), 10(3):262–276.
3. Liang J, Anter E, Dixit S. Ablation of Ventricular Outflow Tract Tachycardias, in Huang S K S, Miller J (Eds). Catheter Ablation of Cardiac Arrhythmia. 4th Edition. (2020), pp 440–466.
4. Iwai S, Jacobson J. Evaluation and Management of Wide QRS Complex Tachycardia, in Camm A J, Lucscher T F, Maurer G, Serruys P W (Eds). ESC Textbook of Cardiovascular Medicine. 3rd Edition. (2019), pp 2256–2259.
5. Buxton A E. Classification and Treatment of NSVT, in Camm A J, Lucscher T F, MaurerG, Serruys P W (Eds). ESC Textbook of Cardiovascular Medicine. 3rd Edition. (2019), pp 2259–2265.

25 Preoperative, Perioperative and CCU Care in Primary Electrical Disorders of the Heart

Madhav Krishna Kumar Nair, Arshad Jahangir, and Praloy Chakraborty

1. What are the primary electrical disorders of the heart?

Primary electrical disorders of the heart result from isolated dysfunction of cardiac ion channels without any demonstrable pathology of the myocardium or heart valve (1). The ion channel dysfunction is usually familial, and patients present with brady arrhythmias or tachyarrhythmias. A significant percentage of unexplained sudden cardiac death (SCD) in the young and otherwise healthy population is contributed by these disorders (1, 2). Congenital long QT interval syndrome (LQTS) and Brugada syndrome (BrS) are the most common primary electrical cardiac disorders, reported to be present in 1 in 2,500 live births for LQTS and 1 in 5,000 to 1 in 2,000 for BrS. Other conditions include catecholaminergic polymorphic ventricular tachycardia (CPVT), idiopathic ventricular fibrillation (IVF), early repolarization syndrome (ERS), short QT syndrome (SQTS), familial sick sinus syndrome and familial atrial fibrillation (AF). Except for familial sick sinus syndrome and familial AF, all other disorders could present as a life-threatening ventricular arrhythmia that predisposes to syncope, cardiac arrest or SCD (1, 2).

2. How are these disorders diagnosed?

Patients may remain asymptomatic for a long time or present with a spectrum of symptoms, from palpitations or lightheadedness to syncope or malignant arrhythmia and cardiac arrest. A family history of sudden death is suggestive. The diagnostic pattern in a 12-lead ECG is often confirmatory. In the absence of diagnostic ECG patterns, exercise ECG and drug provocation tests may unmask the diagnosis. Imaging studies (echocardiography, cardiac MRI and cardiac CT) can be used to rule out valvopathy (arrhythmogenic mitral valve prolapse), subclinical cardiomyopathy or coronary artery origin anomaly as the possible arrhythmogenic substrate in the young presenting with syncope or cardiac arrest.

3. How do you describe the pathogenesis of LQTS and BrS?

LQTS comprises a heterogeneous group of disorders, characterized by prolonged ventricular repolarization (QT interval) in the structurally normal heart with a high risk of malignant ventricular arrhythmias. The key electrical pathophysiology in both LQTS and BrS is abnormal ventricular repolarization. The normal action potential configuration of ventricular myocardium is described in **Figure 25.1**. The rapid upstroke, or phase 0, is due to activation of a fast sodium current (I_{Na}). Rapid inactivation of the Na^+ current along with temporary activation of the repolarization current (transient outward current, or I_{to}) is associated with transient rapid repolarization, or phase 1 of the action potential. The plateau phase, or phase 2 of the action potential, results from a balanced activity between depolarizing I_{Na} (slow Na^+ current) and Ca^{2+} current (I_{Ca}) and repolarizing K^+ currents (I_{Kr} and I_{Ks}). Inactivation of the depolarizing current with unopposed activation of repolarizing potassium currents leads to a rapid repolarization, or phase 3 of the action potential, until the resting membrane potential (RMP), or phase 4 action potential, is achieved. The QT interval in the ECG correlates with the overall action potential duration (APD). As described in **Figure 25.1**, prolongation of the APD and QT interval can occur due to potentiation of the depolarizing current (I_{Na} or I_{Ca}) or reduction of the repolarization current (I_K) (**Figure 25.1** and **Figure 25.2**). With APD prolongation or a delay in repolarization, predisposition to early after-depolarization (EAD) increases that can result in an early coupled premature ventricular complex (PVC), which under conditions of increased heterogeneity of myocardial refractoriness can initiate polymorphic ventricular tachycardia (torsades de pointes [TdP]) (3). The accentuation of the transmural dispersion of APD in LQTS may manifest on ECG as an increased T_{peak} to T_{end} interval and T-wave alternans (TWA) with beat-to-beat alternation of cellular repolarization, a marker for a high risk of SCD (4, 5). The heterogeneity of cardiac repolarization forms a substrate for functional re-entry manifesting as polymorphic ventricular tachycardia (VT) that can degenerate into ventricular fibrillation (VF) (4, 5). Loss-of-function mutations in I_K channel genes or gain-of-function mutations in I_{Na} or I_{Ca} channel genes are associated with congenital LQTS.

BrS results from a disbalance of action potential (AP) configuration within the myocardial layers, with accentuated repolarization of the epicardial surface of the right ventricular outflow

DOI: 10.1201/9781003027584-25

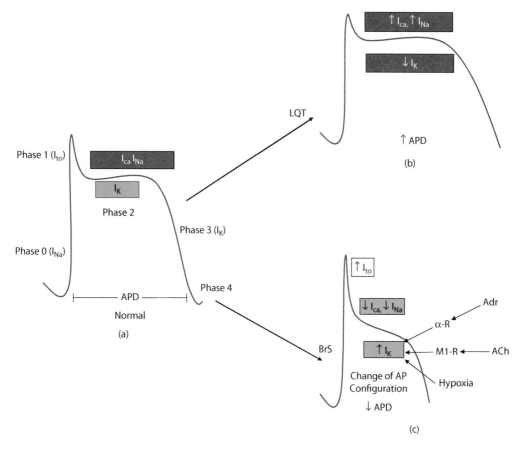

Figure 25.1 Action potential configuration of ventricular myocardium. (a) Normal myocytes, (b) LQTS and (c) BrS.

Note: I_{Ca} and I_{Na} cause prolongation *(red bar)* and I_K causes shortening *(green bar)* of Phase 2 (plateau phase) and APD.

Decreased activity of I_K ($\downarrow I_K$) or increased activity of I_{Na} ($\uparrow I_{Na}$) or I_{Ca} ($\downarrow I_{Ca}$) is associated with APD prolongation ($\uparrow$APD) in LQTS.

Increased activity of I_{to} ($\uparrow I_{to}$) along with the increased activity of I_K ($\uparrow$IK by ACh or ischaemia) or decreased activity of I_{Na} ($\downarrow I_{Na}$ by sodium channel antagonists or hyperthermia) or I_{Ca} ($\downarrow I_{Ca}$ by α-adrenergic agonists, CCB or ACh) is associated with loss of the dome and shortening of APD ($\downarrow$APD) in BrS.

Abbreviations: ACh: Acetylcholine, APD: Action potential duration, BrS: Brugada syndrome, CCB: Calcium channel antagonists, LQTS: Long QT syndrome, I_{Ca}: Calcium current (entry of Ca^{2+} ion), I_{Na}: Sodium current (entry of Na^+ ion), I_K: Potassium current (exit of K^+ ion), I_{to}: Transient outward current, M1-R: Muscarinic receptor 1.

tract (RVOT). The characteristic abnormalities include the accentuation of the phase 1 notch and the loss of phase 2 (dome of the AP) in the epicardial layers without significant change in the endocardium or mid-myocardium, thus creating a potential transmural gradient with a variable change in APD (6, 7). This characteristic abnormality can be precipitated by activation of I_{to} (with higher expression in the epicardium) along with decreased I_{Na} or I_{Ca} or accentuation of the I_K current (**Figure 25.1**). The change in AP configuration on the epicardium with the normal configuration in the endocardium leads to a transmural electrical gradient that produces the characteristic ST elevation pattern localized to the right precordial ECG leads (**Figure 25.2**). The same repolarization heterogeneity is responsible for phase 2 re-entry that can trigger malignant ventricular arrhythmia. Despite the recognition of >20 genes associated with BrS in different families, only the *SCN5A* gene coding for the sodium channel (INa) was found to have a definite causal association with BrS in a systematic, evidence-based evaluation (8).

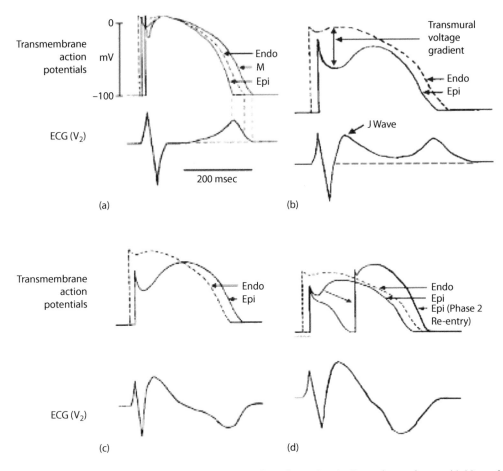

Figure 25.2 Progressive changes of action potential configuration in Brugada syndrome. (a) Normal – Despite the presence of mild accentuated Phase 1 notch in the RVOT epicardium, the ST segment is isoelectric due to the absence of a voltage gradient in Phase 2. The mild transmural voltage gradient in Phase 3 (epicardial repolarization is shorter than the endocardial and mid-myocardial repolarization) is responsible for an upright T wave. (b) Pathological accentuation of phase 1 notch and development of a transmural voltage gradient are responsible for ST-segment elevation. An abbreviated APD in the epicardium compared to the endocardium is responsible for the upright T wave. (c) Further accentuation of the phase 1 notch is associated with prolongation of the epicardial APD. Reversal of the voltage gradient (epicardial voltage is higher than endocardial voltage) during late repolarization is responsible for inversion of the T wave along with ST elevation (Type 1 Brugada pattern). (d) Initiation of fresh AP in the area of the epicardium with abbreviated APD, when the rest of the myocardium is still in the repolarization phase from the previous AP leads to the formation of early coupled PVC, the trigger for arrhythmia. The change in AP configuration in the epicardium is not spatially uniform (Epi 1 versus Epi 2). The transmural and epicardial heterogeneity in repolarization creates a substrate for functional re-entry and VF. *Abbreviations*: AP: Action potential, Endo: Endocardial, Epi: Epicardial, M: Mid-myocardial, RVOT: Right ventricular outflow tract. (With permission from Antzelevitch C. The Brugada syndrome: ionic basis and arrhythmia mechanisms. *J Cardiovasc Electrophysiol*. 2001;12(2):268–272).

4. How is long QT diagnosed?

Patients may present with symptoms like lightheaded spells, syncope, seizure-like episodes, cardiac arrest or polymorphic VT (9, 10). In 10%–15% of patients with LQTS, SCD could be the initial presentation. Some asymptomatic patients may be diagnosed incidentally during routine 12-lead ECG, rhythm monitoring or on family screening (9). Prolongation of the QT interval corrected for the heart rate (QTc) beyond 500 ms (480 ms with symptoms), in the absence of provocable factors (hypokalaemia, hypomagnesemia or QT-prolonging drugs) suggests a diagnosis of LQTS (**Figure 25.3a**). Usually, QTc >450 ms in males and >460 ms in females is considered a long QT (11). A clinical scoring system based on ECG findings, clinical history and family history has been

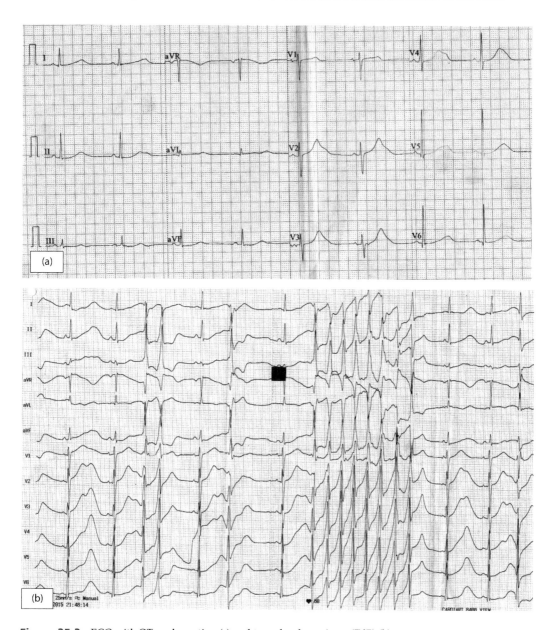

Figure 25.3 ECG with QT prolongation (a) and torsades des pointes (TdP) (b).

developed by Schwartz et al. (9). A score of ≥3.5 on the Schwartz scoring system (**Table 25.1**) suggests a high probability of LQTS (9). Secondary causes of QT_C prolongation, however, should be excluded before considering a diagnosis of congenital LQTS. LQTS types 1–3 account for the majority of genetically confirmed disease, despite 17 genes reported in different families being associated with the autosomal dominant form of this disorder, which is not associated with any congenital hearing abnormality, previously referred to as Romano-Ward syndrome (12, 13). QT prolongation associated with congenital neural deafness is seen in families with the autosomal recessive form of the disease, referred to as Jervel Lange-Nielsen syndrome, which is associated with excessive prolongation of the QT interval and high risk of sudden death at a young age in children born to parents, each carrying a mutation that may or may not manifest as prolonged QT (14). No causative mutation is identified in 20% of patients undergoing genetic testing with the LQTS phenotype (12). Mutations in LQTS are found to modify the repolarization phase of the ventricular myocardial AP (9, 15). Loss of function of potassium channels (I_{Ks} channel in

Table 25.1: Schwartz Score for Diagnosis of Long QT Syndrome

Features		Points
QTc (ms)	≥480	3
	460–479	2
	450–459	1
	QTc fourth minute of recovery from exercise stress ≥480 ms	1
Torsades de pointes		2
T-wave alternans		1
Notched T wave in three leads		1
Low heart rate for age		0.5
Syncope	With stress	2
	Without stress	1
Congenital deafness		0.5
Family history	Family member with definite LQTS	1
	Unexplained sudden cardiac death aged <30 yr among intermediate family members	0.5

LQTS1 and I_{kr} channel in LQTS2) or gain of function of the sodium current (*SCN5A* in LQTS3) are associated with QT prolongation with characteristic T-wave morphology described for the three LQTS subtypes. Up to 25% of individuals may carry pathogenic mutations for LQTS with normal QTc on resting ECG, referred to as concealed LQTS (16). QT prolongation in this group can be unmasked during the early recovery phase of the graded exercise stress test (17). The isoprenaline or epinephrine challenge test can also be used for provocation of QT prolongation in this group that can help differentiate LQTS1 due to a loss-of-function mutation in the gene coding for I_{ks} (paradoxical prolongation of QT with increased heart rate) from LQTS2 (loss of function in I_{kr}) or LQTS3 (gain of function in I_{Na}) that usually exhibits normal shortening of the QT interval with exercise or epinephrine.

5. What are the precipitating factors for arrhythmias in LQTS?

Although primary dysfunction of ion channels leads to congenital LQTS, a host of medications can cause or potentiate QTc prolongation by inhibition of the K⁺ current. Serum electrolytes can also affect the repolarization, and QT prolongation is also precipitated by hypokalaemia, hypocalcaemia and hypomagnesemia. Hypothermia can prolong repolarization duration and potentiate transmural heterogeneity. A sympathetic surge may trigger TdP by β1 adrenergic stimulation, more commonly seen with LQTS1 with a loss-of-function mutation of I_{ks}. Sudden auditory stimuli or startling precipitates TdP in LQTS2, while arrhythmic events during sleep or rest are more common in LQTS3. Postpartum arrhythmic events are more common in women with LQTS2.

6. How is Brugada syndrome diagnosed?

Brugada syndrome (BrS) is diagnosed by characteristic ST-segment elevation in ECG, localized to the right precordial leads (V1–V3) (7). Depending on the severity of electrical heterogeneity, the ST elevation may exhibit different patterns, classified as type 1 (pathognomonic of BrS) or type 2 (suggestive of BrS) (**Figure 25.2**) (18). Due to anatomical proximity with the right ventricle, especially the right ventricular outflow tract (RVOT), the ECG changes are localized in the right-sided lead (V1–V3) and placed in the standard or superior position (up to the second intercostal space) (18). The type 1 Brugada pattern is characterized by concave or straight ST-segment elevation ≥2 mm, followed by a negative and symmetric T wave (**Figure 25.4a**). The type 2 Brugada pattern, or "saddleback type" ST elevation, is characterized by convex ST-segment elevation of ≥0.5 mm (generally ≥2 mm in V2) (**Figure 25.4b**). Current guidelines recommend a diagnosis of BrS by the presence of a type 1 Brugada pattern in any one of the right-sided leads, standard or superior position (19). Even a transient type 1 Brugada pattern during fever or provocation by sodium channel blocker (procainamide, ajmaline or flecainide) is diagnostic of BrS (19).

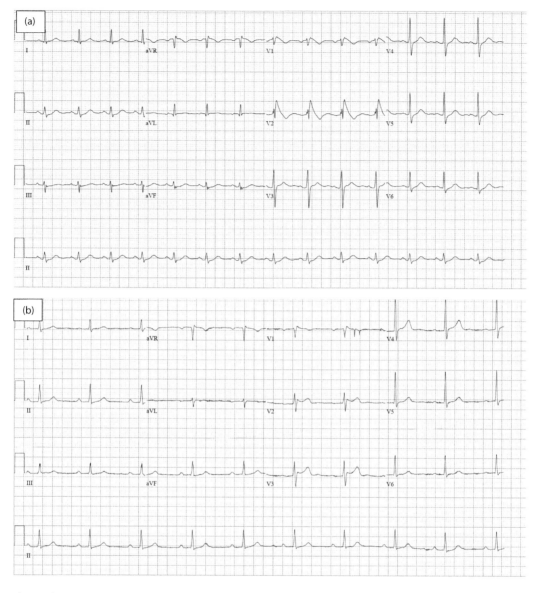

Figure 25.4 Electrocardiographic patterns in Brugada syndrome. (a) Type 1 Brugada electrocardiogram pattern showing a concave ST-segment elevation ≥2 mm followed by a negative T wave. (b) Type 2 Brugada electrocardiogram pattern showing a convex ST-segment elevation followed by a positive T wave.

7. What are the precipitating factors of arrhythmias in BrS?

Loss of the AP dome pattern and shortening of the APD in the epicardium are associated with accentuation of ST elevation and risk of arrhythmia precipitation in BrS patients. Reduction of the depolarizing current (I_{Na} or I_{Ca}) or increase in the repolarizing current (I_K) are associated with a change in AP configuration (**Figure 25.1**), leading to a type 1 Brugada pattern in the ECG.

The precipitating factors include (7, 20–22):

1. Na$^+$ channel blockers and an increase in core temperature by Na$^+$ channel dysfunction.

2. Acetylcholine (ACh) via M1 receptor stimulation and L-type Ca^{2+} channel blocker by inhibition of $I_{Ca.}$

3. α-Adrenergic receptor stimulation by increasing intracellular Ca^{2+} and promoting the repolarizing current.

4. Potentiation of I_K by ACh (activation of I_{KAch}) and ischaemia (activation of I_{KATP}).

5. Dyselectrolytemia (hypokalaemia, hyperkalaemia, hypercalcaemia) can potentiate the repolarization heterogeneity in BrS patients.

6. Parasympathetic stimulation is arrhythmogenic in BrS due to the effect of ACh through the M1 receptor.

7. Glucose-insulin infusion.

8. Why is the risk of arrhythmia higher during the perioperative period?

In a cohort of 429 patients with a normal QT interval, significant perioperative QT prolongation was demonstrated in 80% of patients (23). In a small cohort of BrS patients, ST elevation was associated with the anaesthesia use (24). Life-threatening arrhythmias and sudden death are reported in patients with unremarkable medical history during anaesthesia and the perioperative period (25). However, the perioperative adverse events in patients with channelopathies are not systematically studied and are described in case-based reports. Physiological changes in the perioperative period frequently exaggerate the electrophysiological heterogeneity of the ventricle and predispose to malignant ventricular arrhythmias. The perioperative factors include (15, 16, 26–28):

1. Electrolyte imbalance

   a. Hypokalaemia, hypocalcaemia and hypomagnesemia can prolong APD and precipitate EADs and TdP in LQTS.

   b. Hypokalaemia, hypercalcaemia, hyperkalaemia and hyponatraemia can precipitate a type 1 Brugada pattern and VF.

2. Changes in body temperature

   a. QT prolongation and TdP are associated with hypothermia.

   b. Arrhythmia in BrS is precipitated by an increase in body temperature.

3. Autonomic tone

   a. EADs and TdP are associated with sympathetic stimulation in LQTS patients.

   b. ST elevation and VT in BrS patients can be precipitated by an increase in parasympathetic activity

4. Medications

   a. Potassium channel blockers prolong the QT interval, and sympathomimetic agents promote EADs and are torsadogenic in LQTS.

   b. Sodium channel blockers and parasympathomimetic agents may be arrhythmogenic in BrS.

9. What are the objectives of the preoperative evaluation in channelopathy patients?

The objectives of the preoperative evaluation of channelopathy patients include:

1. Identification of previously undiagnosed patients from family history or 12-lead ECG

2. Identification of high-risk patients with LQTS or BrS

3. Identification of high-risk steps during anaesthesia and surgery (medications, autonomic tone)

4. Identification of medications related to precipitation of phenotype and triggers for arrhythmia:

   a. *For LQT drugs*: https://www.crediblemeds.org/

   b. *For Brugada drugs*: https://www.brugadadrugs.org/

5. Assessment of serum electrolytes

6. Plan for anaesthesia

7. Strategy for ICD/pacemaker adjustment

8. Postoperative monitoring of rhythm, electrolytes, endogenous catecholamines and cholinergic influences, hypoxemia (sleep apnoea), temperature and medications

10. How do you identify high-risk patients?

High-risk features of LQTS (29, 30) and BrS (7, 12, 18) are described in **Table 25.2**.

Table 25.2: Comparison between Long QT Syndrome and Brugada Syndrome high risk patients

LQTS	BrS
1. Baseline QTc ≥500 ms 2. Adult female (in childhood, the risk is higher in males in LQT1) 3. Prior syncope, cardiac arrest or documented spontaneous torsades 4. Genotype: Highest risk in LQT3 followed by LQT2 and minimum with LQT1 5. Presence of T-wave alternans 6. C-loop mutation of *KCNQ1* (LQT1) and pore-loop mutation in *KCNH2* (LQT2)	1. Spontaneous type 1 ECG pattern 2. Male sex 3. Combination of *SCN5A* mutation and family history of premature sudden cardiac arrest 4. Syncopal episodes 5. Nocturnal agonal respiration 6. Previous ventricular tachycardia/ventricular fibrillation 7. AF or sinus node dysfunction 8. Prolonged QRS (QRS duration in V2 ≥120 ms, V6 ≥90 ms, deep S wave in lateral leads, R wave in aVR ≥0.3 mv, R/q ≥0.75 in aVR) 9. Fragmented QRS complex 10. Repolarization abnormalities like QTc in V2 ≥460 ms, presence of T-wave alternans, prolongation of T-peak–T-end interval or augmentation of ST elevation during recovery phase of exercise test 11. Ventricular refractory period <200 ms (identified at invasive electrophysiology study) 12. Early repolarization pattern in inferolateral leads

---

11. What are the high-risk steps in anaesthesia/surgery?

Anaesthesia/surgical steps that are associated with parasympathetic stimulations or change in body temperature are high risk for BrS patients (26, 28):

1. Deep anaesthesia

2. Pneumoperitoneum

3. Bowel handling

4. Neck surgery

5. Hyperthermia

Anaesthesia/surgical steps that are associated with sympathetic stimulations or changes in body temperature are high risk in LQTS (15, 16):

1. During intubation

2. Hypoxia or hypercarbia

3. Inadequate anaesthesia

4. Valsalva manoeuvre

5. Raised intrathoracic pressure

6. Recovery from anaesthesia

7. Perioperative and postoperative pain

8. Intracranial events

9. Hypothermia

12. How do you manage cardiovascular implantable electronic devices (CIEDs) during surgery?

A significant number of patients with cardiac channelopathy receive an implantable cardiac defibrillator (ICD) or pacemaker. Electrocautery during a surgical procedure may be associated with electromagnetic interference (EMI), leading to malfunction of the ICD or pacemaker. To protect the CIEDs from EMI, the following steps should be followed (16, 26):

1. ICD therapy should be disabled during the procedure.

2. If the patient is pacemaker dependent, the pacemaker should be kept in asynchronous mode (DOO/VOO).

3. In patients with a risk of brady-dependent torsades (i.e., in LQTS3 or drug-induced torsades), the pacing rate should be kept high (90–110 bpm).

4. If the programmer for the CIED is not available, placement of a magnet over the CIED will disable the ICD (preventing inappropriate therapies) and put the pacemaker in asynchronous mode (continuous pacing) in pacemaker-dependent patients.

13. How should these patients be monitored during the perioperative period?

The following precautions should be taken in the operating room (15, 16, 26, 28):

1. Continuous ECG monitoring, preferably 12 lead

2. Placement of external defibrillation/pacing pads

3. Intra-atrial blood pressure monitoring

4. Monitoring of oxygen saturation (SpO$_2$) and carbon dioxide tension (TCO$_2$)

5. Monitoring of depth of anaesthesia by bispectral index

6. Protection from hypothermia or hyperthermia and maintenance of body temperature around 37°C

7. Monitoring the degree of neuromuscular block

8. Avoidance of cholinergic medications for BrS patients and sympathomimetics in LQTS patients

14. Which perioperative medications are torsadogenic in LQT patients?

Perioperative medications include preanesthetic medications, vasoactive agents, vasodilators, intravenous anaesthetics, volatile anaesthetics, neuromuscular blocking agents, reversal agents, anticholinergic agents and pain medications. Potential torsadogenic mechanisms of these agents include QT prolongation, generation of EADs (calcium loading) and/r adrenergic stimulation (**Table 25.3**).

Table 25.3: Perioperative Drugs and Their Torsadogenic Significance in Relation to LQTS

Medication Category	Name of Medication	Mechanism
α-2-adrenergic agonists	Dexmedetomidine	QTc prolongation in children
Analgesics	Methadone	QTc prolongation
	Sufentanil	QTc prolongation
	Ketamine	Sympathetic stimulation
Antiemetics	Droperidol	QTc prolongation
	Domperidone	QTc prolongation
	5-HT3 receptor antagonists	QTc prolongation
Vasoactive agents	Adrenaline, noradrenaline (norepinephrine), isoprenaline, ephedrine	QTc prolongation
IV Anaesthesia	Etomidate	QTc prolongation
Volatile anaesthetics	All halogenated agents	QTc prolongation
	Nitric oxide (NO)	Sympathetic stimulation
Neuromuscular blocking agent	Succinylcholine	QTc prolongation
	Pancuronium	QTc prolongation
Anticholinergic	Glycopyrrolate and Atropine	QTc prolongation
Local anaesthesia	Mixing with epinephrine	QTc prolongation

15. Which perioperative medications are safe in LQTS patients?

The perioperative medications which can be used safely in patients with LQTS are listed in **Table 25.4**.

Table 25.4: Safe Drugs in Relation to LQTS

Medication Category	Name of Medication	Comments
α-2 adrenergic agonists	Clonidine	Can be used to treat pressor response during intubation
Analgesics	Fentanyl, buprenorphine, IV lidocaine	
Antiemetics	Phenothiazines and dexamethasone	
Vasoactive agents	Metaraminol, phenylephrine	
IV anaesthesia	Midazolam, propofol, thiopental	Thiopental increases QTc but reduces dispersion, propofol is associated with QTc reduction
Volatile anaesthetics	Isoflurane	Although all halogenated anaesthetics can prolong QT, the safety of isoflurane is documented in several case reports
Neuromuscular blocking agents	All except succinylcholine and pancuronium	
Reversal agent	Sugammadex	
Local anaesthesia	Long-acting agents like bupivacaine, levobupivacaine and ropivacaine	

16. Which perioperative medications can provoke the Brugada ECG pattern?

The use of some perioperative medications may exaggerate the ST elevation in patients with BrS. The potential mechanisms include inhibition of I_{Na}, I_{Ca}, α-adrenergic stimulation or parasympathetic stimulation. The agents are listed in **Table 25.5**.

Table 25.5: Precipitators of Arrhythmia in Brugada Syndrome

Medication Category	Name of Medication	Mechanism
α-2 adrenergic agonists	Clonidine, dexmedetomidine	α-adrenergic stimulation, parasympathetic stimulation
Analgesics	Tramadol	Na+ channel block
Antiemetics	Metoclopramide, dimenhydrinate and phenothiazines	Na+ channel block
Blood sugar control	Glucose-insulin infusion	—
Vasoactive agents	Norepinephrine, methoxamine, phenylephrine	α-Adrenergic stimulation
Vasodilators	Calcium channel blockers, nitrates	Inhibition of L-type calcium current
IV anaesthesia	Propofol	
Volatile anaesthetics	Halogenated anaesthetics	No effect on Brugada ECG pattern but affects QTc
Reversal agents	Cholinesterase inhibitors	Parasympathetic stimulation
Local anaesthesia	Long-acting agents like bupivacaine, levobupivacaine and ropivacaine	Na+ channel block
Surface anaesthesia	Cocaine	Na+ channel block

17. Which perioperative medications are safe in patients with BrS?

The perioperative medications that can be used safely in patients with LQTS are listed in **Table 25.6**.

Table 25.6 Safe Drugs in Brugada Syndrome

Medication Category	Name of Medication	Comments
Analgesics	All except tramadol	–
Antiemetics	Droperidol and 5-HT3 receptor antagonists	–
Vasoactive agents	Dobutamine and ephedrine	–
IV anaesthesia	Thiopental, midazolam and low-dose propofol for short duration	Thiopental increases QTc but reduces dispersion, propofol is associated with QTc reduction
Volatile anaesthetics	NO, sevoflurane	–
Neuromuscular blocking agents	All agents	–
Reversal agent	Sugammadex, combination of cholinesterase inhibitors and muscarinic receptor antagonist	–
Local anaesthesia	Mixing with epinephrine	–

18. What is propofol infusion syndrome (PRIS)?

Long-duration administration of high-dose propofol is associated with PRIS in some patients (26). PRIS is characterized by metabolic acidosis and cardiac dysfunction, along with at least one of the following: Rhabdomyolysis, hypertriglyceridemia or renal failure. Cardiac manifestations include wide QRS complex, Brugada type 1 ECG pattern, ventricular tachyarrhythmias, cardiogenic shock and asystole. Reduction of the Na^+ and Ca^{2+} currents along with autonomic imbalance (β-adrenergic inhibition and cholinergic stimulation) by propofol may contribute to myocardial dysfunction (26).

Administration of propofol is reported to be associated with significant ST elevation in patients with BrS (**Figure 25.5**) (31). Use of high dose (>4 mg/kg/hr) and long-duration (≥48 hr) propofol

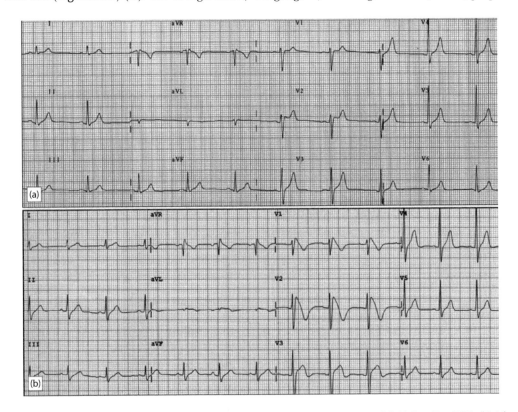

Figure 25.5 ECG showing provocation of the Type 1 Brugada pattern by propofol. (a) Baseline ECG. (b) After long-term administration of high doses of intravenous propofol. (With permission from Dendramis G et al. Anesthetic and perioperative management of patients with Brugada syndrome. *Am J Cardiol.* 2017;120:1031–1036.)

should be avoided in BrS patients, especially those with high-risk features (**Table 25.2**). If propofol needs to be used in high doses for a long duration for this population, arterial blood gas, serum lactate and creatine kinase should be monitored frequently (32).

19. What precautions are needed during the perioperative period for LQTS patients?

The following precautions should be followed during the perioperative period in patients with suspected or confirmed LQTS (4, 15, 16, 33):

1. Continue β-adrenergic antagonists.

2. Avoid provoking agents.

3. Liberal use of sedatives and analgesics (reduce endogenous catecholamines).

4. Lidocaine (1.5 mg/kg) can be used intravenously during induction in high-risk LQTS.

5. Pressor response during intubation can be treated with alfentanil, esmolol, clonidine or topical lidocaine.

6. Intra-operative hypoxia, hypercarbia and dyselectrolytemia should be avoided. Hypoxia and hypercarbia may lead to sympathetic stimulation. Serum K^+ should be more than 4.5 mmol/L and Mg^{2+} should be more than 2.0 mg/dL.

7. A quiet operating room.

8. Avoid hypothermia and maintain temperature around 37°C.

9. Recovery from anaesthesia should be managed with adequate beta-blockade.

10. Liberal pain medications for postoperative pain control.

20. What precautions are needed during the perioperative period for BrS patients?

The following precautions should be followed during the perioperative period in patients with suspected or confirmed BrS (18, 28):

1. Avoid the routine use of prophylactic β-adrenergic antagonists.

2. Avoid provoking agents.

3. Close monitoring of intra-operative acid-base and electrolyte balance.

4. Depth of anaesthesia should be monitored closely – very deep anaesthesia is associated with vagal stimulation and accentuation of ST elevation.

5. Avoid hyperthermia and maintain the temperature around 37°C.

6. Avoid unintentional parasympathetic stimulation.

21. How do you manage intra-operative TdP?

The TdP in LQTSs is usually recurrent, ill sustained and associated with haemodynamic deterioration. The treatment of choice for sustained TdP is defibrillation. The drug of choice for TdP is intravenous magnesium sulphate (IV $MgSO_4$) (34). Irrespective of serum level, $MgSO_4$ should be administered as an IV bolus (30 mg/kg) followed by infusion of 2–4 mg/kg (4, 35). The bolus dose can be repeated every 15 min. Magnesium infusion does not affect the QT interval but prevents TdP by reducing the repolarization heterogeneity. Intravenous lidocaine may also be used; however, amiodarone or drugs with potassium channel–blocking properties should be avoided. In drug induced TdP with acquired QT prolongation, isoproterenol or dobutamine can be used to increase the heart rate and helps shorten repolarization. Overdrive pacing through a temporary or permanent pacemaker can be used to increase the ventricular rate (90–110 bpm) in bradycardia-dependent TdP (4, 15, 16).

22. How do you manage intra-operative electrical storms in BrS?

Unlike in LQTS, VF in BrS is sustained and requires electrical defibrillation. For VF storm, defined as more than two episodes of VT or VF in 24 hr, isoprenaline is the treatment of choice to reverse ST-segment elevation and suppress arrhythmic storms (26, 28, 36). The starting dose of intravenous isoprenaline infusion is 0.003 µg/kg/min. Dose titration to increase the heart rate by 20% of the baseline is usually successful in suppressing arrhythmia. Supportive management includes aggressive management of pyrexia, optimization of fluid-electrolyte balance and discontinuation of provocative agents. Quinidine is an alternative for IV and oral use. Bepridil and cilostazol are other second-line oral agents. In refractory cases, identification and ablation of the arrhythmogenic substrates on the RVOT and right ventricular (RV) anterior wall could eliminate VF storm (18).

REFERENCES

1. Kaufman ES. Mechanisms and clinical management of inherited channelopathies: Long QT syndrome, Brugada syndrome, catecholaminergic polymorphic ventricular tachycardia, and short QT syndrome. Heart Rhythm. 2009;6(8 Suppl):S51–5.
2. Blayney LM, Lai FA. Ryanodine receptor-mediated arrhythmias and sudden cardiac death. Pharmacol Ther. 2009;123(2):151–77.
3. Weiss JN, Garfinkel A, Karagueuzian HS, Chen PS, Qu Z. Early afterdepolarizations and cardiac arrhythmias. Heart Rhythm. 2010;7(12):1891–9.
4. Booker PD, Whyte SD, Ladusans EJ. Long QT syndrome and anaesthesia. Br J Anaesth. 2003;90(3):349–66.
5. Whyte SD, Nathan A, Myers D, Watkins SC, Kannankeril PJ, Etheridge SP, et al. The safety of modern anesthesia for children with long QT syndrome. Anesth Analg. 2014;119(4):932–8.
6. Antzelevitch C. The Brugada syndrome: Ionic basis and arrhythmia mechanisms. J Cardiovasc Electrophysiol. 2001;12(2):268–72.
7. Antzelevitch C, Patocskai B. Brugada syndrome: Clinical, genetic, molecular, cellular, and ionic aspects. Curr Probl Cardiol. 2016;41(1):7–57.
8. Hosseini SM, Kim R, Udupa S, Costain G, Jobling R, Liston E, et al. Reappraisal of reported genes for sudden arrhythmic death: Evidence-based evaluation of gene validity for Brugada syndrome. Circulation. 2018;138(12):1195–205.
9. Schwartz PJ, Crotti L, Insolia R. Long-QT syndrome: From genetics to management. Circ Arrhythm Electrophysiol. 2012;5(4):868–77.
10. Shah SR, Park K, Alweis R. Long QT syndrome: A comprehensive review of the literature and current evidence. Curr Probl Cardiol. 2019;44(3):92–106.
11. Schwartz PJ, Stramba-Badiale M, Crotti L, Pedrazzini M, Besana A, Bosi G, et al. Prevalence of the congenital long-QT syndrome. Circulation. 2009;120(18):1761–7.
12. Priori SG, Wilde AA, Horie M, Cho Y, Behr ER, Berul C, et al. HRS/EHRA/APHRS expert consensus statement on the diagnosis and management of patients with inherited primary arrhythmia syndromes: Document endorsed by HRS, EHRA, and APHRS in May 2013 and by ACCF, AHA, PACES, and AEPC in June 2013. Heart Rhythm. 2013;10(12):1932–63.
13. Nakano Y, Shimizu W. Genetics of long-QT syndrome. J Hum Genet. 2016;61(1):51–5.
14. Jervell A, Lange-Nielsen F. Congenital deaf-mutism, functional heart disease with prolongation of the Q-T interval and sudden death. Am Heart J. 1957;54(1):59–68.
15. O'Hare M, Maldonado Y, Munro J, Ackerman MJ, Ramakrishna H, Sorajja D. Perioperative management of patients with congenital or acquired disorders of the QT interval. Br J Anaesth. 2018;120(4):629–44.
16. Levy D, Bigham C, Tomlinson D. Anaesthesia for patients with hereditary arrhythmias; part 2: Congenital long QT syndrome and arrhythmogenic right ventricular cardiomyopathy. BJA Education. 2018;18.
17. Sy RW, van der Werf C, Chattha IS, Chockalingam P, Adler A, Healey JS, et al. Derivation and validation of a simple exercise-based algorithm for prediction of genetic testing in relatives of LQTS probands. Circulation. 2011;124(20):2187–94.
18. Brugada J, Campuzano O, Arbelo E, Sarquella-Brugada G, Brugada R. Present status of Brugada syndrome: JACC State-of-the-Art Review. J Am Coll Cardiol. 2018;72(9):1046–59.
19. Priori SG, Blomström-Lundqvist C. 2015 European Society of Cardiology Guidelines for the management of patients with ventricular arrhythmias and the prevention of sudden cardiac death summarized by co-chairs. Eur Heart J. 2015;36(41):2757–9.
20. Litovsky SH, Antzelevitch C. Differences in the electrophysiological response of canine ventricular subendocardium and subepicardium to acetylcholine and isoproterenol. A direct effect of acetylcholine in ventricular myocardium. Circ Res. 1990;67(3):615–27.
21. Miyazaki T, Mitamura H, Miyoshi S, Soejima K, Aizawa Y, Ogawa S. Autonomic and antiarrhythmic drug modulation of ST segment elevation in patients with Brugada syndrome. J Am Coll Cardiol. 1996;27(5):1061–70.
22. Nogami A, Nakao M, Kubota S, Sugiyasu A, Doi H, Yokoyama K, et al. Enhancement of J-ST-segment elevation by the glucose and insulin test in Brugada syndrome. Pacing Clin Electrophysiol. 2003;26(1p2):332–7.
23. Nagele P, Pal S, Brown F, Blood J, Miller JP, Johnston J. Postoperative QT interval prolongation in patients undergoing noncardiac surgery under general anesthesia. Anesthesiology. 2012;117(2):321–8.
24. Kloesel B, Ackerman MJ, Sprung J, Narr BJ, Weingarten TN. Anesthetic management of patients with Brugada syndrome: A case series and literature review. Can J Anaesth. 2011;58(9):824–36.
25. Tabib A, Loire R, Miras A, Thivolet-Bejui F, Timour Q, Bui-Xuan B, et al. Unsuspected cardiac lesions associated with sudden unexpected perioperative death. Eur J Anaesthesiol. 2000;17(4):230–5.
26. Dendramis G, Paleologo C, Sgarito G, Giordano U, Verlato R, Baranchuk A, et al. Anesthetic and perioperative management of patients with Brugada syndrome. Am J Cardiol. 2017;120(6):1031–6.
27. Sorajja D, Ramakrishna H, Poterack AK, Shen WK, Mookadam F. Brugada syndrome and its relevance in the perioperative period. Ann Card Anaesth. 2015;18(3):403–13.
28. Levy D, Bigham C, Tomlinson D. Anaesthesia for patients with hereditary arrhythmias part I: Brugada syndrome. BJA Education. 2018;18(6):159–65.
29. Barsheshet A, Dotsenko O, Goldenberg I. Genotype-specific risk stratification and management of long QT syndrome. Ann Noninvasive Electrocardiol. 2013;18(6):499–509.
30. Priori SG, Schwartz PJ, Napolitano C, Bloise R, Ronchetti E, Grillo M, et al. Risk stratification in the long-QT syndrome. N Engl J Med. 2003;348(19):1866–74.

31. Inamura M, Okamoto H, Kuroiwa M, Hoka S. General anesthesia for patients with Brugada syndrome. A report of six cases. Can J Anaesth. 2005;52(4):409–12.
32. Flamée P, De Asmundis C, Bhutia JT, Conte G, Beckers S, Umbrain V, et al. Safe single-dose administration of propofol in patients with established Brugada syndrome: A retrospective database analysis. Pacing Clin Electrophysiol. 2013;36(12):1516–21.
33. Owczuk R, Wujtewicz MA, Sawicka W, Piankowski A, Polak-Krzeminska A, Morzuch E, et al. The effect of intravenous lidocaine on QT changes during tracheal intubation. Anaesthesia. 2008;63(9):924–31.
34. Khan IA. Clinical and therapeutic aspects of congenital and acquired long QT syndrome. Am J Med. 2002;112(1):58–66.
35. Staikou C, Chondrogiannis K, Mani A. Perioperative management of hereditary arrhythmogenic syndromes. Br J Anaesth. 2012;108(5):730–44.
36. Priori SG, Wilde AA, Horie M, Cho Y, Behr ER, Berul C, et al. Executive summary: HRS/EHRA/APHRS expert consensus statement on the diagnosis and management of patients with inherited primary arrhythmia syndromes. Heart Rhythm. 2013;10(12):e85–108.

26 Electrical Storm

Sunandan Sikdar and Deepak Padmanabhan

1. What is an electrical storm?

A cardiac electrical storm (ES) is characterized by three or more discrete episodes of ventricular arrhythmia within 24 hr or incessant ventricular arrhythmia for more than 12 hr. In patients with an implantable cardiac defibrillator (ICD), this condition is defined as the occurrence of three or more appropriate device therapies within a 24-hr period, separated from one another by at least 5 min.

2. What is the prognosis in ES?

ES is a medical emergency with a mortality rate of 14% in the first 48 hr with poor outcomes related to progressive heart failure and sudden death, and there is increased possibility of heart transplant. In the case of automatic implantable cardioverter defibrillator (AICD) patients, after an initial episode, a recurrent storm may occur in 50%–80% of patients over the subsequent year. ES causes sympathetic stimulation that starts a vicious cycle of further ventricular fibrillation (VF), further shocks, shock-induced left ventricular (LV) dysfunction and progressive heart failure. The risk of death is maximum in the first 3 months of ES. It is unclear whether ES has a causal role in increased mortality or is a marker of end-stage heart disease.

3. What are the reversible triggers of ES?

Acute myocardial ischaemia, electrolyte derangements (e.g., hypokalaemia), sepsis, decompensated cardiac failure, non-compliance with heart failure and/or antiarrhythmic medication, QT prolongation, hyperthyroidism, fever, infections and drug toxicity are some of the reversible triggers, though frequently they may not be found.

4. What is the mechanism of ES?

ES requires:

a. *Substrate*: Ischaemic heart disease, cardiomyopathies, LV dysfunction, channelopathies (long QT, Brugada, catecholaminergic polymorphic ventricular tachycardia [CPVT], idiopathic ventricular fibrillation [IVF]).

b. Triggers

c. Autonomic imbalance

5. What are the causes of ES?

The cause of ES has significant implications on therapy and requires early recognition. Sometimes multiple causes may be at work, e.g. ischaemia + hypokalaemia or dilated cardiomyopathy + drug-induced QT prolongation.

A. *With structural heart disease*

a. With ischaemia – acute – acute coronary syndromes, chronic – old myocardial infarction (MI)

b. Without ischaemia – acute – myocarditis, chronic – dilated cardiomyopathy, hypertrophic cardiomyopathy, arrhythmogenic right ventricular (RV) dysplasia, sarcoidosis

B. *With normal heart*

a. *Primary*: Brugada syndrome (BrS), Long QT syndrome, Short QT syndrome, IVF, CPVT

b. *Secondary*: Electrolyte abnormality, drug/toxin induced, pacing on T wave

6. What are the electrophysiological patterns of ES?

Two groups are evident:

a. *Monomorphic ventricular tachycardia (VT)*: The vast majority of ES is caused by monomorphic VT due to heterogenous scar tissue. The substrate in such cases is usually ischaemic or non-ischaemic cardiomyopathy.

b. *Polymorphic VT/VF*: Occurs in acute ischaemia, channelopathy and IVF.

DOI: 10.1201/9781003027584-26

7. What are the strategies to manage ES?

The following strategies are utilized (often escalating and using some of them simultaneously).

a. *Pharmacological therapy*: Antiarrhythmics and treating reversible causes like ischaemia or electrolytes

b. Sedation + ventilation

c. Neuraxial modulation

d. Catheter ablation

e. Device programming

f. *Circulatory support*: Intra-aortic balloon pump (IABP), extracorporeal membrane oxygenation (ECMO) or ventricular assist devices (refractory cases with shock).

8. What are pharmacological treatments for ES?

The cornerstone of therapy is beta-blockers. Amiodarone, sotalol, phenytoin and lidocaine are other important drugs. For an extended discussion about drugs, refer to the chapter on cardiac drugs.

Beta-blocker: Increased sympathetic drive, including shock-induced anxiety and hyperadrenergic state, lies at the heart of the storm. In chronic heart failure cases, there is a downregulation of beta-1 receptors, so non-specific beta-blockers like propranolol may be better in some cases. Because of its lipophilicity, its penetration of the blood-brain barrier may be an advantage to counter the centrally mediated sympathetic state. Propranolol has been shown to decrease the time to arrhythmia termination, improve the arrhythmia-free period and reduce the hospital stay compared to metoprolol when administered in addition to amiodarone. The dose of intravenous propranolol is 1–3 mg every 5 min to a total of 5 mg – however, it is seldom available or used. Though a beta-blocker forms the mainstay of therapy in congenital long QT syndrome (LQTS) and outflow tract VT, in acquired LQTS, it may worsen bradycardia-induced torsades.

Amiodarone: Universally used in ES due to structural heart disease, the drug can terminate ventricular arrhythmias in 40%–60% of cases alone. When used in conjunction with beta-blockers, the conversion rate is higher. Intravenous amiodarone has predominantly class III properties but class I, II and IV properties are also present, and it also reduces sympathetic drive. Its advantage is its lack of negative inotropic effect and less predisposition to torsades in spite of QT prolongation. Along with beta-blockers it reduces ICD shocks, but the drug unfortunately raises the defibrillation threshold. Amiodarone reduces ES frequency fourfold in 2-year follow-up. Owing to long-term multiple side effects, its use must be carefully considered in every case. The loading dose is 150 mg, then 1 mg/min in 6 hr followed by 0.5 mg/min for 18 hr.

Sotalol: In racemic form, it has both nonselective beta-blocker activity and class III actions. It reduces the defibrillation threshold. It reduced death and ICD shocks by 48%. However, its QT prolongation is a concern in ES with structural heart disease.

Lidocaine: Being a fast sodium channel blocker (class 1B) with use dependence, lidocaine works better during tachycardia, especially in ischaemic settings. Its effectivity is primarily in ischaemia, and the conversion rate may be 8%–30%. It does not cause QRS or QT prolongation, though bradycardia can occur. Often lidocaine and amiodarone have been given together, sometimes on top of a beta-blocker. The dose is 0.5 mg/kg initially, with another repeat bolus after 10 min then maintenance infusion 2 mg/min.

Mexilitine: Used orally after control of ES in the maintenance phase, this class IB drug is used when amiodarone plus a beta-blocker is unable to prevent breakthrough ICD shocks. It also finds usage in Type 3 LQTS-related ES, provided the genotype is known.

Verapamil: The injectable form may be useful in fascicular VT–related ES. Verapamil may also be useful in LQTS not responding to beta-blockers.

Magnesium: It finds a specific role in (1) correction of hypokalaemia or hypomagnesemia and (2) ES-related polymorphic VT, especially in LQTS.

9. What are the non-pharmacological treatments of ES with structural heart disease?

Catheter ablation (CA): If ES is resistant to pharmacotherapy and the substrate is *structural heart disease* without any reversible trigger, early catheter ablation is the best way forward. In ES with a *normal heart*, especially in BrS, if ES is being triggered by premature ventricular contractions (PVCs) with similar morphology (in Holter/bedside monitor/12-lead ECG), catheter ablation, especially in the right ventricular outflow tract (RVOT) region, may be tried. In the VANISH trial, catheter ablation in ES resulted in reduction of death, ES and appropriate shocks from ICD. There was a 34% reduction of ES recurrence by CA compared to antiarrhythmic drugs. Overall acute success in VT elimination occurs in 70% and reduction in VT burden occurs in a further 20%.

Neuroaxial modulation (NM): NM has a proven benefit in LQTS and CPVT. However, structural heart disease, including VT storm after MI, also responds favourably. NM involves:

a. *Thoracic epidural anaesthesia (TEA)*: This is done by percutaneous administration of a local anaesthetic into the thoracic epidural space: Injection of 1 mL of 0.25% bupivacaine followed by an infusion at 2 mL/hr, which can be uptitrated according to the arrhythmic response.

b. *Stellate ganglion block (SGB)*: SGB involves percutaneous injection of local anaesthetic into the left or both stellate ganglia. Reducing sympathetic outflow to the heart via blockade of afferent and efferent neurons, SGB achieves an immediate success of nearly 90% and gives a temporary method in stabilizing ES until permanent techniques are implemented.

c. *Cardiac sympathetic denervation (CSD)*: CSD surgically removes the lower half of the left or bilateral stellate ganglia and the T2–T4 thoracic ganglia. Bilateral CSD is better than unilateral CSD with higher survival free of ICD shocks. CSD has an important role in ES due to LQTS and CPVT and in some refractory cases of structural heart disease.

d. *Renal Sympathetic Denervation (RSD)*: The role of catheter ablation of neural plexuses around the renal adventitia to reduce sympathetic afferent traffic and thus reduce the hyperadrenergic state to treat ES is an evolving area.

Intubation and ventilation: Ventilation is often an effective way to break the vicious cycle of anxiety, hypersympathetic state and consequently more ICD shocks in ES. After ventilation and deep sedation (propofol or benzodiazepine), pharmacotherapy may become more effective.

Overdrive pacing: Using a temporary pacing wire (those who do not have an ICD) or keeping the ICD at a lower rate of 100–120/min may suppress ES triggering PVC in many cases and reduce the arrhythmia episodes. Overdrive pacing with a temporary wire is especially important in bradycardia-dependent polymorphic VT in LQTS and in some cases of drug-induced QT prolongation (until the time the drug washes away).

Revascularization: Polymorphic VT due to active ischaemia must undergo emergent cardiac catheterization and revascularization. Treatment of ischaemia can dramatically reverse an ES and must be ruled out in all cases.

IABP/ECMO: ES with haemodynamic instability with or without ischaemia not responding to pharmacotherapy is a candidate for IABP. The mechanism of benefit with IABP for improving ventricular arrhythmia may be (1) improved coronary perfusion and (2) unloading of the LV with reduction in wall stress. IABP offers the opportunity for proceeding confidently to revascularization/catheter ablation by improving haemodynamics. ExtraCorporeal Membrane Oxygenator (ECMO) or an assist device may be an option in refractory cases.

10. How do you treat ES in BrS/channelopathies?

The first step is to recognize that the aetiology of the ES is a channelopathy – specifically BrS and Idiopathic VF (BrS is channelopathy most commonly related to ES). A young male of less than 40 years with recurrent AICD shocks (**Figures 26.1** and **26.2**) or recurrent syncope with a suggestive baseline ECG (see the channelopathy chapter) with a normal heart on echocardiogram forms the classic substrate. The BrS-ES is caused by reduced inward Na and Ca currents and an accentuated outward K current (Ito), especially in the RVOT epicardium with transmural dispersion of repolarization causing electrical heterogeneity. The protocol of management of BrS-ES is markedly different from other ES, and hence its recognition is crucial:

a. Start the isoprenaline infusion @ 0.004 mcg/kg/min (often a dosage in the range of 1–2 mcg/min is required). Ampoules are available containing 2 mL (1 mg/mL) of the drug, which is dissolved in 50 mL normal saline (NS) and started at 1–1.3 mL/hr, keeping a heart rate target >20% above baseline or about 100–120/min. Usually VF/appropriate shocks subside immediately. Isoprenaline increases L-type Ca currents and reduces electrical heterogeneity.

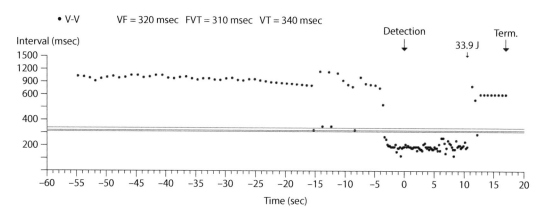

Figure 26.1 RR interval vs time plot showing sudden shortening of RR at onset of electrical storm, its detection and shocking by AICD device.

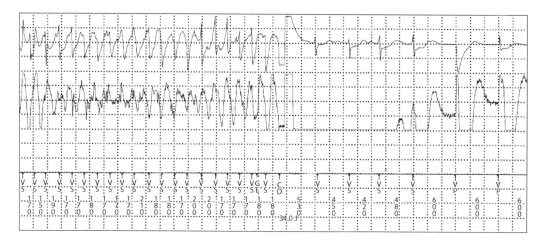

Figure 26.2 Device electrograms during VF and after shock.

b. *Alter the precipitating factors/triggers*: Sedate and give paracetamol if febrile. Vagal responses, e.g., cold exposure on the face, are also known to be triggers.

c. Wait for complete suppression of VF, adding 2–3 event-free days on isoproterenol before starting to taper the drug. While tapering, oral drugs should be added, usually in combination – some are orphan drugs and are unavailable locally. The preferred combination may be quinidine + cilostazol. Quinine may be used if quinidine is not available. In case of unavailability of quinine/quinidine, disopyramide is useful.

d. Switch to oral drugs.

Ito-blockers

i. *Quinidine*: 300–400 mg once daily and **quinine** sulphate (quinine sulphate as high as 300 mg thrice daily has been used as per case reports; the side effects of cinchonism can be mitigated by tryptophan-rich diets like meats and nuts) are the drugs of choice. Though it is also a Na channel blocker, its beneficial effects are principally by Ito blockade, an effect not available in the commonly used sister drugs chloroquine and hydroxychloroquine. But gastrointestinal side effects of quinine are common. These drugs are not easily available in most countries (in India, it is available but with some difficulty).

ii. *Disopyramide*: 150 mg/day is a drug which is usually available. It is also an Ito blocker like quinine but less potent. Owing to Na channel blockade, ST-segment elevation of the

BrS ECG may accentuate, but it reduces the frequency of VF by increasing the initiation threshold.

iii. *Biperidil*: (200 mg/day) acts by Ito blockade but is unavailable in India.

Ca current enhancers

i. *Cilostazol*: An oral phosphodiesterase III inhibitor, 100 mg twice daily, has been given in combination to reduce the frequency of VF by enhancing the Ca current.

ii. *Orciprenaline*: An oral therapy (45 mg/day in divided doses) has been used to reduce VF via Ca current enhancement.

iii. *Denopamine*: A combined alpha- and beta-agonist; at a dose of 30 mg/day is a particularly useful drug which acts by increasing the Ca current but is unavailable in India.

11. What are the antiarrhythmics to be avoided in BrS?

Amiodarone and procainamide are pro-arrhythmics in the BrS setting and hence avoided. Though in theory beta-blockers and Ca channel blockers are also harmful, in usual therapeutic doses, adverse effects are not observed.

12. What is the prognosis in BrS-ES?

Most patients are at risk for VF or another bout of BrS-ES admission, especially if they reduce their antiarrhythmics due to side effects.

FURTHER READING

1. Steinberg Chirstian, Zachary W M L, Krahn A D. Idiopathic Ventricular Fibrillation, in Zipes D, Jalife J, Stevenson W G (Ed). Electrophysiology from Cell to Bedside. Seventh Edition. Elsevier, pp 925–931.
2. Geraghty L, Santangeli P, Tedrow U, Shivakumar K, et al. Contemporary Management of Electrical Storm. Heart, Lung and Circulation (2018), https://doi.org/10.1016/j.hlc.2018.10.005
3. Sikdar S, Bera D, Kumawat K, Jahangir A, Chakraborty P. An Unusual Genetic Observation in a Case of Short-Coupled PVC-Triggered Ventricular Fibrillation. J Am Coll Cardiol Case Rep (2022),101651 (https://doi.org/10.1016/j.jaccas.2022.09.018)

27 Permanent Pacemakers and Defibrillators

From Basics to Troubleshooting

Sunandan Sikdar and Dilip Kumar

1. What are the different types of cardiac implantable electronic devices?

Therapeutic devices

- *Pacing* (**Figure 27.1**)

  - *Endocardial*: Right ventricular (RV) apical/His bundle/left bundle (single/dual chamber)

  - Endocardial leadless pacing (RV apical) (**Figure 27.1b**)

  - *Epicardial pacing*: Done by cardiac surgeons

- *Resynchronization*: Cardiac resynchronization therapy pacemaker (CRT-P), His bundle optimized-CRT (HOT-CRT), cardiac resynchronization therapy defibrillator (CRT-D) (**Figure 27.1 a, b**)

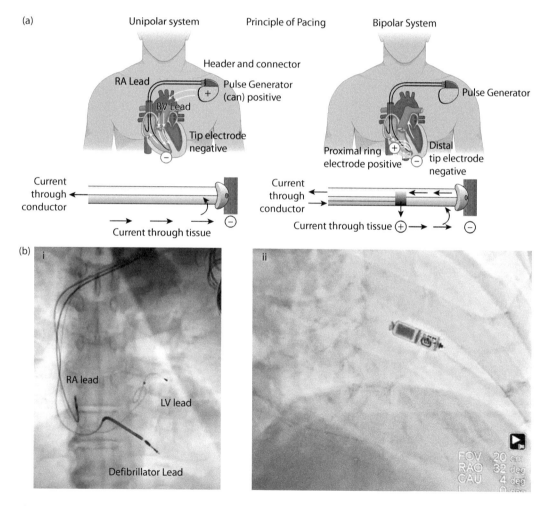

Figure 27.1 (a) Pacing systems and their principles. Unipolar systems have one conductor, while bipolar systems have two. Current flow is from the anode (positive) to cathode (negative). Conventionally, the actual flow of electrons is opposite to that of the current. (b) Pacing: Examples of devices (i) CRT-D and (ii) leadless (RV) pacing.

DOI: 10.1201/9781003027584-27

■ *Defibrillation*:

- Endocardial automatic implantable cardiac defibrillator (AICD): Dual chamber/single chamber

- Subcutaneous AICD

Monitoring devices: Implantable loop recorder

2. What are the components of a pacing/AICD system?

A. *Pulse generator*

   i. Outer titanium casing

   ii. Battery

      - *Pacemaker*: Lithium iodide

      - *AICD*: Lithium silver vanadium oxide

   iii. Output circuit

   iv. Sensing circuit

   v. Timing circuit

   vi. Telemetry coil

   vii. Header and connector – where the lead connects with the pulse generator (For AICD, additionally there is a capacitor for storing a charge.)

B. *Lead*

   i. Outer insulation (silicone, polyurethane or a mixture)

   ii. Inner conductor (coaxial inner and outer cables in bipolar systems)

   iii. Electrodes at the tip (previously unipolar, nowadays all bipolar – cathode at tip, anode at ring, usually 10 mm proximal to it)

   iv. *Fixation mechanism*: Active (screw)/passive (tines)

■ For AICD there will be additional shocking coil(s) – Dual-coil design, (superior vena cava [SVC] and RV) with DF-1 pin, or single-coil design (RV) with DF-4 pin

   - For CRT, there is an additional left ventricular (LV lead that is ideally placed in the postero-lateral vein of the coronary sinus.

3. What is the North American Society of Pacing and Electrophysiology (NASPE) coding for pacemakers?

Table 27.1: Pacemaker Codes

I	II	III	IV	V
Chamber paced	Chamber sensed	Response to sensing	Programmability	Multisite Pacing
O (None)	O (None)	O (None)	O (None)	O (None)
A (Atrium)	A (Atrium)	I (Inhibit)	R (Rate Response)	A (Atrial)
V (Ventricle)	V (Ventricle)	(Triggered)	P (Simple Programmable)	V (Ventricle)
D (Dual)	D (Dual)	D (I +T)	M (Multiprogrammable)	D = Dual (A+V)
S (Single)	S (Single)		C (Communicating)	

In the first version developed in 1987, the fifth position belonged to antitachycardia pacing. In the revised version (2001) this was altered to Multisite pacing.

The two most common modes are:

VVIR – Ventricle paced, ventricle sensed with rate response

DDDR – Dual paced, dual sensed with rate response

4. What are the parameters normally used to check a pacemaker?

Mode: See the NASPE coding of pacemakers. The indication for pacing is also to be enquired.

Pacing (capture) threshold: It is the minimal energy required by the lead (usual surface area 1–5 mm²) to depolarize the "local" myocardium in diastole to initiate a self-propagating impulse (called a capture) and ensure contraction of the chamber concerned. It is determined by the voltage applied, and the duration of the current (the longer the duration, smaller the voltage required – can be plotted as a voltage-duration curve). The usual voltage in ventricular leads is <1.0 V in acute implants and <2.5 V in chronic implants. The corresponding values for atrial leads are <1.5 V and <2.5 V. The duration is usually 0.4 msec (0.4–1 msec). Increasing the duration beyond 0.7 msec may not significantly reduce the voltage threshold due to the hyperbolic nature of the voltage (strength) duration curve. In the first few months after implant (usually 6 weeks), there is a rise in the pacing threshold. However, an abnormally increased threshold indicates lead dislodgement or lead fracture. Scar, hypothyroidism, use of flecainide and hyper/hypokalaemia are other causes. Because the pacing threshold is linked to battery usage, but the safety margin of pacing is also to be ensured, the output is initially set at to thrice and then at 2–3 months at twice the pacing threshold.

Electrogram (EGM): A bipolar EGM displays the electrical potential difference between the electrodes situated at the lead tip and the proximal ring as a function of time. In the case of a unipolar EGM, the lead tip and the pacemaker can serve as the electrodes. Because of the bigger circuit, the unipolar EGM is prone to recording noises like myopotentials. EGM recording non-local signals is called far-field EGM.

Sensing threshold: Ability to detect intrinsic cardiac electrical activity gives rise to the property of sensing and is based on a recording of the EGM (**Figure 27.2**), its processing, amplification and presentation to the sensing circuitry. The atrial (P wave) and ventricular signal (R wave) (EGM) amplitude (measured from base to peak) is 1–5 mV and 5–20 mV, respectively. The frequency content of the T wave (1–10 Hz) is lower and that of electromagnetic interference signals (5–50 Hz) much higher than the QRS. Thus, bandpass filtering is used to prevent non-essential signals from being picked up by the sensing circuit and inhibiting pacing output. Thresholds can be as small as 2 mV for ventricular and 0.3–0.6 mV for atrial channels. A minimum ventricular EGM (R wave) of 5 mV is essential at implant to ensure proper sensing.

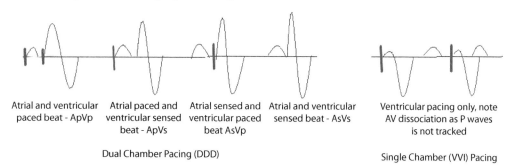

Atrial and ventricular paced beat - ApVp   Atrial paced and ventricular sensed beat - ApVs   Atrial sensed and ventricular paced beat AsVp   Atrial and ventricular sensed beat - AsVs

Dual Chamber Pacing (DDD)

Ventricular pacing only, note AV dissociation as P waves is not tracked

Single Chamber (VVI) Pacing

Figure 27.2   Pacemaker-related notation.

Impedance: It is the resistance offered by the lead to current flow – by Ohm's law, Voltage = Current (I) × Resistance (R). A smaller lead tip surface results in reduced current drain and a better signal-to-noise ratio. On the other hand, this results in poor sensing quality. This is countered by creating a fractal geometry at the tip by coating some leads with iridium. Normal impedance is 250–1200 ohms. A rise in impedance (>1200 ohms) occur with lead fracture, and fall (<250 ohms) occurs with insulation breaks.

Battery voltage: Stable output, low self-discharge rates and long life characterize lithium iodide batteries. Longevity varies with manufacturer but is usually 7–12 years for single-chamber and 6–12 for dual-chamber pacing. The initial battery voltage is 2.8 V. Elective/relative replacement indicators (ERI/RRT) are reached when the voltage is 2.1–2.4 V. When the battery reaches end of life/service (EOL/EOS), the voltage is usually <2.1 V.

Battery impedance: As the battery ages, impedance rises, starting from 100 ohms at implant to 10,000 ohms toward EOS. Battery voltage is estimated from impedance by the programmer.

Percentage of pacing: The percentage of atrial pacing (Ap) and ventricular pacing (Vp) is important and is obtained from the programmer. Vp >40% leads to LV dysfunction over the long term. Further, whether a patient is dependent on Vp most of the time can be estimated from this parameter.

AV delay (for dual-chamber pacing): The time duration after an atrial sensed or paced signal when the ventricular channel gives its impulse. A sensed atrioventricular (AV) delay (about 150 msec) is usually kept shorter than the paced AV delay (200 msec) to accommodate for the extra time taken in sensing. In order to minimize Vp, different algorithms are used (AV search hysteresis, minimum ventricular pacing) that search routinely for intrinsic conduction.

Lower rate limit: It is the lowest rate at which intrinsic conduction is allowed and is usually kept at 60/min. It is applicable for both for single- and dual-chamber pacemakers.

Blanking period: After a sensed or paced beat, the channel in the respective chamber turns off its sense amplifier for a fixed period (20–250 msec).

Refractory period: After the blanking period, this is a programmable period when sensed events do not reset a timing cycle but may be detected and used in features like mode switch. Thus, there is a ventricular refractory period (VRP, both in VVI and DDD) and an atrial refractory period (ARP, in AAI and DDD).

Post-ventricular atrial refractory period (PVARP) (**Figure 27.3**): This interval starts with the ventricular paced or sensed event and extends to the time when the atrial channel is kept refractory to an atrial sensed event (programmable duration). The PVARP prevents atrial sensing of the retrograde P wave from a premature ventricular contraction (PVC), thus starting pacemaker-mediated tachycardia (PMT). Hence in PMT, PVARP should be increased.

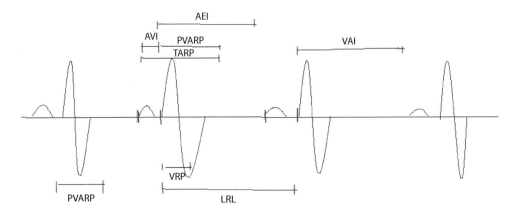

Figure 27.3 Pacemaker timing cycles. *Abbreviations*: AEI: Atrial escape interval, AVI: Atrio-vent interval, LRL: Lower rate limit, PVARP: Post-vent atrial refractory period, TARP: Total atrial refractory period, VAI: Vent atrial interval, VRP: Vent refractory period.

Upper rate limit (URL): In DDD pacing, this limit determines the maximum rate to which the ventricular channel will respond to a rising atrial rate, i.e., the rate at which P wave will be tracked. One of the factors determining this rate is PVARP. Above this rate, every alternate P wave may fall in the PVARP and is not sensed. On ECG, the rhythm looks like a 2:1 AV block, as an alternate P will not have its ventricular counterpart.

Mode switch: In DDD/VDD pacing modes, occurrence of atrial tachyarrhythmia leads to atrial tracking and ventricular pacing up to the URL. This can be avoided if mode switch is turned on. When atrial tachyarrhythmia occurs, the pacemaker reverts to VVI mode.

Rate responsiveness: The physiologic increase in heart rate with physical and emotional activity has been partially achieved by using rate response sensors, with an accelerometer (tracks body movement) being the most common. Sinus node disease and chronotropic incompetence are the two conditions where it is most useful.

5. What is hysteresis?

Hysteresis allows the pacemaker to refrain from pacing until a special lower rate (often 50/min), known as the hysteresis rate, is reached. Once this is reached, the pacer will pace at a selected rate (usually at a lower rate limit, e.g., 60 beats/min). The objective is to reduce the pacer requirement.

6. What are fusion and pseudo-fusion beats?

Pseudo-fusion beats are a superimposition of an ineffectual pacemaker stimulus on the surface QRS complex originating from a single focus (**Figure 27.4**). The intrinsic morphology (especially the ST segment) is not deformed and looks like the spontaneous beat if a pacemaker artefact occurs late enough.

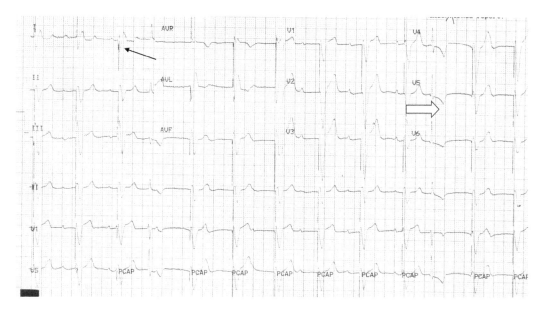

Figure 27.4   ECG from a VVI pacemaker showing pseudo-fusion *(black arrow)* and inverted (memory) T wave following a normal beat *(white arrow).*

In case of fusion beats, the ventricles are depolarized simultaneously by spontaneous and pace-maker-induced activity. As a result, the ST segment is markedly different from the spontaneous beat.

Both can occur in the presence of absolutely normal sensing.

7. What are the different types of pacemaker malfunction?

Pacemaker malfunctions are summarized in **Table 27.2**. The cardinal rule is that oversensing causes underpacing. For any apparent lack of pacing, look at the lead malfunction and any issues related to sensing (**Figure 27.5**).

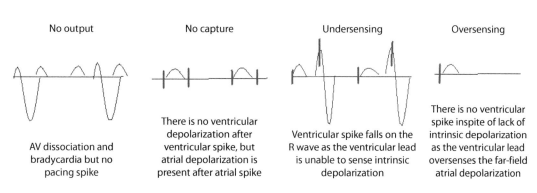

No output	No capture	Undersensing	Oversensing
AV dissociation and bradycardia but no pacing spike	There is no ventricular depolarization after ventricular spike, but atrial depolarization is present after atrial spike	Ventricular spike falls on the R wave as the ventricular lead is unable to sense intrinsic depolarization	There is no ventricular spike inspite of lack of intrinsic depolarization as the ventricular lead oversenses the far-field atrial depolarization

Figure 27.5   Pacemaker malfunction.

Table 27.2: Pacemaker Malfunctions and Interpretations

Problem	Characteristics	Causes	Comments
Failure to pace	No spike but bradycardia with HR <60 min consistently	• Oversensing • Battery EOL • Lead fracture	• If on placing magnet spike appears, oversensing • If impedance is high, then fracture

Failure to capture	Spike present but no succeeding QRS	• Lead dislodgement
		• Lead fracture
		• Lead insulation break
		• Hyperkalaemia or scar
		• EOS
			• Impedance
			  • Normal – dislodgement
			  • Increased – fracture
			  • Decreased – insulation break

Failure to sense (undersensing)	Spike on ST segment or just after QRS	Lead malfunction	• Differentiate from fusion or pseudo-fusion • Treated by increasing sensitivity
Oversensing	Apparent lack of pacing	Senses extrinsic electrical signals or intrinsic (far field) signals from another chamber	• *Cross-talk*: Sensing of atrial signal by ventricular channel leading to lack of ventricular output • Treated by decreasing sensitivity or by blanking
Electromagnetic interference	High frequency, low amplitude signals	Electromagnetic apparatus nearby	Can cause oversensing and thus underpacing
Pseudo-malfunction	• Hysteresis • Mode switch • Upper rate behaviour	Due to specific programming issues	Alteration of program is the solution

8. Can the site of a ventricular lead be inferred from the ECG?

ECG clues are given in **Table 27.3**.

Table 27.3: Site of Pacing and ECG Characteristics

Site	ECG	Comments
RV apex	Left axis, LBBB, −ve QRS II, III, aVF	• Depolarization from inferior to superior • QS or Rs may occur in V5, V6
RVOT pacing	Inferior axis, LBBB qR or QR in I, aVL	May be a narrower QRS complex
LV-only pacing	Right axis, RBBB	• With basal location, leads V5, V6 are +ve • With apical location, they are −ve
His bundle (HBP) (Figure 27.6a)	Paced QRS may be narrower than baseline QRS	Selective and nonselective HBP are possible
Left bundle pacing (LBP)	RBBB V1, sometimes near-normal QRS duration	Peak LV activation time (pLVAT) <80 msec in V5, V6 suggests LB capture
Biventricular pacing, RV lead in apex, LV lead in posterolateral vein	Right superior axis, RBBB V1, Qr I, aVL	• RVOT lead may cause LBBB • LV lead in middle cardiac vein may cause LBBB

9. What are the causes of a dominant R wave in V1 in a "routine pacemaker"?

a. Ventricular fusion with intrinsic right bundle branch block (RBBB) complexes

b. Lead in RV apex but ECG recorded from one intercostal space higher

c. LV pacing – Epicardial or endocardial

d. RV lead perforation with LV stimulation

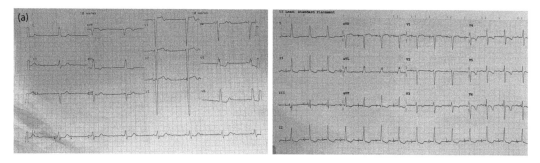

Figure 27.6   (a) ECG narrowing by conduction system pacing before *(left)* and after *(right)*.

10. How do you know whether CRT is functioning properly?

Characteristics of the ECG in a normally functioning CRT (Figure 27.6(b)) include the following:

a. RBBB on V1.

b. Qr in I and aVL. If Q disappears, suspect dislodgement of the LV lead.

c. Narrow QRS at the time of initial implant.

d. Negative QRS in leads II, III and aVF.

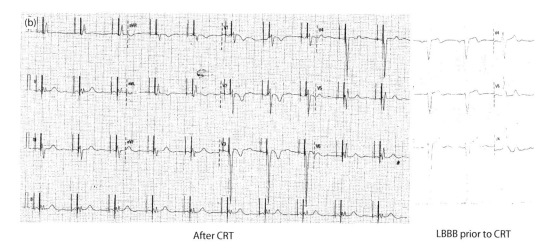

After CRT   LBBB prior to CRT

Figure 27.6   (b) QRS narrowing by CRT. Note q in I, aVL.

If the LV lead dislodges, then V1 will become like a left bundle branch block (LBBB), lead I will become positive (R) and lead III negative. The LBBB pattern in V1 may also occur if LV lead is in the middle cardiac vein by choice.

11. How do you calculate the QT interval in a paced rhythm?

In a patient with a paced rhythm or intraventricular block, the formula for the corrected QT is:

$$QTc = QTc - (QRS\ duration - 100\ msec)$$

Another option is to use the JT interval and thus the corrected JT interval in such cases.

If there is a prolongation of QTc by >25% or by >60 msec from the baseline on starting a drug, it should be discontinued.

12. What are the indicators for replacement Recommended Replacement Time (RRT) of a pacemaker?

Once RRT is reached, the pacemaker should be replaced in 3 months. The indicators are:

i. Percent or fixed decrease in pacing rate on magnet application

ii. Change to simpler pacing mode

iii. Elevated battery impedance

iv. Restricted programmability

In a suspected case of End of Life (EOL) or End of Replacement Indicators (ERI), avoid using a magnet, as it leads to sudden current drain and potential asystole in a dependent patient.

13. How are magnets used with a cardiovascular implantable electronic device (CIED)?

The magnetic field effect of the clinical magnet is directly proportional to the strength of the magnet and inversely proportional to the distance of the magnet from the device. A magnetic field effect of ≥10 Gauss aligned with the magnetic reed switch is required to activate the magnetic switch in order to alter the device function. Available clinical magnets usually have the strength of ≥90 Gauss. In obese individuals, more than one magnet may be needed to change the function of the device. The magnet should be properly placed over the device. In St. Jude ICDs, the position of the magnet is recommended to be placed off-centre with the curve of the magnet over the bottom or top end of the ICD.

i. Application of a magnet leads to asynchronous pacing (no sensing of intrinsic beats) due to application of the reed switch (if the reed switch malfunctions, magnet mode may not turn on, but this is rare). Magnet application may be useful in emergency situations when sensing difficulties cause underpacing or electromagnetic interferences occur in operation theatres causing lack of output from the pacemakers and bradycardia. Pacemaker-mediated tachycardia, where retrograde V-A conduction after a V-paced beat leads to activation and triggering of the atrial and ventricular channels, is terminated on magnet application. This is because the retrograde P wave is not sensed.

ii. *Identification of battery status*: For Medtronic devices, the magnet rate is 85/min with a normal device (in some, the initial three beats may be at 100/min) and 65/min at ERI. For St. Jude/Abbott devices, the magnet rate is 100/min in asynchronous mode normally, which reduces to 85/min at ERI. For Boston Scientific pacers, the magnet rate is 100/min and 85/min at ERI.

iii. Suspends all anti-tachycardia therapies of most AICDs without affecting the pacing mode.

iv. Magnet application can also be used to identify manufacturers based on the specific magnet-induced pacing rate of each mode.

v. In the case of the AICD delivering inappropriate shocks due to electromagnetic interference, a loose set screw, T-wave/myopotential oversensing or in supraventricular tachycardia (SVT), the magnet application may be lifesaving.

vi. With the AICD, an auditory response to the magnet may reveal the manufacturer. Medtronic devices have magnet-activated alert tones that warn the patient about any device-related urgency.

- If a magnet is placed over an AICD, programming should be done as soon as possible because older models from some manufacturers may change their functioning.

- If a magnet is applied but a response is not observed, then there are any of three possibilities:

i. Magnetic field is too weak to reach the device

ii. Pacemaker EOL

iii. Pacemaker programmed to ignore the magnet

14. What are the causes of electromagnetic interference (EMI) in a pacemaker?

Medical: MRI, radiofrequency (RF) ablation, defibrillation, electrocautery, lithotripsy, electroshock therapy, radiation therapy

Environment: High power lines, wielding, metal detectors

Personal: Mobile phones

15. What are the pacemaker responses to EMI?

a. *Oversensing*: EMI in the atrial lead may lead to misdiagnosis of atrial arrhythmia by the device and a mode switch to non-tracking mode or speeding up the ventricular rate to the URL. EMI in the ventricular lead may lead to inhibition of ventricular output in dependent patients and syncope. Noise reversion mode is activated automatically by the device to protect itself from EMI.

b. *Power reset*: Pacemakers reset to factory settings in response to strong EMI like defibrillation or electrosurgery because the programmable memory (random access memory [RAM]) disconnects from pre-stored read-only memory (ROM). Zenner diodes are used to protect the circuitry from excessive voltage.

16. What is the impact of surgery on a pacemaker?

Coagulation mode (up to 10 kV) has a higher EMI than cutting mode (<2 kV) and hence the former should be used sparingly. Further, bipolar systems affect a smaller amount of tissue and should be preferred over unipolar systems. The device should be interrogated before operation and switched to VOO/DOO mode if the surgical field is nearby. Postoperative check-up of the device is essential to switch back to VVI/DDD mode and monitoring of parameters.

17. What is the impact of radiation?

As in surgery, device interrogation is required. If the cumulative dose <2 Gy, the risk of EMI is low.

18. What are the different types of therapy available on an AICD?

AICDs offer three types of therapies:

a. Defibrillation

b. Anti-tachycardia pacing

c. Back-up bradycardia pacing

19. How is anti-tachycardia pacing different from bradycardia pacing?

Bradycardia pacing involves a quiescent myocardium in diastole, and the current requirement is smaller. On the other hand, anti-tachycardia pacing involves progressive penetration by trains of beats (3–10, usually 8) into the excitable gap of the ventricular tachycardia occurring at a site remote from the stimulus site, and this requires a higher current. The trains may be given in bursts (fixed rate in the same train of beats) or in a ramp (progressively faster in the same train of beats). Almost 80% of ventricular tachycardias (VTs) can be converted to a sinus rhythm, especially slower VTs.

20. How is defibrillation different from pacing?

While pacing is a local phenomenon, defibrillation requires a sufficiently strong electric field to depolarize the entire heart at a point in time, which is partially refractory due to ongoing ventricular fibrillation (VF). Hence, defibrillation coils are larger with a greater surface area than pacing leads. The field strength (1 V/cm vs 3–5 V/cm), shock energy (voltage) and pulse duration (0.3–0.6 msec versus 6–12 msec) are all smaller in pacing compared to defibrillation. A biphasic waveform is used with the RV coil as the anode and the AICD can as the cathode in the first phase and the reverse in the second phase. Placing the AICD can in the left pectoral region requires less defibrillation energy (as the vector from the coil can pass through a larger myocardial mass), and hence this is the usual implantation site. Further, while the nature of the relation between the strength of stimulus and myocardial depolarization in pacing is deterministic, that between shock energy and defibrillation is probabilistic. Hence, a stimulus more than the pacing threshold will always depolarize, and a shock energy above the defibrillation threshold (DFT) is more likely to, but will not surely, cardiovert. A 12-joule shock may fail to defibrillate in the first attempt but may be successful in the second. DFT may be increased by scarring, electrolyte imbalance and drugs (amiodarone). It may be decreased by sotalol. In most AICD implantations for the primary prevention of sudden death, DFT determination is not done, as it requires VF to be repeatedly induced (binary search protocol) by R-on-T low-energy shocks (vulnerable period toward the end of the ST segment) and defibrillated, which has inherent risks. DFT determination is done still in some centres for secondary prevention cases.

21. How do you program AICDs?

Appropriate shock: Shock given for sustained VT/VF (**Figure 27.7**)

Avoidable shock: If given for self-terminating VTs

Inappropriate shock: Shock given for any other rhythm

Parameter Summary					Type	ATP Seq	Shocks	Success	ID#	Date	Time hh:mm	Duration hh:mm:ss	Avg bpm V	Max bpm V	Activity at Onset
Mode	VVI	Lower Rate	40 bpm		VT-Mon				1496	14-Oct-2021	15:03	:18	135	136	Rest
					VT-Mon				1495	14-Oct-2021	15:02	:51	137	140	Rest
					VF	0	35J	Yes	1494	14-Oct-2021	11:37	01:02:38	375	375	Rest
Detection		**Rates**	**Therapies**		VT-Mon				1493	14-Oct-2021	10:31	:15	135	136	Active
VF	On	>188 bpm	35J × 6		VF	0	35J	Yes	1492	14-Oct-2021	10:30	01:07:15	353	375	Active
FVT	via VF	188–194 bpm	Burst(1), Ramp(2), Ramp+(2), 16J, 25J, 35J		VT-Mon				1491	14-Oct-2021	09:14	:39	140	143	Rest
VT	On	176–188 bpm	Burst(3), Burst(2), Ramp+(1), 20J, 30J, 35J		VF	0	35J,35J	Yes	1490	14-Oct-2021	09:13	:50:31	333	375	Rest
					VF	0	35J	Yes	1489	14-Oct-2021	04:50	:14	333	333	Rest
					VF	0			1488	13-Oct-2021	23:46	:28	300	300	Rest

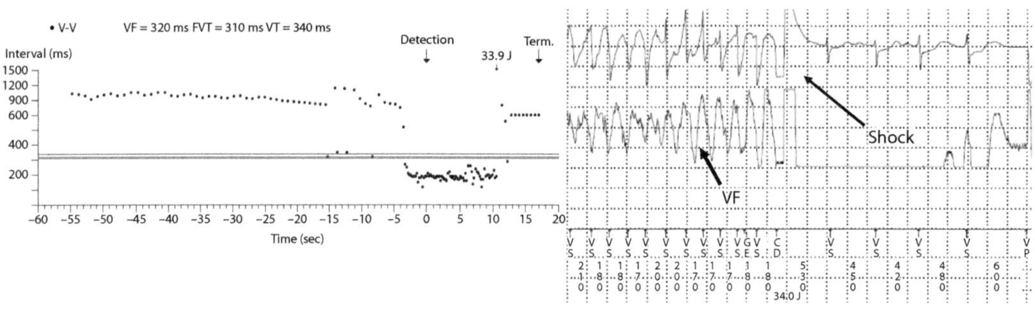

Figure 27.7   AICD interrogation showing multiple VF episodes in a single day, the majority terminated by a 35-J shock.

The entire exercise of programming is to ensure the delivery of appropriate shocks and minimize avoidable and inappropriate shocks.

Sensing: When a filtered signal crosses a pre-set amplitude, it must be sensed. The timing of sensed events can be seen in the marker channel (marked as Vs for sensed ventricular beats, Ts for ventricular tachycardia sense and Fs for ventricular fibrillation sense). It must be remembered that the annotation applied by the device is as determined by the algorithm and may differ from the clinical event.

Detection: The process by which the ICD algorithm counts and classifies a sequence of sensed signals to decide what therapy to deliver. This is based on what is already programmed into the device.

Zones: Setting zones is the basic exercise of programming. For primary prevention indication when VT/VF is a rare occurrence but sudden fast VT/VF is more common, a sinus, a fast VT and a VF zone are enough. A rate threshold of 185–200/min with a detection duration of 6–12 sec (delayed detection at 30 sec favourably reduced shocks in the MADIT-RIT trial) is usual. A minimum delay of >2.5 sec or >30 intervals prior to shocking is recommended. For secondary prevention indication where self-terminating VT or slower VT is more common, three zones are required – VT (kept about 10 beats less than clinical VT), fast VT and VF. The threshold is kept higher at 200/min so that ATP can be applied. Slower VTs often terminate by this form of therapy. Most of the time for VT/VF, before or during charging, the ATP therapy continues. The device takes a final look at the rhythm before giving a shock.

Bradycardia pacing: In order to minimize ventricular pacing and consequent worsening of LV function, especially for single-chamber AICD, keep the lower rate limit at 40/min.

Discriminators: Though rate is one of the discriminators between SVT vs VT, other discriminators are required for reducing therapy.

Rate and duration: The rate for primary prevention is >200/min. This is just below the clinical VT rate in secondary prevention.

Sudden onset: Once a tachycardia has been detected, the device measures the difference between the shortest RR interval before the onset of the tachycardia and that at the beginning of the tachycardia. VT is declared if this difference is greater than the programmed value. This parameter differentiates VT from sinus tachycardia.

Stability: VT, in contrast to atrial fibrillation (AF), has a more stable RR interval usually. This is usually set at <40 msec variability in the RR interval. The combination of sudden-onset and stability criteria performs well at ventricular rates less than 190 bpm, and accuracy deteriorates with faster heart rates. The rate and duration rider are important in order to diagnose VT with variable RR.

Template match: Immediately at implant the device creates a morphology template from the sinus rhythm QRS. With the onset of VT, the device matches the new QRS morphology with the stored QRS. However, this parameter is also not fool-proof as tachycardia morphology may change due to an increased rate. Usually, the template match threshold is kept at 65%.

Atrial lead criteria (for dual-chamber AICD): Two inputs are crucial: (1) Whether the tachycardia started with a V or an A, – if V, it is a VT and (2) whether the number of V > A, which implies VT. If the number of A > V, then it is SVT. If number of V = A, then other discriminators are required. In the case of V = A, VT with retrograde conduction and SVT are the possibilities. If A falls just before or after the V, SVT is likely (AVNRT). If it falls in the first half of VV, it may be VT. If in the second half of VV, then it may be long RP SVT.

Confirmation of therapy: Confirmation of VT takes place after ATP is delivered and the device charges for high-voltage shock as some tachycardias will terminate after ATP or by the time of charging. Then the shock is withheld. These are called noncommitted shocks. On the other hand, in the VF zone where self-termination is remote, the device must give a committed shock, i.e., without rechecking the rhythm. For safety, once the first shock is given to terminate the tachycardia, the device looks at (this is called *redetection*) the rate only without going into SVT-VT discriminators.

Programming the ATP: Usually three sets (typically 8 beats) of ATP are given, each progressively more aggressive (faster) than the previous one in either the "burst" or "ramp" protocol explained previously. Slower VTs often terminate, but there is always a risk that faster VTs may accelerate.

Programming the shock: The shock strength is determined by DFT or kept at the highest energy available from the device if DFT is not done. The shock is usually biphasic (RV coil anode in the first phase, reverse in the second phase), the tilt (initial voltage – truncated voltage/truncated voltage) is kept at 65% and the number of shocks at 6 (a larger number of shocks does not improve success rates).

22. What aesthetic agent is best used during cardiac rhythm device (CRMD) implants?

In the case of shorter-duration procedures (pacing, AICD), fentanyl is commonly used. For longer-duration procedures (CRT, CRT-D) in patients with severe LV dysfunction, where local anaesthesia only is insufficient and deep sedation is required, etomidate has been *proposed* to be preferred over propofol, as the incidence of hypotension is low. A side effect of etomidate is adrenal suppression, and it should be avoided over prolonged periods.

23. What are the AICD-related malfunctions?

A. *Sensing problems – Oversensing*:

- Intra-cardiac – cyclic oversensing (i.e., in sync with the ventricle) – T-wave/P-wave oversensing (leading to double count of the heart rate [HR] and assigning them in the VT zone), lead malfunction.

- Extracardiac – usually non-cyclic – e.g., EMI and lead-header problem (non-physiological signal).

B. *Impedance problems*: These may occur at either the pacing/sensing conductor or the high voltage (shocking) conductor

  a. *Pace sense problem – Increase*: Sudden >50% increase in impedance implies a lead fracture or lead header problem

    Gradual: If no oversensing, means lead maturation

    Decrease – Sudden: RV perforation

    Gradual: Insulation break

  b. *High-voltage impedance problem – Sudden increase*: Fracture.

    Decrease: Insulation break

C. *Lead failure*: Occurs in 1.3/100 lead years. Oversensing (e.g., pectoral myopotentials/unexplained EMI) with normal pacing impedance is the most common. Impedance changes or lack of capture may occur. Shocking conductor malfunction may present with an abnormal non-physiologic signal on EGM, impedance changes or defibrillation failure. Get a chest X-ray (CXR) always to look for lead integrity.

24. What would you do in a patient presenting with recurrent shocks?

Step 1. Were there any symptoms during shock?

Was there palpitation/syncope? What was the activity that precipitated it? An absence of symptoms increases the possibility of inappropriate shocks.

Step 2. Inspect the device site and interrogate the device

Check stored EGMs and far-field ECG – if the events match and whether there was tachycardia or oversensing. If tachycardia, then the signals will be cyclical and correspond with the QRS in the far-field ECG. If a non-cyclical, non-physiologic signal (high frequency, low amplitude) are seen, it is likely that they are oversensed.

Step 3. Was the shock appropriate?

If true tachycardia occurred, then check whether SVT versus VT was correctly assigned by the device. Check the discriminators.

Step 4. If inappropriate, what was the cause and how can you fix it?

If oversensing was the problem, check whether it is due to T or P oversensing or EMI. For T-wave oversensing ventricular sensitivity, the sensing bandwidth and sensing bipole can be changed. Specific algorithms are available with some manufacturers. If lead failure is the issue, it must be replaced.

Step 5. If appropriate, was there a reversible cause?

If VT/VF occurred, check electrolyte, ischaemia, drugs (e.g., QT-prolonging drugs) and other causes.

Step 6. If no reversible cause, is drug therapy or ablation required?

If recurrent PVC is the trigger, then class III drugs (amiodarone/mexiletine/sotalol) can be chosen as per substrate. PVC ablation may also be considered.

Step 7. How do you reduce appropriate shocks in the future?

You may program ATP or add drugs or consider ablation.

25. How do drugs modify shocks?

a. *Reduce defibrillation energy requirement*: Sotalol, dofetilide

b. *Increase defibrillation energy requirement*: Amiodarone, flecainide, verapamil

c. *Slows VT rate and delays recognition*: Amiodarone, flecainide

d. *Increases SVT rate and makes it look like VT*: Flecainide by 1:1 conduction

e. *Makes SVT irregular*: Amiodarone, flecainide

f. *Increases frequency of VT*: QT-prolonging drugs

g. *Reduces frequency of VT*: Beta-blocker, amiodarone

26. What are the precautions in a pacing/AICD patient undergoing MRI?

Risks of MRI on an electrical device include (1) magnetic field-induced movement of the device (lead dislodgement, perforation, tamponade) or altering its functionality (increase in capture threshold, runaway pacemaker), (2) magnet field-induced electric current generation causing arrhythmias and (3) heating effect.

At present, medical devices are categorized into one of three groups by the American Society for Testing and Materials: (1) MR-safe: An item that poses no known hazards in an MR environment; (2) MR conditional: An item that has been demonstrated to pose no known hazards in a specified

MR environment with specified conditions of use; and (3) MR-unsafe: An item that is known to pose hazards in all MR environments. CRMDs are usually classified as MRI-conditional.

The following may be excluded: Patients with newly implanted (<6 weeks), abandoned or epicardial leads; temporary pacing wire; and pacemaker-dependent patients with ICD devices. Those devices without "MRI-conditional features," a pacemaker prior to 1996 or an AICD before 2000 may be also excluded. Passive fixation leads need to be dealt with using caution. The strength of the magnetic field permitted on the device must be adhered to (1.5 Teslas versus 3 Teslas).

Pre-scan and post-scan lead parameter check, and restoration of the original programming settings should be done. The MRI-safe algorithm is turned on. An inhibited pacing mode is programmed for the duration of the MRI scan, and if the device is an ICD, tachycardia therapies are disabled. In pacemaker-dependent patients, an asynchronous mode is chosen to minimize the risks of inappropriate pacing inhibition. Magnet response, rate response and sensing are disabled. During MRI pulse, BP and oxygen saturation are preferably checked. After the scan, recheck programming and reset to the necessary parameters. Long-term follow-up 3–6 months after MRI should be conducted to ensure no significant chronic changes in device parameters have occurred.

FURTHER READING

1. Ellenbogen K A, Willkof B L, Kay G N, Lau C P, Auricchio A (Ed). Clinical Cardiac Pacing, Defibrillation, and Resynchronization Therapy. Fifth Edition (2017). Elsevier.
2. Barold S S, Stroobant R X, Sinnave A F (Ed). Cardiac Pacemakers and Resynchronisation Step by Step: An Illustrated Guide. Second Edition (2010). Wiley Blackwell.

28 Cardiomyopathies

Sunandan Sikdar, Arijit Ghosh, and Subhasis Roy Chowdhury

1. How do you classify cardiomyopathies?

European Society of Cardiology (ESC) classifications (2008)

   a. Hypertrophic cardiomyopathy (HCM)

   b. Dilated cardiomyopathy (DCM)

   c. Arrhythmogenic right ventricular cardiomyopathy (ARVC)

   d. Restrictive cardiomyopathy (RCM)

   e. Unclassified

World Heart Federation Classification (MOGES)

   Morpho-functional: HCM, DCM, RCM, ARVC, left ventricular non-compaction cardiomyopathy (LVNC)

   Organ system: Heart, muscles, nervous system, liver, kidney

   Genetics: Autosomal dominant (AD), autosomal recessive (AR), X-linked recessive (XLR), X-linked dominant (XLD)

   Aetiology: Genetic, myocarditis

   Stage: American Heart Association (AHA) stages A–D, New York Heart Association (NYHA) classes I–IV

2. What is ARVC?

ARVC is an inherited (usually AD with variable penetrance) cardiomyopathy that is characterized by ventricular arrhythmias (presenting as effort syncope/palpitation), an increased risk of sudden death and right-sided heart failure due to abnormalities of right ventricular (RV) structure and function. The usual onset is between the second and fifth decades. Vigorous exercise can worsen the condition and lead to earlier development of the phenotype. Although structural involvement of the RV predominates, a left-dominant form of ARVD has been described (usually involving the posterolateral wall) without RV involvement. The pathologic hallmark of ARVC is RV myocyte loss with fibrofatty replacement. Wall thinning, aneurysms and global dilation of the RV are specific features. Mutations in desmosomal proteins (intercellular adhesion molecules) have been identified in most cases (pathogenic mutations are present in >50%). This mutation causes myocyte mechanical and electrical uncoupling between cells under heavy exertion, especially in the thin-walled RV, leading to inflammation, fibrosis and electrical instability. Among the first group of mutated genes to be identified was the palakoglobin gene, causing the rare autosomal recessive ARVC with woolly hair (Naxos disease). The commonly found mutated genes related to classical ARVC are plakophilin-2 (45%) and desmoglein-2 (9%). A mutation due to desmoplakin genes leads to the left ventricular (LV) type of ARVC (Carvajal syndrome), which has AR inheritance.

3. What is the natural history of ARVC?

It passes through four phases: (1) A long asymptomatic phase, (2) a phase of overt electrical instability, (3) a phase of RV failure and (4) a phase of biventricular failure. Heart failure develops 4–8 years after development of right bundle branch block (RBBB) on ECG and may be indistinguishable from DCM. Sudden death occurs as the first manifestation in 50% of afflicted individuals due to accelerated ventricular tachycardia (VT) degenerating into ventricular fibrillation (VF).

4. What are the ECG findings in ARVC?

The ECG is normal in 50% of ARVC cases. The ECG findings in typical cases include (**Figures 28.1 and 28.2**): (1) RBBB, (2) epsilon wave at the end of QRS – a marker of late RV free wall activation, (3) T-wave inversion in precordial leads and (4) localized QRS widening (>110 ms in V1); however, in the presence of RBBB, this localized prolongation is defined, as QRS V1–V3 is more wide compared

DOI: 10.1201/9781003027584-28

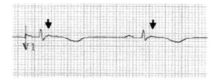

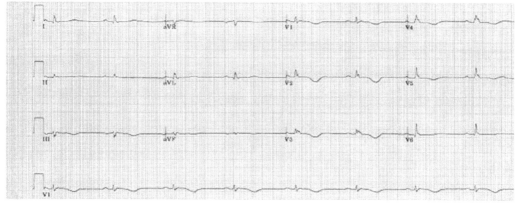

Figure 28.1 ARVC without RBBB: Note T-wave inversion V1–V3 with epsilon wave in V1 *(inset)*. (With permission from Jain R et al. ECG features of ARVD. *Circulation*. 2009;120:477–487.)

to V6 by >25 ms. In addition, (5) the QRSd ratio (V1 + V2 + V3)/(V4 + V5 + V6) >1.2 and (6) there is a fragmented QRS (defined as four or more notches/spikes in a single QRS).

Visibility of the epsilon wave may be improved by using higher amplification (voltage calibration 20 mV), double paper speed (50 mm/sec), filtering at 40 Hz and lead position modification (Fontaine modification) – right arm electrode on the manubrium, left arm on the xiphoid and left leg on V4. The epsilon-like hump may be found in Brugada syndrome, RV infarct and cardiac sarcoidosis.

5. What are the diagnostic criteria of ARVC?

The typical patient presents with palpitation, syncope, and progressive dyspnoea and presents to intensive care unit with VT/VF/recurrent syncope. There are six parameters used in the task force criteria (TFC) for ARVC (2010), and the *major criteria* among them have been summarized and simplified for use in intensive care:

1. Global or regional dysfunction and structural alteration

   Echocardiogram: RV akinesia, dyskinesia or aneurysm with end-diastolic parasternal long axis (PLAX) RV outflow tract (RVOT) diameter >32 mm or PSAX RVOT diameter >36 mm or RV fractional area change <33% (apical four-chamber view)

   Cardiac MRI or RV angiography shows akinesia/dyskinesia/aneurysm

2. Tissue characterization of RV wall

   Pathology: Fibrous replacement (endomyocardial biopsy is usually not available in practice)

3. Repolarization abnormality

   ECG shows T-wave inversion in V1–V4 (in the absence of RBBB, it is a major criteria; in the presence of RBBB, it is a minor criteria)

4. Depolarization abnormality

   Epsilon wave: Reproducible low-amplitude signal (hump) at the end of QRS and onset of a T wave in V1–V2

5. Arrhythmias

   Left bundle branch block (LBBB): Superior axis VT (sustained or non-sustained)
   Premature ventricular contraction (PVC) >500/hr, LBBB – normal axis VT is a minor criterion

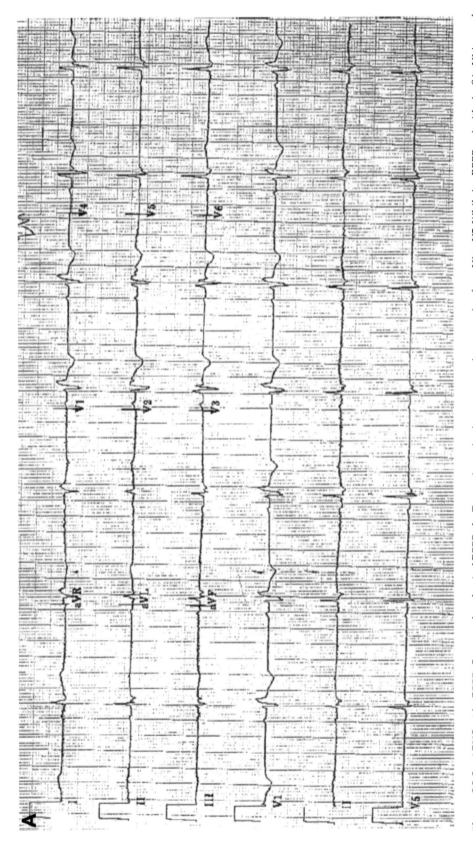

Figure 28.2 ARVC with cRBBB: Compared to classical RBBB, the T-wave inversion is more extensive, occurring from V1 to V5. While in cRBBB rsr' with r' > S in V1 is usual, in ARVC, r' < S occurs. (With permission from Jain R et al. ECG features of ARVD. *Circulation*. 2009;120:477–487.)

6. Family history

Known ARVC in a first-degree relative (In contrast, Premature death <35 years due to suspected ARVC is in minor criteria)

Two major or one major and two minor criteria from different categories are required for a diagnosis of ARVC.

6. What is the differential diagnosis of ARVC?

Echocardiography: Dilated RV can be found in ARVC, athlete's heart, DCM with biventricular involvement and pulmonary hypertension. Specific for ARVC: Trabecular prominence, focal aneurysm and hyper-reflective moderator band.

Arrhythmia: LBBB-VT can have a normal/inferior axis in the classical RVOT VT with a normal heart, and ARVC may mimic this entity in early stages. As the disease progresses multiple VT morphologies may appear, especially LBBB-left superior axis (LBBB-LS) VT. Exercise-induced VT occurs more commonly with ARVC. LBBB-inferior axis VT may be more likely due to ARVC than a normal heart if it does not terminate with adenosine, there is a late precordial transition at V5 and beyond, VT-QRS duration >120 ms in lead I and R < S in lead III *during VT*. PVCs of multiple morphology and precordial T-wave inversion on ECG at baseline are other clues. An electrophysiological (EP) study with inducible VT on programmed stimulation and extensive RV low-voltage area (scar) on 3D electroanatomical mapping are suggestive features of ARVC. Cardiac sarcoidosis may cause similar arrhythmias and can be differentiated from ARVC by cardiac MRI.

7. How do you risk-stratify for arrhythmias in ARVC?

High risk (>10% annual risk of malignant arrhythmia): Aborted sudden cardiac death (SCD)/VF, sustained VT, severe RV (RV ejection fraction [RVEF] <35%)/LV dysfunction.

Intermediate risk (1%–10% annual risk): One or more major risk factors (syncope, non-sustained VT, moderate RV [RVEF 35%–40%]/LV dysfunction).

Low risk (<1% annual risk): No risk factors, healthy gene carriers. Strangely, a family history of arrhythmic events does not influence risk in other family members.

Unexplained syncope is an independent predictor of sudden death.

8. What are the management strategies for ARVC?

Prevention of disease progression: Avoiding exercise/physical strain is paramount. This is particularly useful for those who are diagnosed with a gene mutation in cascade screening of the relatives of the index case, as they are diagnosed early in their natural history. Sports disqualification is lifesaving.

Antiarrhythmic drugs: Given the exertional worsening of the disease, beta-blockers are a mainstay of drug therapy. For those who have recurrent implantable defibrillator device (ICD) shocks due to VT/VF, amiodarone + beta-blockers and in some cases sotalol may be used.

Automatic implantable defibrillator device (AICD): AICD is recommended in all patients satisfying the TFC with any of the following:

a. Sustained VT

b. Arrhythmogenic syncope

c. High degree of ventricular ectopy/non-sustained VT (NSVT)

d. For primary prevention in the high-risk (>10% annual risk) and intermediate-risk (possible benefit) groups described earlier irrespective of arrhythmia status

Incidence of appropriate therapy (those who received ICD shocks due to VT/VF) even for primary prevention indications (i.e., those who did not have a VT before implant) is nearly 50% at the end of 5 years with 20% receiving shocks due to fast VT/VF attesting to the malignant and progressive nature of the disease.

Catheter ablation: Though it is not a curative procedure, ablation (endocardial ± epicardial) reduces the burden of VT-induced ICD shocks. Hence it is indicated in those patients with ARVC who, after being implanted with an ICD, receive recurrent shocks. The efficacy of ablation tends to fall off as newer and newer re-entrant circuits emerge in the fibrosed RV, so that even after a successful ablation, at the end of 1 year nearly half will have a recurrence of VT.

Cardiac transplant: For those with early onset of disease with florid presentation not responding to the previous measures, transplant may be the only option in selected cases.

HYPERTROPHIC CARDIOMYOPATHY

9. What are the HCM phenotypes?

Sarcomeric protein: Beta myosin heavy chain (40%) *mutation*

Myosin-binding protein C (35%)

Troponin T (5%)

Troponin I (3%)

Z disc protein mutation: Ankyrin repeat domain containing protein

Calcium handling protein mutation: Phospholamban, calsequestrin

10. What are HCM phenocopies?

- Phenocopy means like HCM in manifestation but not having a characteristic mutation—HCM here means imaging-based HCM.
- *PRKAG2* mutation (HCM + pre-excitation + conduction disorder)
- Anderson Fabry (alpha-galactosidase gene mutation) (HCM + angiokeratoma + concentric left ventricular hypertrophy [LVH] + stroke in young + proteinuria)
- Pompe disease (glucosidase) (short PR, big QRS compared to LVH)
- Noonan syndrome (HCM + pulmonary valve dysplasia)
- LEOPARD syndrome (HCM + lentiges + conduction abnormality)
- Danon disease (lysosomal-associated membrane protein mutation)
- Mitochondrial disorders (HCM + increased lactate on exercise + stroke)
- Friedrich ataxia (HCM + cerebellar ataxia)

11. What are the indications for genetic testing?

About 40% of HCM cases do not harbour any known mutation. Hence in a clinically suggestive case, a known mutation may not be detected. The role of genetic study is limited to:

1. Cascade screening of relatives if a specific pathogenic mutation is located in the proband
2. To identify a possible treatable syndrome, e.g., Anderson Fabry
3. Unexplained/borderline LVH where HCM is suspected

12. What are the diagnostic features of HCM?

Symptomatology: Angina, dyspnoea, syncope and sudden arrhythmic death.

The diagnosis of HCM is confirmed by cardiac imaging: Wall thickness >15 mm at end diastole in one or more LV myocardial segments, not explained by loading conditions (if measured by echocardiography, M-mode and oblique cuts are avoided and 2D should be used). For children the thickness should be more than twice the standard deviation above the mean value for age (z score >2).

Two-thirds have intraventricular obstruction, mostly at the LVOT and less commonly in the mid-cavity. An outflow gradient >30 mmHg at rest signifies obstruction, which is considered haemodynamically significant if >50 mmHg.

The LVOT gradient is caused by the Venturi effect of blood flow hugging the thickened basal septum during ejection, which draws in the elongated anterior mitral leaflet in the outflow tract, causing systolic anterior motion (SAM) and simultaneously an eccentric mitral regurgitation (MR).

On the other hand, the mid-cavity gradient is often related to papillary muscle hypertrophy. Forty percent of HCM patients have a provocable gradient which is brought out by the Valsalva manoeuvre or multiple sit-ups.

The velocity profile of HCM on continuous wave Doppler (CWD) often has a characteristic dagger shape. The mitral valve apparatus should be inspected for associated abnormalities: (1) Leaflet elongation, (2) abnormal anterior displacement of the papillary muscle and (3) direct papillary muscle insertion to the anterior mitral leaflet.

The HCM morphologic variants include (1) **reversed curvature** (septum convex to LV cavity) – common in the young (commonly sarcomere mutation positive), (2) **neutral** (septum straight), (3) **sigmoid septum** (septum concave to LV cavity) – common in the elderly, (4) **apical hypertrophy** and (5) **others**.

The mid-ventricular obstruction variety has some special features: Absence of SAM, paradoxical reverse flow from the apex to base during early diastole, absence of MR, tendency of apical aneurysm formation and poorer outcomes.

Late gadolinium enhancement (LGE) in HCM may be a marker of SCD.

13. What is the management plan for HCM patients?

Medical management: All drugs used in HCM are symptom modifiers rather than altering the natural history of the disease except diltiazem. Diltiazem may be given to early cases of HCM who are genotype positive but have yet to exhibit the characteristic phenotype. In case of obstructive HCM beta-blockers are the drug of choice followed by disopyramide. For non-obstructive and symptomatic exercise-related LVOT obstruction cases, beta-blockers may be used. For those with resting LVOT obstruction (LVOTO), disopyramide is a better choice. However, disopyramide may cause QT prolongation and may have anticholinergic side effects like dry mouth, difficulty in accommodation and prostatism. Further, the efficacy of disopyramide decreases over time and surgery may be required later.

Heart failure in non-obstructive HCM is caused by disease progression, which is often compounded by diastolic dysfunction, microvascular ischaemia and frequent arrhythmia. Beta-blockers slow the heart rate, reduce oxygen consumption and increase LV filling time and thus control angina and dyspnoea. Verapamil has been used for improving functional status. An important adjunct medication is ranolazine (late sodium current inhibition), which reduces angina and improves myocardial stiffness and arrhythmogenesis. When LVEF <50%, standard guideline-based treatment for heart failure is applied. Five percent of HCM cases progress to advanced heart failure and may benefit from transplant.

Mavacamten is a newly developed cardiac-specific myosin inhibitor that reduces the number of available actin myosin cross-bridges, thus reducing excessive contractility and improving the quality of life. Mavacamten showed a reduction of the post-exercise LVOT gradient, and at least one-third of treated patients showed one class improvement in NYHA symptoms in the EXPLORER HCM trial.

For arrhythmia management, amiodarone and rarely sotalol may be used in certain cases. Some patients have sleep apnoea syndrome which requires early treatment by bilevel positive airway pressure (BIPAP).

Surgery: Ventricular septal myectomy is usually performed via aortotomy on cardiopulmonary bypass. The aim is to debulk the base to the mid-intraventricular septum (IVS), widen the LVOT and eliminate SAM. Two parallel longitudinal incisions are made at the basal IVS, which are extended to the base of the papillary muscles. There is a survival benefit and a reduction of sudden death (and reduction in AICD discharge after the procedure in those already with the device). LBBB is a side effect of myectomy, and hence patients with previous RBBB are at high risk for postoperative pacemaker requirements.

Alcohol septal ablation (ASA): Injection of alcohol (usually <2 mL) in the septal perforators leads to infarction, scarring and thinning of the basal septum, leading to a decrease in gradient. Due to variation in arterial supply, contrast echocardiography through an inflated over-the-wire balloon should be used in most cases during coronary angiogram (CAG), to determine whether the septal perforator supplies the base of the papillary muscles and whether the RV side of the septum is involved. In the presence of these abnormalities septal ablation has been contraindicated. The reduction in gradient follows a biphasic pattern: Initial reduction due to stunning (1–3 days) followed by regaining of gradient followed by permanent reduction of gradient due to remodelling (about 3 months). Most significant complications include RBBB (about 40%), requirement of permanent pacing (complete heart block – about 10%), SCD and late arrhythmia. Because RBBB is a known complication, patients with HCM with pre-existing LBBB are not candidates for ASA, as the chance of heart block is exceedingly high. There is no definite survival benefit, and it is offered to the elderly and in those whose comorbidities prohibit surgery.

14. How do you manage arrhythmia in HCM?

Atrial fibrillation (AF) is the most common arrhythmia in HCM (20%), and its occurrence marks a significant downturn in the natural history, especially in cases of LVOTO and age <50 years. Loss of atrial kick while filling a stiff ventricle causes heart failure symptoms. Any of three drugs may be considered as a part of the rhythm control strategy in paroxysmal AF: Amiodarone, sotalol or disopyramide + a beta-blocker. While amiodarone has the least proarrhythmic side effects, its systemic side effects compel us to limit its dose to about 200 mg once daily (sustained-release form). For those with permanent AF, a beta-blocker or diltiazem may be used for rate control. Digoxin is usually avoided except in cases of non-obstructive HCM with AF and heart failure who require rate control. In recurrent uncontrolled symptomatic episodes of AF, catheter ablation or the surgical maze procedure (e.g., during myectomy) may be considered, though the results are even less durable.

15. What is DCM?

LV or biventricular (BiV) dilation with systolic dysfunction in the absence of abnormal loading conditions (pressure or volume) or coronary artery disease is defined as DCM. Young patients without risk factors are usually affected. DCM may be the end of the road of other cardiomyopathies. It is inherited in one-third and truly idiopathic in half.

16. What are the causes of DCM?

a. *Myocarditis*: Acute, chronic and burnt out

b. *Tachycardia-induced cardiomyopathies*: Atrial tachycardia, flutter, permanent junctional reciprocating tachycardia (PJRT)

c. Catecholamine induced

d. *Toxin/drug induced*: Alcohol, cocaine, chemotherapy

e. Autoimmune diseases and sarcoidosis

f. *Genetic causes*: Family history 5%, genetic screening 20%–30%

  Subtypes

  - Sarcomeric proteins (e.g., myosin heavy chain, troponin, titin)
  - *Cytoskeleton*: Desminopathies, sarcoglycanopathies
  - *Nucleus*: Laminopathies
  - *Desmosomes*: Desminopathy
  - *Ion channel*: Sodium channel mutation
  - Mitochondrial disease

17. What are the aetiological clues?

Mental retardation: Dystrophinopathies, mitochondrial disease

Deafness: Mitochondrial disease

Cataract: CRYAB mutation

Muscle weakness: Dystrophinopathies

Myotonia (involuntary contraction with slow relaxation): Myotonic dystrophy

ECG: AV blocks – Laminopathy, sarcoidosis, myotonic dystrophy

Low P wave: Emery Dreyfuss 1 and 2

Echocardiography: LV non-compaction: Sarcomere mutation

Mild dilation: LMNA mutation, early DCM, myocarditis, sarcoidosis

Posterolateral akinesia: Dystrophinopathy

Wall motion in non-coronary distribution: Myocarditis, sarcoidosis

CT magnetic resonance (CMR): Short T2 (on T2 mapping): Haemochromatosis

Mid-LV wall patchy LGE: Post-myocarditis, dystrophinopathy

Infero-/posterolateral LGE: Muscular dystrophy

Akinesia and LGE in anterobasal septum (transmural/subepicardial) and papillary muscle: Sarcoidosis

T1-weighted fat saturation suggesting fatty replacement in the LV wall: Left-dominant ARVC

- T1 mapping provides an idea about interstitial fibrosis

18. What is the prognosis for DCM?

Now with medical management, the 8-year survival in DCM is more than 80%, adverse events are 2% and sudden death is 0.5%.

19. What are the arrhythmias in DCM?

Three groups of arrhythmias occur in DCM:

1. AF
2. Ventricular arrhythmias – ventricular ectopy and ventricular tachycardia
3. Conduction disturbances

AF occurs in more than half of DCM cases at some stage of its natural history, with increasing prevalence as the disease progresses. While anticoagulation is indicated if CHA_2DS_2-VASc is 2 or more, in patients with non-compaction and HCM-related LV dysfunction, anticoagulation is even more beneficial. Catheter ablation of AF in cases of DCM with heart failure may lead to greater improvement of symptoms and LVEF compared to medical-only therapy with amiodarone and beta-blockers in selected cases.

Ventricular ectopy with >20% ectopic burden (ectopic beats/total number of beats) on Holter monitoring may have improvement of systolic function with ablation of the ectopic focus. VT may be the cause of 38% of cardiac arrests, while bradyarrhythmias and electromechanical dissociation are responsible for the rest.

AICD/cardiac resynchronization therapy defibrillator (CRT-D) for previous VT or cardiac arrest (secondary prevention) in non-ischaemic DCM is straightforward. In those without such history (primary prevention), in the case of non-ischaemic DCM (with LVEF <35%), the subset of patients who would clearly benefit by a defibrillator is yet to be defined. CMR may have a role in risk stratification. In the DANISH trial which compared non-ischaemic patients with and without a defibrillator (nearly two-thirds received CRT in either arm), there was no mortality benefit by adding a defibrillator.

Catheter ablation is useful in secondary-prevention defibrillators with recurrent ventricular arrhythmias. Especially in case of the of bundle branch re-entry VT (LBBB morphology with left axis), catheter ablation of the right bundle is curative.

In DCM conduction abnormalities are frequent: LBBB (nearly 40%), PR prolongation (23%), RBBB (6%) and intraventricular conduction disturbances (4%) may occur. Patients with lamin A/C mutations and those with neuromuscular disorders like myotonic dystrophy are especially prone to conduction disturbances. The former is prone to ventricular arrhythmias also. Patients requiring pacing with LBBB (QRS >150 ms) with LVEF <35% qualify for CRT. Those with higher LVEF but a pacing requirement of >40% in a day also qualify for CRT. For non-LBBB QRS >150 ms, CRT may be offered but the response may be lower. For the lamin mutation, the threshold for a defibrillator is low.

20. What are the medical management options in DCM?

Anti-heart failure therapies are also the medications of choice: Beta-blockers, angiotensin-converting enzyme inhibitors/angiotensin receptor blockers (ACEIs/ARBs), angiotensin receptor/neprilysin inhibitors (ARNIs) and mineralocorticoid receptor antagonists.

Carvedilol, bisoprolol and metoprolol have also been shown to reduce sudden arrhythmic death, as do ARNIs and spironolactone. Statins have not shown any benefit in non-ischaemic DCM but do have a role in preventing sudden death in ischaemic cardiomyopathy.

Though amiodarone is inferior to a defibrillator in preventing sudden death, in those who are high risk and not willing to use the device, amiodarone can be used to reduce sudden death. For 1000 patients on this drug, 26 sudden deaths are averted at the cost of 32 thyroid, 14 lung, 13 bradyarrhythmia and 11 liver side effects. However, if the dose is limited to 200 mg/day, many of the side effects are reduced.

21. What is RCM?

Myocardial disease with restrictive filling of the ventricles with near-normal wall thickness and preserved systolic function.

22. What are the symptoms?

The symptoms include dyspnoea (diastolic dysfunction, raised LV end-diastolic pressure [LVEDP]), fatigue (limited cardiac output), limited exercise capacity, palpitation (arrhythmia) and thromboembolism.

23. What are the causes?

Genetic/Familial: Mutation in troponin I and in other sarcomeric contractile proteins and desmin-related proteins (DES, CRYAB). Haemachromatosis and Anderson-Fabry disease (XLD, more severe in males) are other rarer causes.

Acquired causes: Amyloidosis, endomyocardial fibrosis, sarcoidosis.

24. How do you differentiate constrictive pericarditis (CCP) vs RCM by echocardiography?

Both lead to dyspnoea and anasarca, and both have restrictive diastolic physiology as their common feature, and in some cases, it may be difficult to differentiate them without cardiac CT/MRI or a catheterization study. Subtle echocardiographic features (**Figures 28.3** and **28.4**) may give a clue (**Table 28.1**).

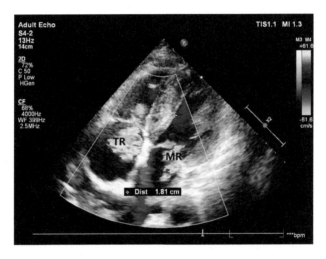

Figure 28.3   RCMP: Hypertrophied ventricle with biatrial enlargement with MR and TR.

Table 28.1: Echocardiography in Differentiating CCP from RCMP

Parameter	CCP	RCMP
Atrium	Normal	Dilated
Pericardium	Thick, bright	Normal
Septal motion	Bounce/paradoxical, left shift with inspiration	Normal
Restrictive mitral inflow	Present	Present
Annular velocity on TDI	Medial E' > lateral E'	Medial E' < lateral E'
Respiratory variation of mitral E velocity	>25% expiratory increase	<25%
Pulmonary hypertension	Rare	Frequent
Hepatic veins	Systolic antegrade flow increased in inspiration	Diastolic flow > systolic flow
Regurgitation in AV valves	Nil	Common (TR > MR)

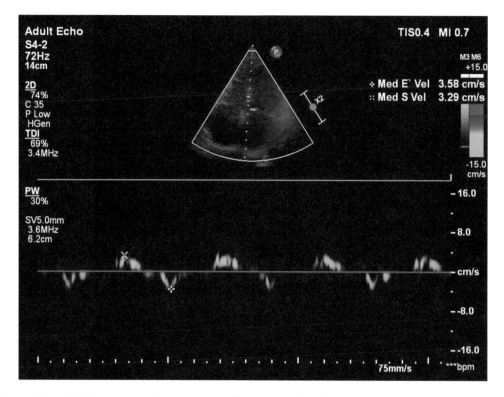

Figure 28.4   TDI in a patient with restrictive cardiomyopathy: Note low E' velocities.

25. What are the types of cardiac amyloid?

AL: Precursor protein from clonal plasma cell (bone marrow)

ATTR: Precursor protein from transthyretin by liver (transports thyroxine and retinol binding protein)

AA: From serum amyloid A

Rare types: Beta-2 microglobulin, gelsolin

26. What are the clinical features?

Amyloidosis is the prototype for RCM and is often under-recognized (**Figure 28.5** and **Table 28.2**).

AL: Heart failure with macroglossia, periorbital purpura, hepatomegaly, autonomic and peripheral neuropathy and nephropathy. Heart failure with periorbital purpura is a clue to this diagnosis.

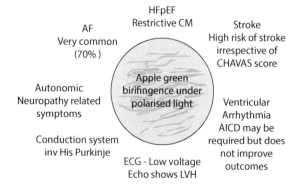

Figure 28.5   Cardiac amyloidosis – Features.

Table 28.2: Clues to Amyloidosis

Cardiac Manifestation	Extracardiac Manifestation
Anti-hypertensive or anti-heart failure medication can cause hypotension	Sensorimotor polyneuropathy
Discordance between QRS voltage on ECG and wall thickness on echocardiography	Autonomic dysfunction (orthostatic hypotension, alternating constipation and diarrhoea)
Thickening of atrial wall, RV or LV wall	Carpal tunnel syndrome
Unexpected AV blocks/pacemaker requirement	Biceps tendon rupture
Persistent low-level troponin elevation	Lumbar stenosis

ATTR (hereditary): Heart failure with peripheral and autonomic neuropathy. Family history is present in half of the patients.

ATTR (wild type): Heart failure, AF common, carpal tunnel syndrome, biceps tendon rupture, spinal stenosis.

27. What are the diagnostic modalities in cardiac amyloidosis?

ECG: Low voltage (<5 mm) in limb leads and poor precordial R-wave progression occur in half of those affected (**Figure 28.6**). Discordance between low voltage in ECG and ventricular hypertrophy on echocardiography (often mimicking HCM) is a clue to this diagnosis.

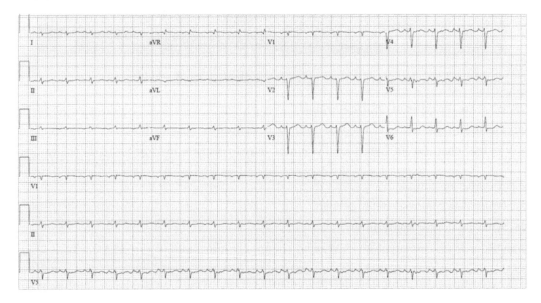

Figure 28.6 Cardiac amyloidosis: The characteristic ECG signature of AL amyloid: Low voltage in limb leads with poor R progression in chest leads. (With permission from Falk R H et al. *JACC*. 2016;68:1323–1241.)

Echocardiography: Increased LV wall thickness (>14 mm) with a small cavity, thickened valves (especially aortic), a granular sparkling appearance of the myocardium, thickened interatrial septum and often RV wall, biatrial dilation, pericardial effusion, diastolic dysfunction with small A wave (decreased atrial contractility) with normal deceleration time, characteristic strain pattern: Decreased longitudinal strain in basal and mid-LV segments with apical sparing ("bull's eye pattern") and reduced atrial strain (**Figure 28.7**).

MRI: Elevated native T1 values, difficulty nulling the myocardium and abnormal delayed enhancement.

Nuclear (bone) scintigraphy: Tc-DPD and Tc-HMDP uptake by the myocardium in ATTR amyloidosis. Uptake intensity ratio of the heart compared to the contralateral chest (ribs) is >1.5. This characteristic uptake differentiates it from AL amyloidosis (**Figure 28.8**).

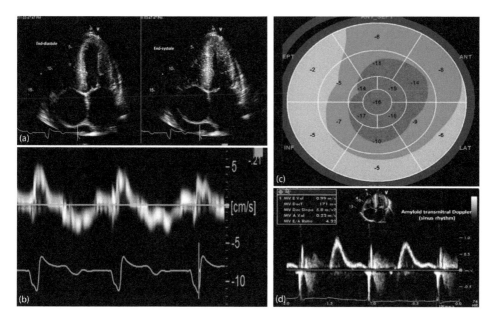

Figure 28.7 Cardiac amyloidosis echocardiography findings summarized: The hypertrophic septum with increased echogenicity, biatrial enlargement with reduced atrial contraction (a), reduced tissue Doppler velocity in spite of normal ventricular contractility (b), reduced ventricular basal and preserved apical strain (c), transmitral inflow Doppler showing small A wave due to reduced atrial contraction despite a normal E-wave deceleration time (d). (With permission from Falk R H et al. *JACC*. 2016;68:1323–1341.)

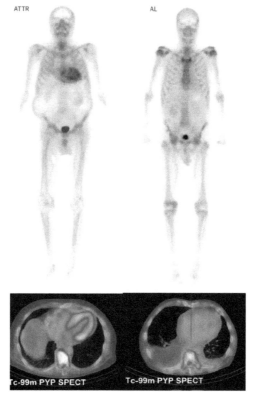

Figure 28.8 Cardiac amyloidosis: Tc-99m pyrophosphate SPECT can differentiate TTR vs AL amyloidosis. In TTR *(top)* there is cardiac uptake of radiotracer, in AL *(bottom)* there is no uptake in spite of severe cardiac involvement. (With permission from Falk RH et al. *JACC*. 2016;68:1323–1341.)

Blood tests: Serum and urine protein electrophoresis with immunofixation and serum-free light chains (**Figure 28.9**).

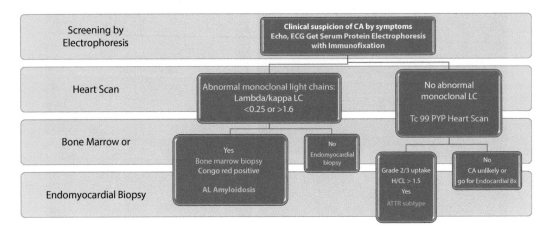

Figure 28.9 Simplified algorithm for diagnosis of cardiac amyloidosis.

28. What is the treatment for AL amyloidosis?

Chemotherapy and autologous stem cell transplantation are the treatments of choice, with those achieving remission having better outcomes. Patients in advanced stages (IV) have a grim prognosis (6 months) (**Figure 28.10**).

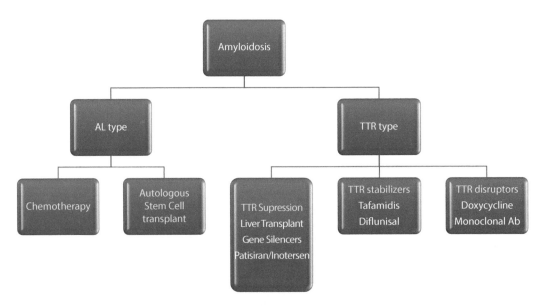

Figure 28.10 Treatment of cardiac amyloidosis.

29. What is the treatment for ATTR amyloidosis?

Treatment of TTR amyloid cardiomyopathy is useful before the onset of class III symptoms. Three groups of drugs have shown promise: TTR silencers, TTR stabilizers and TTR disruptors. TTR silencers patisiran (an siRNA) and inotersen (an antisense oligonucleotide) degrade TTR mRNA and reduce the blood level of the TTR protein. TTR stabilizing agents tafamidis and diflunisal (an NSAID) are entering clinical use, with tafamidis already FDA approved (ATTR-ACT trial). TTR disruptors like doxycycline have yet to prove their efficacy. Though liver transplant or heart-liver transplant are options, recurrence due to deposition of wild-type TTR can occur (**Figure 28.10**).

30. What are the challenges in treating heart failure in cardiac amyloidosis?

The toxic nature of amyloid deposits in the myocardium leads to a lack of reverse remodelling on beta-blocker or ACEI therapy. These agents are poorly tolerated. Further, diastolic dysfunction, hypotension and autonomic neuropathy add to the difficulty in getting optimum response. There is a concern that owing to digoxin binding to AL amyloid, a risk of sudden death and digoxin toxicity may occur. Amiodarone is a better agent for rate and rhythm control in the case of atrial arrhythmias, which are more common in cardiac amyloidosis. AF, which may occur in nearly 70% of amyloid patients, is both poorly tolerated and difficult to control, often requiring direct current cardioversion (DCCV). The risk of thromboembolism is higher than in the control population. Ventricular arrhythmias and sudden death occur, and the benefit of AICD in this population in reducing mortality is unclear.

31. What are the prognostic markers in TTR cardiac amyloidosis?

Based on troponin I and NT-pro-BNP, the Mayo and UK staging systems have been developed. Troponin I >0.05 ng/mL and NT-pro-BNP >3000 pg/mL portend a poor prognosis with survival <2 years.

FURTHER READING

1. Marcus F I, Mackenna W J, Sherill et al. Diagnosis of ARVC/D. Circulation 2010;121:1533–1541.
2. Falk R H, Alexander K M, Liao et al. AL Cardiac Amyloidosis: JACC 2016;68:1323–1341.
3. Kittelson M M, Maurer M S, Ambardekar A S, et al. Cardiac Amyloidosis: Evolving Diagnosis and Management. Circulation 2020;142:e7–e22.

29 Myocarditis

Sunandan Sikdar and Subhajit Das

1. What is myocarditis?

Myocarditis is defined as inflammation of the heart following an injury occurring as a result of exposure to either discrete external antigens, such as viruses, bacteria, parasites, toxins or drugs, or internal triggers, such as autoimmune activation against self-antigens. Acute myocarditis has an onset of symptoms to presentation within 1 month.

Following is simplified version of available criteria for diagnosis of myocarditis:

Biopsy-based: Histologic, immunohistochemical and immunologic criteria when a biopsy is available (the criteria of the World Health Organization/European Society for Cardiology [WHO/ESC]).

Histological – Dallas criteria: Inflammatory infiltrates with myocyte degeneration and necrosis (non-ischaemic) in the myocardium

Immunohistochemical: >14 WBC/mm^2 including up to 4 monocytes/mm^2 with CD3-positive T cells >7 cells/mm^2

Immunological criteria: Viral polymerase chain reaction (PCR) +ve or cardiac autoantibodies +ve

Clinical-based: Diagnosis is one or more clinical presentations + one or more diagnostic criteria + exclusion criteria satisfied

If asymptomatic (clinical presentation absent), then two or more diagnostic criteria are required.

Clinical Presentation

a. *Acute coronary syndrome*-like – with or without global or regional wall motion abnormality and/or right ventricular (RV) dysfunction on echocardiogram or Cardiac magnetic resonance (CMR) with or without increased troponin. Chest pain is present in >90% of patients. Flulike symptoms may or may not be present (18%–80% in different studies).

b. *New-onset or worsening heart failure* not explained by any other cause.

c. *Life-threatening arrhythmia*/cardiogenic shock (8% cases) or sudden death.

Diagnostic Criteria

I. *ECG*: (a) Abnormal Q wave, (b) low voltage QRS, (c) frequent premature ventricular contractions (PVCs), (d) ventricular tachycardia/ventricular fibrillation (VT/VF), (e) supraventricular tachycardia/atrial fibrillation (SVT/AF), (f) sinus arrest, (g) atrioventricular (AV) block, including third-degree AV block (more common in sarcoidosis, Chagas disease and immune checkpoint inhibitor anti-cancer drugs), h) bundle branch block, i) ST changes and j) sinus tachycardia (usually the most common abnormality). ST elevation may be present in nearly two-thirds, especially in inferior and lateral leads.

II. *Cardiac troponin*: Raised.

III. *Imaging – Echocardiography*: Global or regional wall motion abnormality, ventricular dilation, pericardial effusion, endocavitary thrombi.

IV. *Tissue characterization – Cardiac MRI (CMRI)*: Late gadolinium enhancement

Endomyocardial biopsy as described previously.

Exclusion criteria: (1) Obstructive lesion (>50%) on cardiac angiogram (CAG) excluded and (2) pre-existing diseases (valvular/congenital) excluded.

2. What is the aetiology of myocarditis?

Infectious – Viral – RNA virus: Coxsackie A and B, coronavirus including COVID-19, influenza A and B, chikungunya, dengue, hepatitis C, measles, mumps, HIV.

Bacterial: Staphylococcal, streptococcal, pneumococcal, *Mycoplasma*, *Mycobacterium*

Spirochaetal: *Borrelia* (Lyme disease), *Leptospira* (Weil's disease)

 DOI: 10.1201/9781003027584-29

Immune mediated: Autoantigen induced: Giant cell myocarditis, lymphocytic myocarditis, sarcoidosis, connective tissue disease

Vaccine induced: Tetanus toxoid induced

Drug-induced immune reaction: Penicillin, furosemide, isoniazid, methyldopa, phenytoin, thiazide

Toxin mediated – Drugs: Anthracycline, cyclophosphamide, trastuzumab, fluorouracil, catecholamines, lithium, cocaine, ethanol, IL-2, amphetamine

Heavy metal: Copper, iron

Miscellaneous: Pheochromocytoma, snake and scorpion bite

3. What is the natural history of myocarditis?

Fifty percent of acute myocarditis cases will recover spontaneously, 25% will progressively worsen to end-stage heart failure and 25% will continue to have left ventricular (LV) systolic dysfunction.

4. What are the characteristic features of giant cell myocarditis (GCM)?

GCM is a particularly devastating form of autoimmune myocarditis with a transplantation-free survival of only 5 months. It may present with cardiogenic shock, with the rate of death or cardiac transplantation of nearly 90%. Of those who survive, on follow-up nearly a third of GCM patients developed VT and 15% developed less advanced AV block and 8% complete heart block. Endomyocardial biopsy is necessary for confirming the diagnosis. If diagnosed early, the disease can be stabilized by immunosuppression while waiting for a transplant. Even if recovery occurs, there is chance of recurrence (nearly 25%), and even after transplanting it is known to occur in donor hearts. Recurrence is treated with intensified immunosuppression.

5. What are the characteristics of eosinophilic myocarditis (EM)?

Myocarditis associated with hypereosinophilia may present with biventricular heart failure evolving over weeks to months. Rarely arrhythmias may cause sudden death. It may be associated with malignancy, parasite infection and early endocardial fibrosis.

6. What are the characteristics of hypersensitivity myocarditis (HSM)?

Often drugs or toxins are the offenders. The long list includes azithromycin, benzodiazepines, clozapine, cephalosporins, dapsone, *dobutamine*, gefitinib, lithium, *loop diuretics*, methyldopa, *mexiletine*, NSAIDs, penicillins, phenobarbital, tetanus toxoid, tetracycline, *thiazide diuretics* and tricyclic antidepressants. The toxins include snake bite and scorpion bite.

HSM may present with sudden death, rapidly progressive heart failure and a more chronic presentation like cardiomyopathy.

Withdrawal of offending drugs and immunosuppression are cornerstones of therapy.

7. What is the presentation of sarcoidosis?

Sarcoid granuloma has a predilection for involving the LV free wall, posterior interventricular septum, papillary muscles, atria and RV. Conduction system involvement can cause bradyarrhythmia or tachyarrhythmia and, rarely, sudden death.

Sudden development of arrhythmia (AV blocks and/or VT) or heart failure in a patient with sarcoidosis may indicate the development of myocarditis.

Due to focal involvement, the yield of endomyocardial biopsy may be low, and CMRI/positron emission tomography (PET) may be more appropriate in most cases.

8. What are the imaging features of myocarditis?

Echocardiography may be the most important investigation in intensive care in these cases where haemodynamic instability precludes CMRI. Echocardiographic findings in patients with acute myocarditis include LV systolic/diastolic dysfunction, regional wall motion abnormality, non-specific changes in image texture, intracardiac thrombi, secondary mitral regurgitation (MR) and/or tricuspid regurgitation (TR) and coexistent pericardial involvement. In fulminant myocarditis, the chamber dimensions may be normal with increased septal thickness (caused by inflammation). Septal thickness may resolve as the inflammation resolves. Contrast echocardiography may demonstrate perfusion defects not matching the coronary artery territory. Global longitudinal strain reduction may be related to inflammation.

CMRI: Though motion artefacts and arrhythmia are its limitations, superior tissue delineation has made CMRI an attractive imaging modality in myocardial diseases (**Figures 29.1** and **29.2**). Two chamber, four chamber and short axis are imaged. A technique used for better endothelial identification is steady state free presession (SSFP). Those for tissue characterization include three basic sequences (Lake Louis criteria for myocarditis): **T2-weighted imaging** for myocardial **oedema**, contrast-enhanced fast spin echo **T1-weighted images** for **hyperaemia** and **delayed gadolinium enhancement** for necrosis or **fibrosis**. If at least two of the three tissue-based criteria are positive, myocarditis can be predicted or ruled out with a diagnostic accuracy between 59% and 92%, and in acute presentations typically around 85%. Subtle wall motion abnormalities in the inferolateral region missed by echocardiography may be picked up by CMR.

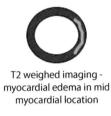 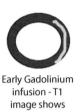 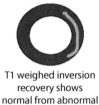

T2 weighed imaging - myocardial edema in mid myocardial location

Early Gadolinium infusion - T1 image shows enhancement

Late Gd enhancement s/o necrosis

T1 weighed inversion recovery shows normal from abnormal

Native T1 mapping shows increased values of T1 in the indicated area

Native T2 mapping shows increased values

Figure 29.1 CMRI findings in myocarditis.

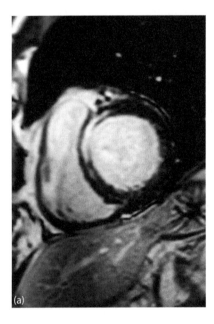 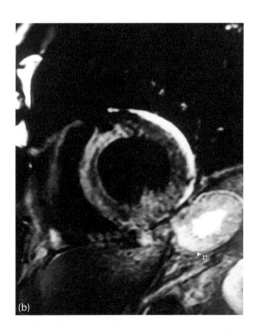

Figure 29.2 COVID myocarditis cardiac MRI images: (a) Short axis delayed enhancement sequence showing mid-myocardial enhancement in the septum, seen in COVID myocarditis. (b) Short axis STIR sequence showing patchy areas of myocardial oedema predominantly in the septum. (Image courtesy Dr Subhajit Das, consultant cardiac radiologist, NH RTIICS, Kolkata.)

Myocarditis typically presents with regional and/or global high signal intensity on T2 mapping, which usually equals or exceeds that of skeletal muscle as an internal reference by a factor of 2 and is reported as the signal intensity (SI) ratio. An increased SI ratio in acute myocarditis is a good predictor of functional recovery.

Black blood fast spin echo (T1 mapping) early after gadolinium (between 20 sec and 3 min after contrast) shows increased uptake due to inflammation, which is caused by a combination of hyperaemia, capillary leakage and necrosis. This finding is also common in Chagas disease, sarcoidosis and doxorubicin toxicity. T1 mapping may be more predictive in acute myocarditis and T2 in chronic myocarditis.

Delayed gadolinium (Gd) enhancement (>10 min after contrast with inversion recovery gradient echocardiography sequence) with increased uptake (bright areas) suggests necrosis in acute stages and scar in chronic cases. Hyperenhancement in myocarditis has two important characteristics: It does not follow coronary distribution and the endocardium is spared. This helps to differentiate it from ischaemic aetiology. LGE imaging in myocarditis has indicated two common patterns of myocardial injury: Either an intramural, rim-like pattern involving the septum or a patchy epicardial distribution involving the lateral free wall of the LV. LGE in the anteroseptal wall doubles the risk of major cardiac events. Findings in relation to Gd enhancement may resolve in 2–4 weeks.

9. What is the role of endomyocardial biopsy (EMB)?

EMB should be considered in (1) heart failure with cardiogenic shock, (2) arrhythmias: AV blocks and VT and (3) failure to respond to guideline-based treatment for >2 weeks. The right jugular vein is the commonly used access, and RV EMB is more commonly performed. Major complications (e.g., perforation) occur in 0.64% of LV EMBs and 0.82% of RV EMBs. Minor complications (including postprocedural pericardial effusion) may occur in up to 2.89% of LV EMBs and 5.10% of RV EMBs. Because of the fear of complications, and also due to the paucity of pathological centres interpreting cardiac biopsy, EMB is infrequently used.

10. What are the prognostic factors?

Poor prognostic factors include severe LV or biventricular systolic dysfunction, syncope, a prolonged QRS duration, left bundle branch block, pulmonary hypertension and New York Heart Association (NYHA) class III or IV heart failure symptoms. Patients with GCM have a substantially worse prognosis.

11. What are the management protocols in myocarditis?

General management

General management of heart failure (**Figure 29.3**) and cardiogenic shock is started as per the clinical situation (discussed in the chapters on acute decompensated heart failure [ADHF] and cardiogenic shock). Angiotensin-converting enzyme inhibitors/angiotensin receptor blockers (ACEIs/ARBs), beta-blockers (carvedilol has been used in myocarditis trials) and eplerenone may be used. Mechanical circulatory support with vasopressors, intra-aortic balloon pump (IABP), extracorporeal membrane oxygenation (ECMO) or Impella device may be required in cases of shock. Arrhythmias may be treated with amiodarone. Temporary pacing support may be required in AV blocks. In case of sarcoidosis or Chagas myocarditis, definitive treatment with steroids (for sarcoidosis) and antibiotics (intravenous ceftriaxone followed by oral amoxicillin and doxycycline for 4 weeks for Chagas) may preclude the use of a permanent pacemaker. On the other hand, in case of tachyarrhythmias like VT in cases of sarcoidosis, GCM and eosinophilic myocarditis, an automatic implantable cardiac defibrillator (AICD) may be considered. Intravenous immunoglobulin therapy may have a benefit in Kawasaki disease-related myocarditis and in a selected paediatric population. Trials of immunosuppression in dilated cardiomyopathy (DCM) in adults in the initial 6 months were not shown to be beneficial compared to longer-duration trials, probably because in the placebo arm with acute myocarditis less than 6 months subjects largely recovered spontaneously. Up to 40% of patients with chronic DCM will have immunohistochemical evidence of myocardial inflammation, defined by human leukocyte antigen (HLA) or cell-specific antigen expression on endomyocardial biopsy. But administration of immunosuppression in these cases only alters LV volume and ejection fraction to a limited extent, without improving death, hospitalization or readmission. Thus, except in specific cases mentioned later, the role of immunosuppression and antiviral therapy in acute myocarditis is yet to be determined.

Specific Treatment

- **Giant Cell Myocarditis** (*GCM*): Antithymocyte globulin (100 or 275 mg in 0.9% normal saline [NS] for 24 hr) for 1–5 days (or 1–3 days in a different protocol).

  - *Methylprednisolone*: 1 mg/kg starting after 4 weeks then decrease by 10 mg and then reduce by 10 mg every 2 weeks until the 5- to 10-mg maintenance dose is achieved. Continue for a year.

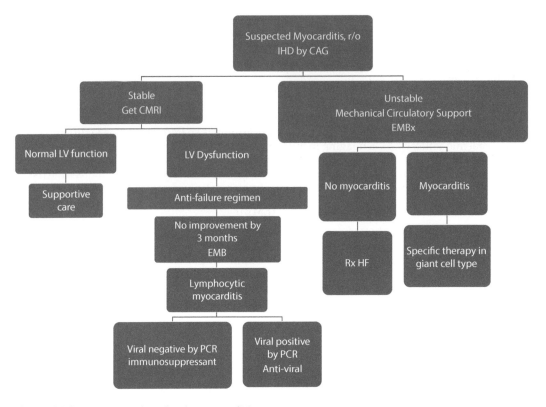

Figure 29.3 Treatment algorithm for myocarditis.

- *Cyclosporin*: 100 mg twice daily for one year. Another common regimen is tacrolimus + mycophenolate mofetil.

■ *Cardiac sarcoidosis*: Methylprednisolone in the dose stated earlier. *Duration*: 6 months.

■ *Eosinophilic Myocarditis (EM)*: Methylprednisolone in the dose stated earlier. *Duration*: 6 months.

  - *Azathioprine*: 50 mg twice daily orally for 6 months.

  - *Chronic autoimmune myocarditis*: Methylprednisolone in the dose stated earlier. *Duration*: 6 months.

  - *Azathioprine*: 50 mg twice daily orally for 6 months.

■ *Enteroviral/Adenoviral cardiomyopathy*: Interferon beta: 4 million U SC every 48 hr for the first week then 8 million U SC every 48 hr starting the second week for and 6 months.

■ *HHV-6*: Ganciclovir 1000 mg/24 hr IV × 5 days.

  - *Valganciclovir*: 900 mg/24 hr orally for 6 months.

CASE STUDY 29.1: ANECDOTAL CASE

A 22-year-old woman presented in emergency with pulmonary oedema with hypotension for which she was ventilated and started on inotropic support and intravenous diuresis with furosemide. She had a history of treatment for infertility. Her ECG showed sinus tachycardia with LV enlargement. Her chest X-ray showed pulmonary oedema with cardiomegaly. Her troponin T was 0.1 ng/mL (normal <0.01 ng/mL). An echocardiogram revealed global hypokinesia with severe LV systolic dysfunction and an LV ejection fraction (LVEF) of 25%. Her routine biochemical investigations were normal except a borderline creatinine of 1.5 mg%, which was attributed to a prerenal cause. She had a haemoglobin of 7.5 gm% which was microcytic,

---

hypochromic and was attributed to iron deficiency. After she was off inotropic support and weaned from the ventilator, she showed psychotic behaviour. She was transferred out of the intensive care unit but had persistent psychotic behaviour. Her urinalysis was normal. In view of her multiple unrelated systemic involvement, the possibility of autoimmune disease was considered. Antinuclear antibody and ds-DNA were positive with a high titre of 250 and 192 IU/mL. Her complement C3 and C4 were low at 66 mg/dL and 9 mg/dL, respectively (normal range 90–180 and 10–40 mg/dL). Her lactate dehydrogenase (LDH) was 416 U/L. Her Coombs direct and indirect tests were negative. A diagnosis of systemic lupus with myocarditis and cerebral involvement was made. She was started on intravenous methylprednisolone 1 g daily for a week. Her ejection fraction, which did not respond to the standard regimen of carvedilol, ramipril and spironolactone, showed a dramatic improvement from 25% to 38%. Subsequently, she was started on oral prednisolone 1 mg/kg/day and hydroxychloroquine 200 mg/day. By 2 weeks she was free of orthopnoea and though her neuropsychiatric symptoms had improved, they were not entirely gone. At 1-month follow-up, echocardiography showed a normal LV systolic function. She has neither dyspnoea nor any neuropsychiatric symptoms at 1-month follow-up.

FURTHER READING

1. Ghosh K, Sikdar S, Ghosh S, et al. Heart Failure in a Young Lady: A Reversible Cause. *Journal of Diagnostics.* 2015, 2(1): 1–4.
2. Pollack A, Kontrovitch A R, Fuster V, et al. Viral Myocarditis – Diagnosis, Treatment Options, and Current Controversies. *Nat. Rev. Cardiol.* Advance online publication 21 July 2015; doi:10.1038/nrcardio.2015.108
3. Ammirati E, Frigerio M, Adler E, et al. Management of Acute Myocarditis and Chronic Inflammatory Cardiomyopathy: An Expert Consensus Document. *Circ Heart Fail.* 2020: 663–687
4. Caforio A P, Pankuweit S, Arbustini E, et al. Current state of knowledge on aetiology, diagnosis, management, and therapy of myocarditis: A position statement of the European Society of Cardiology Working Group on Myocardial and Pericardial Diseases. *Eur Heart J* (2013), 34: 2636–2648.

30 Stress Cardiomyopathy

Sunandan Sikdar, Soumik Basu, and Sumanta Chatterjee

1. How do you diagnose stress cardiomyopathy or Takotsubo syndrome (TTS)?

Diagnostic criteria for stress cardiomyopathy include:

Population: Common in postmenopausal women.

Triggers—Common triggers: Emotional, neurologic (cerebrovascular accident [CVA], subarachnoid haemorrhage), pheochromocytoma, seizures.

Rarer triggers: Obstructive airway disease and respiratory failure (most common physical trigger), urosepsis, operation, fracture, malignancy.

Time course: Transient

Complete recovery of ventricular systolic function within days to weeks.

Morphology: Left ventricular wall motion abnormality – hypokinesia, akinesia, or dyskinesia presenting as apical ballooning or midventricular, basal or focal wall motion abnormalities.

Right ventricular involvement (in one-third of cases).

Transitions between all types can exist.

The regional wall motion abnormality usually extends beyond a single epicardial vascular distribution.

Rare cases can exist where the regional wall motion abnormality is present in the subtended myocardial territory of a single coronary artery (focal TTS).

Evidence of cardiac injury: ECG changes: ST-segment elevation, ST-segment depression, T-wave inversion and QTc prolongation

Biomarkers: Moderate elevation of troponin and brain natriuretic peptide (BNP)

Exclusions: Potential coronary lesion (i.e., no critical stenosis, no unstable plaque)

Myocarditis

Table 30.1 provides the **interTAK** diagnostic criteria.

Table 30.1: Diagnostic Criteria for Stress Cardiomyopathy

Parameter	Score	
Female sex	25	Low/Intermediate probability, Score <70
Emotional stress	24	
Physical stress	13	
ST-segment depression	12	High probability Score >70
Psychiatric disorder	11	
Neurologic disorder	9	
QT prolongation	6	

2. What is the etiopathogenesis of TTS?

Epicardial spasm: Sympathetically mediated epicardial spasm of multiple vessels has been described.

Microcirculatory dysfunction: Due to catecholamines acting on $\alpha 1$, and an endothelin type A receptor has been described.

Catecholamine toxicity on cardiomyocytes: Increased catecholamines lead to adrenergic receptor-mediated calcium overload and cellular dysfunction. In mammalian hearts left ventricular (LV) β-adrenergic receptor density is highest in the apex, while sympathetic innervation is the lowest.

DOI: 10.1201/9781003027584-30

Studies have found that β2 receptors predominate in the apex and β1 predominate in the base. Increased catecholamine may cause a switch from a β2 Gs (positive inotropic) to β2 Gi (negative inotropic) state. Activation of the β2 Gi pathway also leads to oxidative stress by the peroxynitrite pathway and cellular dysfunction selectively in the apical segment.

Hormonal factors: The preponderance of postmenopausal women can be explained by the fact that oestrogens can attenuate catecholamine-mediated vasoconstriction and decrease the sympathetic response to mental stress.

Survival pathways: Hypokinesia has been theorized as a way of reducing energy requirements and minimizing cellular damage.

3. What are the types of TTS?

There are four types: Based on LV angiography morphology (RAO view) or echocardiography (**Figure 30.1**):

1. *Apical TTS* (80%): Most common and the classical form of TTS. Systolic apical ballooning of the LV – it looks like a Japanese octopus pot with a narrow neck and wide base used for trapping octopuses. There is hyperkinesia of the base with hypokinesia of the mid and apical segments.

2. *Midventricular TTS* (15%): The mid-ventricle is predominantly affected.

3. *Basal TTS* (2.2%): This is often called basal hypokinesia with apical sparing. It is found more commonly with pheochromocytoma, epinephrine-induced TTS or subarachnoid haemorrhage. This pattern warrants investigation for these causes.

4. *Focal TTS* (1.5%): Usual focal pattern, often in the anterolateral segment.

5. *Global*: Rare presentation.

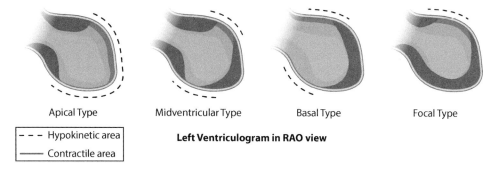

Left Ventriculogram in RAO view

Apical Type   Midventricular Type   Basal Type   Focal Type

- - - Hypokinetic area
—— Contractile area

Figure 30.1   Stress cardiomyopathy: Morphologic types based on ventriculogram.

4. What are the ECG changes in TTS?

a. *ST elevation*: Nearly half of the patients have ST elevation. This ST elevation is predominant in the anterior, lateral and apical leads (V4–V6, I). In contrast in case of anterior wall myocardial infarction (MI), ST elevation dominates in V1–V3, I and aVL. *An ST depression in aVR and ST not elevated in V1 is a specific ECG feature of TTS. In general, reciprocal ST depression is rare* – another fact that differentiates TTS from acute coronary syndrome/ST-segment MI (ACS/STEMI). There is rapid evolution of these changes in 1–3 days.

b. *Q waves*: May be present – marker of myocardial oedema and not necrosis.

c. Transient left bundle branch block (LBBB) may occur.

d. *Deep T-wave inversion*: Within 2 days the changes noted earlier frequently change into deep T inversion (also common in subarachnoid haemorrhage – the mechanism may be similar). T-wave inversion may be the presenting finding and may persist for months. It may be evidence of stunning.

e. *QT prolongation occurs with T inversion*: It is a substrate for torsades, ventricular fibrillation (VF) and sudden death in this disease.

ECG monitoring of the QT interval is thus mandatory in the cardiac care unit (CCU) for TTS. The highest risk for torsades occurs in the second to fourth day of onset and occurs more frequently in those with a QT interval of >500 msec.

5. What are the changes in biomarkers?

Troponin is raised in >90% of patients with TTS. A characteristic of biomarkers in TTS is the low troponin, high BNP pattern, unlike in ACS where it is just the opposite. The moderate rise of troponin is enigmatic because it does not seem to correlate with the wide extent of regional wall motion abnormality (RWMA) recorded in the echocardiogram. A serum BNP to troponin ratio >502 identifies TTS with 100% specificity. Since creatinine phosphokinase (CPK) is negligibly raised compared to troponin, a troponin/CPK MB ratio also has some value.

6. What are the echocardiographic findings of TTS?

Echocardiography is the first non-invasive imaging modality.

a. *RWMA* in a circumferential pattern not conforming to coronary territories. Usually in an apical ballooning pattern in the majority, but hypokinesia may also occur in the midventricular or basal segments in a few cases.

b. *Left ventricular outflow tract obstruction (LVOTO)*: It occurs in the acute phase in 20% of the population, usually in elderly women, with a septal bulge, systolic anterior motion (SAM) of the mitral valve and basal hypercontractility.

c. *Mitral regurgitation (MR)*: Reversible moderate to severe MR is found in 20% of cases of TTS because of tethering of mitral leaflets, displacement of papillary muscles and SAM.

d. *Apical thrombus* may occur due to apical hypokinesia.

7. What is the role of coronary angiography (CAG) and ventriculography?

Since the differentiation between TTS and ACS by non-invasive tests may not be accurate, CAG is mandatory to rule out critical epicardial stenosis and establish a diagnosis of TTS. Slow flow may be present. Non-critical coronary plaque may also occur. Ventriculography in the RAO view shows any of the four different morphologic types of wall motion described earlier. Since these abnormalities are transitory, documenting the wall motion by ventriculographic cine frames is important for future reference.

8. What is the role of cardiac magnetic resonance (CMR) in TTS?

Specific CMR criteria for TTS diagnosis at the time of acute presentation include the combination of typical RWMAs, oedema and the absence of evidence of irreversible tissue injury (late gadolinium enhancement [LGE]). However, CMR is more useful in the subacute phase of TTS when the clinical condition stabilizes. While LGE is usually absent and predicts complete normalization of LV function, subtle fibrosis may indicate worse outcomes. In most TTS patients, myocardial oedema is present in regions with abnormal systolic function possibly due to inflammation, increased wall stress and/or transient ischaemia and is indicative of the extent and severity of tissue injury.

9. How do you treat TTS?

a. *Antiplatelets, statins and antithrombotics* are administered as in ACS in the emergency room. So are the anti-heart failure therapies. After CAG shows no critically obstructive lesion, aspirin and statin may continue. Intravenous fluid is given in LVOTO.

b. *Levosimendan*: The difference from ACS occurs in the use of vasopressors during hypotension. Because TTS is a hyperadrenergic state, **all vasopressors and inotropes are contraindicated in the TTS shock state except levosimendan**. Its use, however, is limited to those patients with impaired systolic function, without LVOTO and with systolic blood pressure >90 mmHg. Levosimendan should be infused for 24 hr at a dose of 0.1 µg/kg/min, without a loading dose. During infusion, the patient should be haemodynamically and ECG monitored for the risk of hypotension and arrhythmias.

c. *Beta-blockers*: Useful and important cornerstone of therapy, especially in prolonged QT, LVOTO and catecholamine storm. Start with short-acting agents and with lower doses.

d. *Ivabradine*: TTS patients with LVOTO may benefit from the I_f channel inhibitor ivabradine.

e. *Angiotensin-converting enzyme inhibitor/angiotensin receptor blocker (ACEI/ARB)*: Useful in heart failure and preventing recurrences.

f. *Nitrates*: If angina is the presenting symptom and epicardial spasm is suspected, use nitrates. Avoid in LVOTO.

g. *Mechanical circulatory support (MCS)*: Impella has been claimed as the best MCS in TTS with shock, as it overcomes LVOTO and improves MR. An intra-aortic balloon pump (IABP) may increase the transaortic gradient in LVOTO. Extracorporeal membrane oxygenation (ECMO) reduces preload and increases end-organ perfusion at the cost of increased afterload, causing a possible rise in the transaortic gradient and worsening of MR.

Long-term treatment: ACEIs/ARBs should be continued as they prevent recurrence. However, beta-blockers have not been shown to reduce recurrence. The role of oestrogen supplementation in postmenopausal women is not clear.

10. What are the complications of TTS?

Common: Acute heart failure, LVOTO, MR, cardiogenic shock.

Rare: Atrial fibrillation, LV thrombus, cardiac arrest (4%–6%), AV block ~5%, tachyarrhythmia, bradyarrhythmia, torsades de pointes (2%–5%), death (1%–4.5%) and ventricular tachycardia/fibrillation (~3%).

11. What are the determinants of the prognosis?

Markers of adverse in-hospital outcome: Male, physical trigger, acute neurologic or psychiatric diseases, initial troponin >10 upper reference limit, and admission LVEF <45%.

Long-term adverse outcomes are dependent not on the morphologic variant per se but on atrial fibrillation, LVEF<45% and neurologic disease. In the largest TTS registry to date, death rates are estimated to be 5.6% and the rate of major adverse cardiac events (MACEs) 9.9% per patient-year.

Recurrence may take place after as little as 3 weeks or as late as several years after the initial event. Most adverse events take place in the first year.

FURTHER READING

1. Ghadri J.-R., Wittstein I. S., Prasad A. et al. International Expert consensus document on Takotsubo syndrome (part II): Diagnostic workup, outcome, and management. *European Heart Journal*, 2018 (39). 2047–2062.
2. Templin C., Ghadri J. R., Diekmann J. et al. Clinical features and outcomes of Takotsubo (stress) cardiomyopathy. *New England Journal of Medicine* 2015 (373): 929–938.

31 Acute Decompensated Heart Failure

Sunandan Sikdar and Munna Das

1. What is heart failure (HF)?

It is a clinical syndrome characterized by symptoms and signs due to a cardiac abnormality, resulting in a reduced cardiac output and/or elevated intracardiac pressures at rest or during stress.

2. What are the types of HF?

The European Society for Cardiology (ESC) 2016 guidelines have classified HF into the following types (**Table 31.1**).

Table 31.1: Classification of Heart Failure

Type	HF with Reduced EF (HFrEF)	HF with Mildly Reduced EF (HFmrEF)	HF with Preserved EF (HFpEF)
Signs + symptoms	Present	Present	Present
LVEF	<40%	41%–49%	50% and above
BNP/NT-pro-BNP	Not required	Raised	Raised
Diastolic dysfunction	Not required	Present or LAE	Present or LAE

3. What are the stages of HF?

American Heart Association (AHA) stages include the following:

Stage A: High risk for development of HF but no structural disease

Stage B: Structural disease present but no symptoms

Stage C: Structural disease with symptoms of HF (or under treatment)

Stage D: End-stage disease requiring specialized therapies

4. What are the common causes of HF?

The common causes of heart failure are listed in Table 31.2.

Table 31.2: Causes of Heart Failure

Basic Mechanism	Broad Category	Examples
Myocardial disease	• Ischaemia • Toxin • Infiltrative • Genetic	• Post-infarction • Alcohol • Amyloidosis • HCM, DCM, ARVC Non-compaction
Abnormal loading condition	• Hypertension • Valvular disease • High-output states	• Hypertensive crisis • Aortic stenosis and regurgitation • Anaemia, thyrotoxicosis
Arrhythmia	• Tachyarrhythmia • Bradyarrhythmia	• Atrial flutter, PJRT complete heart block

5. What is the role of ECG in heart failure?

An absolutely normal ECG is rare in acute decompensated HF (ADHF), and tachycardia is the most common finding. ECG should be used to rapidly determine: (1) Myocardial infarction, (2) arrhythmia, (3) QRS width, (4) any other specific finding like right ventricular (RV) strain in pulmonary embolism.

6. What are the recommended blood tests for HF?

Arterial blood gas is the initial test to guide therapy on admission for acute decompensation. Others are CBC, creatinine, sodium, potassium, liver function tests, TSH, FBG, and HbA1c. Brain natriuretic

DOI: 10.1201/9781003027584-31

peptide (BNP) or NT-pro-BNP is a marker of importance to confirm diagnosis and also monitor response to therapy. The diagnostic cut-off of BNP for ruling out and ruling in HF is <100 and >400 pg/mL, respectively. The corresponding cut-off values of NT-Pro-BNP for ruling out and ruling in HF are <300 and >450 pg/mL (<50 years), >900 pg/mL (50–75 years) and >1800 pg/mL (>75 years), respectively. Troponin should be used judiciously if the purpose is ischaemia screening. Mild elevations are common in even HF due to non-ischaemic causes and may lead to unnecessary tests.

7. What are the imaging tests?

1. Echocardiography

2. *Chest X-ray*: To rule out pneumonia and parenchymal lung disease and rule in pulmonary oedema

3. *Lung ultrasound*: For B lines, three or more B lines in each of two quadrants (anterior and axillary) bilaterally are suggestive of pulmonary oedema (see lung ultrasound chapter).

4. *Cardiac MRI (after stabilization)*: Transmural contrast enhancement with T1 mapping with a territorial distribution suggests nonviability in ischaemic heart disease and LV dysfunction. Mid-LV wall and epicardial hyperenhancement suggest sarcoidosis, myocarditis and rarely hypertrophic cardiomyopathy (HCM). Global subendocardial hyperenhancement may suggest amyloidosis, systemic sclerosis or post-transplant (**Figure 31.1**).

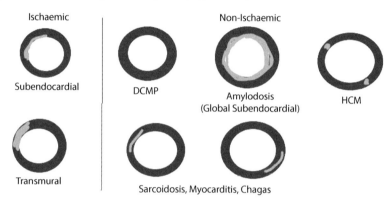

Figure 31.1 CMRI findings in heart failure.

8. What is the indication for a pulmonary artery catheter in HF?

In case of respiratory distress or impaired perfusion whose filling pressure cannot be determined non-invasively. Other less common indications are in patients waiting for heart transplant or mechanical circulatory support and those having pulmonary hypertension and are in line for structural heart intervention. Except in the cardiothoracic unit, use of a pulmonary catheter is uncommon. Clinical and echocardiography clues suffice.

9. What is the indication for a coronary angiogram (CAG) in HF?

If there is a wall motion abnormality on echocardiogram, suggestive clinical history of ischaemic heart disease and the patient is a candidate for revascularization, CAG should be done.

10. What are the triggers for acute HF?

The common causes are acute coronary syndrome, infection, tachyarrhythmia or bradyarrhythmia, hypertension, increased fluid intake, medications like NSAIDs and pregnancy.

11. What are the initial steps of management?

1. *Assess haemodynamics*: Two parameters (perfusion = warm/cold and congestion = wet/dry) and four sets of patients (**Table 31.3**)

   Warm-wet: Hypertensive failure (most common), ischaemic HF

   Warm-dry: Compensated HF, anaemia-related HF, thyrotoxicosis

   Cold-wet: Cardiogenic shock with pulmonary oedema (poorest prognosis)

   Cold-dry: Right-sided failure (e.g., pulmonary embolism)

Table 31.3: Classification of ADHF

Cold-wet	**Warm wet**
Cardiogenic shock with pulmonary oedema	Hypertensive heart failure
Cold-dry	**Warm dry**
Pulmonary embolism	Thyrotoxicosis, anaemia

The ESC guideline has classified Acute Heart Failure into four syndromes - Acute Decompensated Heart failure (ADHF), Acute Pulmonary Edema (example hypertensive heart failure), Isolated right heart failure and Cardiogenic Shock. The first and the last share similarites, especially the presence of reduced LVEF and one may progress to the other.

Indicators of hypoperfusion: Systolic blood pressure (SBP) <90 mmHg, confused patient, lactate >2 mmol/L

First optimize the blood pressure with inotropes/vasopressors. Start arrangement for mechanical circulatory support if not stabilizing with vasopressors.

2. *Assess respiration*: *Indicators of respiratory failure*: SpO_2 <90%, respiratory rate >25/min/use of accessory muscle: Start non-invasive ventilation (continuous positive airway pressure [CPAP] or non-invasive positive pressure ventilation [NIPPV]), especially if normotensive, starting with a positive end-expiratory pressure (PEEP) of 5–7.5 cm H_2O. Complications include anxiety, claustrophobia, dry mucous membranes, worsening RV failure, hypercapnia, pneumothorax and aspiration. In hypertensive crisis with failure, injectable morphine 3 mg IV may be useful. But morphine should be avoided in hypotension, bradycardia, drowsiness and hypercapnia.

    If it does not improve/worsens/the patient is already in severe respiratory failure: pO_2 <60 mmHg, pCO_2 >50 mmHg (in non-COPD patient), pH <7.25 or patient becoming obtunded or is hypotensive (SBP <90 mmHg with vasopressors): Intubation and mechanical ventilation should be strongly considered.

3. *Start pharmacological therapy for HF*: See later.

4. *Address the specific aetiology of HF*: Use the CHAMP acronym of A**C**S, **H**ypertensive emergency, **A**rrhythmia, Acute **M**echanical cause (e.g., acute mitral regurgitation due to ruptured papillary muscle) and **P**ulmonary embolism.

12. What are the poor prognostic markers in ADHF?

The three important prognostic markers of ADHF are hypoperfusion, natriuretic peptide levels and renal dysfunction. Raised lactate >2 mmol/L is also a marker of poor prognosis, as it indicates tissue hypoxia

13. What are the optimal medical therapies for HF?

1. *Loop diuretics*: Since volume overload (congestion) is present in nearly 95% of patients with HF and rapid symptomatic relief is essential, loop diuretics are the first-line drugs. Volume overload is to the tune of 4–5 L, sometimes even more. To improve bioavailability (because gut congestion is common), intravenous bolus plus infusion is common practice. However, there was no outcome difference between continuous infusion versus intermittent bolus doses in the DOSE study. The starting IV dose is 2–2.5 times that of chronic oral therapy in the case of furosemide, the most commonly used diuretic:

    • *Injectable furosemide*: 40–60 mg IV bolus followed by 3–5 mg/hr until congestion is controlled is often adequate.

    • *Oral or injectable torsemide*: 20–50 mg bolus then 5–20 mg/hr.

    Side effects: Activation of the neurohormonal system, worsening renal function and hypokalaemia are common.

2. *Distal tubule diuretics*: Resistance to diuretics is frequent and distal loop diuretics like metolazone 2.5–5 mg PO once daily may be added if congestion (bibasal crepitations or pedal oedema) persists.

3. *Potassium-sparing diuretics*: These agents not only prevent hypokalaemia due to loop diuretics but also reduce mortality on long-term use in HFrEF. Spironolactone 25 mg once or twice daily or eplerenone 25 mg are the preferred agents. The principal side effect is hyperkalaemia, and monitoring potassium regularly in the critical care unit (CCU) is critical. Spironolactone causes gynaecomastia on prolonged (months) use.

4. *Vasodilators*: Vasodilators are the second most important part of therapy. Two commonly used vasodilators are nitroglycerin (NTG) (predominantly a venodilator) and nitroprusside (a balanced, both venous + arterial dilator).

   NTG, in the initial doses, causes venodilation leading to reduced LV filling pressures followed by arterial dilation at higher doses especially if there is underlying vasoconstriction. It dilates the epicardial coronaries and reduces ischaemia. NTG is a nitric oxide donor and increased cellular levels of cyclic guanosine monophosphate (cGMP) causes relaxation of smooth muscles of the vessel wall. NTG is usually started at 20 micrograms/min and titrated upwards with an acute goal of reducing mean arterial pressure (MAP) by 10 mmHg and providing symptom relief. It should be discontinued if SBP <100 mmHg. The principal side effect is nitrate headache (20% in 24 hr) and hypotension (5%), which should be closely monitored. Nitrate-related hypotension resolves rapidly on its own and rarely requires administration of IV fluids, to which it responds promptly. Nitrate-related hypotension is severe if there is concurrent sildenafil use. Hence, nitrates are contraindicated if there is a history of recent usage of a phosphodiesterase type 5 (PDE5) inhibitor. The principal limitation is development of tolerance, which occurs in 24 hr in most cases.

   Sodium nitroprusside (SNP) is a balanced vasodilator that is used in special situations: In LVF with hypertensive crisis or in chronic kidney disease with refractory hypertension or in LVF in the setting of acute mitral regurgitation (MR). It is a prodrug that generates nitric oxide and cyanide. It reduces afterload, wall stress and ischaemia and has a very short half-life. Because of the fear of hypotension and cyanide toxicity (increased in impaired liver and renal function), SNP is often underused. The starting dose is 0.3 mcg/kg/min and should be titrated to a SBP ~100 mmHg (use <4 mcg/kg/min). Since it is photosensitive, the SNP bottle should be covered during infusion. As there is a concern of intramyocardial coronary steal, SNP should not be used in active myocardial ischaemia. Though invasive BP monitoring was previously advocated, non-invasive BP monitoring is often useful in selected subjects.

5. *Inotropes and vasopressors*: See the section on cardiogenic shock.

14. What is the role of ultrafiltration?

Conceptually ultrafiltration should be able to remove a larger amount of isotonic fluid and hence a larger amount of salt in a shorter time without activating the neurohumoral system in comparison to loop diuretics. But studies (UNLOAD and CARRESS) have failed to show benefit in terms of better outcomes. Worsening renal function and dialysis catheter-related complications have been the Achilles heel of this therapy. Ultrafiltration was used at a fluid removal rate of 200 mL/hr in CARRESS. This therapy should be used in HF with advanced renal disease with oliguria where diuretic efficacy is really suboptimum. The rate of fluid removal must be reduced if the MAP is borderline or falls on initiation of ultrafiltration, as these subsets of patients are "sicker" and poorly tolerate hypotension, especially if they have severe LV systolic dysfunction.

15. What drugs are prescribed at discharge?

Principles of management of HFrEF are given in **Figure 31.2**.

Angiotensin-converting enzyme inhibitors (ACEIs): These drugs are the cornerstones of therapy, as there is a 27% relative risk reduction with respect to mortality in HFrEF when compared to placebo over a period of 1 year (enalapril in the CONSENSUS trial). Administration of an ACEI inhibits the conversion of angiotensin I to angiotensin II (results in inhibition of the AT1 receptor pathway) and prevents the breakdown of bradykinin (increased bradykinin causes cough and angioedema – two important side effects of ACEIs). The AT1 receptor pathway is known to cause vasoconstriction, sodium retention and sympathetic activation, which are inhibited by ACEIs. ACEIs are also recommended in patients with asymptomatic LV systolic dysfunction to reduce the risk of HF development, HF hospitalization and death. Enalapril (starting dose 2.5 mg twice daily, target dose 20 mg twice daily) and ramipril (starting dose 2.5 mg once daily, target dose 10 mg once daily) are the two drugs in this class with robust trial evidence. Adverse effects include hyperkalaemia, hypotension and metallic taste. They are contraindicated in pregnancy. Use with caution in renal failure (creatinine >3 mg/dL).

Angiotensin receptor blockers (ARBs): These drugs inhibit the AT1 receptor directly with attendant benefits. Because they do not increase bradykinin levels, unlike ACEI, cough is reduced. Valsartan (Val-HeFT trial, VALIANT trial) was non-inferior to ACEIs and should be used in

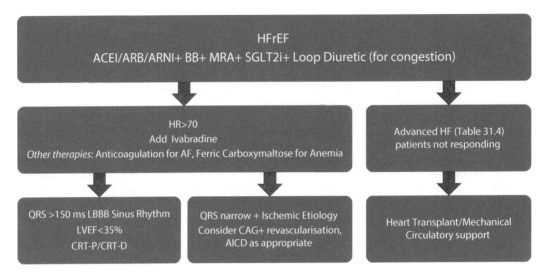

Figure 31.2 Management of HFrEF.

ACEI-intolerant patients (often cough is the cause) with a starting dose of 40 mg twice daily (target dose 160 mg twice daily). Adverse effects and contraindications are similar. *A combination of ACEI and ARB should not be used as they increase hyperkalaemia, hypotension and renal dysfunction without any added benefit.*

Angiotensin receptor–neprilysin inhibitors (ARNIs): Neprilysin is a membrane-bound endopeptidase found predominantly in the kidney, which hydrolyzes natriuretic peptides (ANP/BNP/CNP) and degrades others (urodilantin, adrenomedullin, bradykinin, substance P, etc). The neprilysin inhibitor sacubitril causes increased levels of natriuretic peptide and thereby results in beneficial effects (vasodilation, antifibrosis and antihypertrophy). Since neprilysin also degrades angiotensin II, administration of sacubitril causes increased levels of angiotensin II and consequent activation of the deleterious renin-angiotensin-aldosterone system (RAAS) by the AT1 receptor pathway where angiotensin II binds. Thus, to counteract the RAAS activation by sacubitril, an AT1 receptor blocker valsartan has been added into a single molecule of sacubitril + valsartan (ARNI). The landmark PARADIGM-HF trial showed that administration of ARNI results in a 16% reduction of all-cause mortality, 21% reduction of sudden death and 20% reduction in cardiovascular death and HF hospitalization when compared to its active comparator enalapril (up to then the standard of care in a dose of 10 mg twice daily) in ambulatory HFrEF when given for a median period of 27 months. It has to be started once ADHF settles and SBP crosses 100 mmHg in HFrEF (LVEF<40%), eGFR >30 mL/min/1.73 m^2 and serum potassium <5 mmol/L. The TRANSITION trial supported initiation of ARNI in ADHF patients pre-discharge. Patients previously on ACEIs should be given a washout period of 36 hr before starting an ARNI (not required for ARBs). The starting dose can be 50 mg twice daily (especially those with borderline SBP, the elderly and those with renal impairment) and built up over 2–4 weeks to 100 mg twice daily and finally to 200 mg twice daily if the patient tolerates it (monitor SBP, potassium and creatinine). The side effects and contraindications of ARBs apply to ARNIs too, with a rare occurrence of angioedema, in which case it should be stopped immediately. NT-pro-BNP instead of BNP may be used to monitor therapy during the dose titration phase. As per the ESC 2016 guidelines, the drugs of choice in initiating HFrEF treatment are ACEI + a beta-blocker (class I indication). An ARNI can be used in place of an ACEI if the patient is still symptomatic on ACEIs or intolerant to ACEIs (class I). If there is history of ventricular tachyarrhythmia, an ARNI may be the favoured drug over an ACEI as it reduces sudden death (class I).

Beta-blockers: Beta-blockers inhibit the sympathetic system and RAAS (β1 receptor antagonism), prevent ischaemia, have a beneficial effect on ventricular remodelling and favourably modify myocardial gene expression. Robust data in chronic HFrEF exists for carvedilol (COPERNICUS), bisoprolol (CIBIS), nebivolol (SENIORS) and metoprolol (MERIT–HF) showing a reduction of all-cause mortality (39% in COPERNICUS), HF hospitalization and sudden death (44% in CIBIS II).

However, initiation after an ADHF lacks adequate representation in large trials. Once ADHF settles or in cases of acute LVF where heart rate control is paramount, the beta-blocker should be started in the lowest possible doses and gradually built up, doubling doses after > 2 weeks or as the patient tolerates: Carvedilol 3.125 mg twice daily (target dose: 25 mg twice daily), bisoprolol 1.25 mg once daily (target dose 10 mg once daily), metoprolol XL 25 mg once daily (target dose: 200 mg once daily) and nebivolol 1.25 mg once daily (target dose: 10 mg once daily). Contraindications to beta-blockers include bradycardia <50/min, Mobitz type II block or more advanced heart block and severe obstructive airway disease. Bradycardia and/or hypotension leading to dizziness is common during up-titration of the dosage, especially those who are elderly or those with borderline BP. Fatigue, sexual dysfunction, sleep disturbance and hypoglycaemia unawareness are other subtle effects of long-term therapy. However, sudden withdrawal of a beta-blocker due these concerns is also risky because β1 receptors are up-regulated on chronic beta-blocker usage, and ventricular arrhythmia (catecholamine storm)/ angina may occur. It is better to reduce the dose and continue. For the elderly (>70 years) nebivolol is the favoured beta-blocker based on trial (SENIORS) evidence. For obstructive airway disease, more selective β1 blockers like bisoprolol and nebivolol are preferred. In the case of chronic kidney disease lipophilic beta-blockers like metoprolol, carvedilol and bisoprolol can be used (in that order of preference). Though it looks counterintuitive, trials have failed to show a mortality benefit of beta-blockers in HF with atrial fibrillation (AF) even if the heart rate is uncontrolled at initiation.

Ivabradine: Ivabradine is a selective funny current (I_f) inhibitor in the pacemaker cells of the sinoatrial node reducing the Na and K flow through the *Hyperpolarization-activated Cyclic Nucleotide-gated transmembrane channel* (HCN). It reduces the slope of spontaneous diastolic depolarization and hence slows the heart rate in sinus rhythm. Since it binds to the inner part of the HCN channel in the open state, the drug shows "use-dependence," that is, the faster the heart rate, the more effective it is. Unlike beta-blockers it has no negative inotropic effect and is not contraindicated in asthma (hence, it is the ideal HR-lowering agent in COPD). The SHIFT trial showed that in stable symptomatic (predominantly ischaemic) HF (LVEF<35%) in sinus rhythm (HR >70/min), the addition of ivabradine (started at 5 mg twice daily, target 7.5 mg twice daily, 70% reached target dose) on top of guideline-directed ACEI + BB reduced HF hospitalization by 26% in nearly 2 years (no mortality benefit). Though robust trial data is not available in ADHF, ivabradine can be started once vasopressors have been tapered and HR >75/min, starting at 2.5 mg or 5 mg twice daily. Gradually a beta-blocker is added once SBP improves beyond 100 mmHg. Contraindications include bradyarrhythmias (sick sinus syndrome/AV blocks/ patients dependent on ventricular pacing), use of verapamil/diltiazem and use of cytochrome 3A4 inhibitors. Side effects include visual side effect (flashes) due to retinal I_f blockade and bradycardia. In HF nearly 40% have renal dysfunction, and ivabradine at 2.5 mg or 5 mg twice daily maintains its efficacy in this subset.

Mineralocorticoid receptor (MR) antagonists: RAAS activation in HF causes increased aldosterone level and MR up-regulation. Even RAAS blockage by an ACEI cause "aldosterone escape" by other pathways and continued salt + water retention, vasoconstriction, fibrosis and sympathetic activation. Spironolactone and eplerenone competitively bind the aldosterone-dependent potassium channel in the distal tubule, and their effectivity is determined by the level of aldosterone. Eplerenone, being a more selective antagonist of MR with nonsignificant binding to oestrogen receptors, does not cause gynaecomastia, unlike in the case of spironolactone where this adverse effect causes drug discontinuation. It also has a shorter half-life. The benefit of spironolactone (RALES trial) and eplerenone (EPHUSUS and EMPHASIS trials) demonstrated mortality reduction (~30% in RALES) and rehospitalization in patients with HFrEF. In HFpEF spironolactone had a beneficial effect in only those with raised natriuretic peptide but no mortality reduction. The initiating dose in the case of both drugs is 25 mg once daily and built up to 50 mg once daily. If already on RAAS blockers, a higher dosage is not recommended. Hyperkalaemia is common and requires strict monitoring, especially in the case of concomitant RAAS blockade. Contraindications include advanced renal failure (creatinine >3 mg/dL).

Loop diuretics: In HFrEF the failing heart tries to preserve cardiac output. It compensates for the lack of contractility by increasing preload by intravascular fluid retention (activating RAAS) and increasing HR (activating the neurohormonal system). Diuretics reduce the volume overload state and by a venodilator (both systemic and pulmonary) effect, reduce the preload, and by extension both systemic and pulmonary congestion. Thus, though diuretic use does not translate to improved outcomes or mortality benefit, they give dramatic symptom relief. Loop diuretics are a cornerstone of therapy in this regard. They inhibit the Na-K-Cl transporter in the ascending limb of the loop of Henle, leading to both sodium and water excretion. Torsemide has a higher bioavailability than furosemide, a fact which is important as gut oedema is common. Intravenous furosemide is twice as effective as the oral formulation. The equivalent doses are furosemide 40 mg = torsemide 20 mg = ethacrynic acid 50 mg. *Ethacrynic acid is the diuretic of choice in case of sulphur allergy.* The starting doses are higher in ADHF and gradually they are tapered to maintenance doses (furosemide 40 mg twice or thrice daily usually, torsemide 10 mg twice daily). Higher doses are required in nephropathy and in some cases of severe LV dysfunction. Diuretic use results in neurohormonal/RAAS activation (leading to diuretic resistance, **Figure 31.3**), and they should be given in conjunction with beta-blockers. Other side effects include hypokalaemia (requires monitoring to prevent lethal VT/VF), renal dysfunction (dose reduction if creatinine rises/dehydration occurs), hypotension (dehydration) and ototoxicity (reversible) in higher doses of furosemide/ethacrynic acid. Fluid restriction <1.5 L/day and salt restriction <2 g/day are important lifestyle measures to improve diuretic effectiveness.

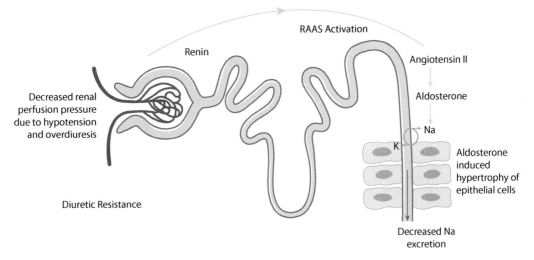

Figure 31.3   Diuretic resistance in heart failure.

SGLT2 inhibitors: Empagliflozin (EMPEROR REDUCED trial) and Dapagliflozin (DAPA-HF trial) are now cornerstones of HF therapy. Addition of these drugs has resulted in nearly 25% reduction in the combined end point of HF hospitalization and cardiovascular (CV) death over optimal medical therapy in patients with New York Heart Association (NYHA) class II–IV and LVEF <40%. Further, empagliflozin resulted in a reduction of eGFR decline.

Digoxin: The role of digoxin has become limited due to its narrow therapeutic window. It is indicated for patients with HF in sinus rhythm to reduce HF hospitalization and in some cases of HF with AF where in spite of other rate-lowering drugs there is a rapid ventricular rate. Digoxin is used to lower the HR to 70–90/min.

Antiplatelets/Anticoagulation: Antiplatelets are used in ischaemic heart disease as per the guideline described in previous chapters. Anticoagulation is used in the case of AF.

Statins: Used in ischaemic heart disease as per guidelines described in previous chapters.

Parenteral iron therapy: Iron deficiency anaemia is common in HF (more than one-third) and regarded as a factor in HF progression. Depleted intracellular iron leads to mitochondrial dysfunction and adverse myocardial energetics. It is diagnosed as absolute iron deficiency (inadequate supply) if serum ferritin <100 mcg/L. It is a functional deficiency (trapped iron) if serum ferritin 100–299 mcg/L with transferrin saturation <20%. As HF involves systemic stress and ferritin is an acute phase reactant, the cut-off values in this condition have been kept higher than in routine iron deficiency anaemia. Intravenous iron as ferric carboxymaltose can be given in the dosage of 500 mg in 100 mL normal saline over 1 hr on 2 consecutive days. On sixth week if Hb <10 gm/dL, another intravenous dose of 500 mg can be given if body weight is <70 kg, and 1000 mg if body weight >70 kg. Total iron deficit is calculated by Ganzoni's formula : body weight × 2.4 × (15 - Hb) + 500 mg. Intravenous iron has been shown to alleviate symptoms and reduce HF hospitalization in patients with LVEF

<45%, a benefit not seen in the case of oral iron. After ADHF settles, HFrEF patients should be actively investigated for iron deficiency even if not anaemic.

16. In terms of non-pharmacological treatment, what should be discussed at discharge?

Indications for cardiac resynchronization therapy (CRT)

a. For symptomatic patients with HF in sinus rhythm with a QRS duration >130 msec (>150 msec receives more benefit) and left bundle branch block (LBBB) QRS morphology (non-LBBB QRS may be offered therapy but with less benefit) and with LVEF ≤35% despite Optimal Medical Therapy (OMT).

b. CRT rather than RV pacing is recommended for patients with HFrEF regardless of NYHA class who have an indication for ventricular pacing and high-degree AV block in order to reduce morbidity. This includes patients with AF.

c. For patients with a QRS duration ≥130 msec, LVEF ≤35% in NYHA class III–IV with AF despite OMT, provided a strategy to ensure biventricular capture (Atrio-ventricular node ablation, for example) is in place, or the patient is expected to return to sinus rhythm.

d. Patients with HFrEF who have received a conventional pacemaker or an implantable cardiac defibrillator (ICD) and subsequently develop worsening HF despite OMT and who have a high proportion of RV pacing (>40% V pacing) – upgrade to CRT.

Indications for an automatic implantable cardiac defibrillator (AICD)

a. *Secondary prevention*: Patients who have recovered from a ventricular arrhythmia causing haemodynamic instability and who are expected to survive for >1 year with good functional status. In the case of a person with ADHF with structural heart disease having a history of a non-reversible cause of VT, they qualify for this therapy after stabilization.

b. *Primary prevention*: Patients with symptomatic HF (NYHA class II–III), and an LVEF ≤35% despite a history of ≥3 months of OMT, provided they are expected to survive substantially >1 year with good functional status, and they have ischaemic heart disease (IHD) (unless they have had a myocardial infarction [MI] in the prior 40 days) or dilated cardiomyopathy (DCM). Patients with this history prior to admission with ADHF are candidates.

Indications for LV assist device

Patients with LVEF <25%, >2 months of severe symptoms on optimum medical + device therapy, >3 hospitalizations in a year and progressive end-organ dysfunction due to reduced perfusion but with adequate ventricular filling (pulmonary capillary wedge pressure [PCWP] ≥20 mmHg and SBP ≤80–90 mmHg or Cardiac Index (CI) ≤2 L/min/m^2), often on inotropes but with an adequate RV function.

Advanced HF (**Table 31.4**) *frequently and recurrently presents as ADHF, and it may be worthwhile to classify them to better explain the prognosis.*

Table 31.4: Criteria for Advanced HF

- NYHA III-IV in spite of OMT

- Severe cardiac dysfunction (*Any of*: LVEF < 30%, RV dysfunction, inoperable cases)

- Recurrent episodes of pulmonary or systemic congestion requiring i,v diuretics or hypotension requiring inotropes

- Exercise capacity 6-min walk test < 300 m or pVO2 <12 mL/kg/min

---

INTERMACS (Interagency Registry for Mechanically Assisted Circulatory Support) stages for classifying patients with advanced HF are presented in **Table 31.5**.

Indications for Heart Transplant

End-stage HF with severe symptoms, a poor prognosis and no remaining alternative treatment options who is adequately motivated for intensive therapy post-transplant. *Contraindications*: Infection, cancer, advanced renal failure, multisystem dysfunction, history of drug/alcohol abuse and inadequate social support.

Table 31.5: INTERMACS Categories of Advanced Heart Failure Patients

Terminology	NYHA	Description	Device	One-Year Survival When LVAD Used
Cardiogenic shock "crash and burn"	IV	Haemodynamic instability in spite of increasing doses of catecholamines/mechanical circulatory support with critical hypoperfusion of target organs (severe cardiogenic shock)	ECMO, IABP	50%
Progressive "downsliding on inotropes"	IV	Intravenous inotropic support with acceptable blood pressure but rapid deterioration of renal function, nutritional state or signs of congestion	ECMO, LVAD	60%
Inotrope "dependent stability"	IV	Haemodynamic stability with low or intermediate doses of inotropes	LVAD	80%
Resting symptom "frequent flyer"	IV	Temporary cessation of inotropic treatment is possible, but patient presents recurrences, usually fluid overload	LVAD	80%
Exertion intolerant "house bound"	IV	Complete cessation of physical activity, stable at rest, but frequently with mild fluid overload and renal dysfunction	LVAD	>90%
Exertion limited "walking wounded"	III	Minor limitation on physical activity and absence of congestion while at rest and easily fatigued by light activity	LVAD optional	-
Placeholder	III	No current or recent fluid imbalance	LVAD optional	-

FURTHER READING

1. McDonagh T A, Metra M, Adamo M, et al. ESC Guidelines for the diagnosis and treatment of acute and chronic heart failure. European Heart Journal (2021) 42: 3599–3726.

32 Valvular Heart Disease and Infective Endocarditis

Sunandan Sikdar, Indranil Dutta, and Arunansu Dhole

Chapter 32 may be accessed online at: www.routledge.com/9780367462215

DOI: 10.1201/9781003027584-32

33 Pericarditis and Pericardial Effusion

Sunandan Sikdar, Anup Khetan, and Biswarup Sarkar

1. What are the types of pericarditis?

Table 33.1: Classification of Pericarditis

Pericarditis	Definition
Acute	Acute inflammation of pericardium (see later)
Incessant	Pericarditis lasting >4–6 weeks but <3 months without remission
Recurrent	Recurrence of pericarditis after documented first episode of acute event and symptom-free interval of 4–6 weeks
Chronic	Pericarditis lasting for >3 months

Pericarditis is classified according to temporal relation of symptoms (Table 33.1).

2. How do you diagnose pericarditis?

Acute pericarditis is diagnosed if any two of the following four criteria are present.

Pericardial chest pain: Retrosternal chest pain which increases on inspiration or on lying down and decreases on sitting up and leaning forward. There is a radiation of the pain to the trapezius ridge. However, presentations like arm radiation and epigastric discomfort may be present. Associated complaints like cough and hiccoughs may occur.

Pericardial rub: The characteristic rub is a leathery squeak which may be triphasic (ventricular systole, diastole and atrial systole) or, more commonly, biphasic. They are usually evanescent and are best auscultated on the lower part of left sternal border on sitting up and leaning forward.

ECG changes: The ST segment is elevated in all leads, especially the inferolateral and anterior leads, but not in aVR and V1 (**Figure 33.1**). The changes are evident only in two-thirds of cases and especially if underlying myocarditis is present. The usefulness of ECG features in differentiating two other important conditions presenting with ST elevation is given in Table 33.2. Spodick defined four stages of ST-segment elevation in pericarditis:

a. PR-segment depression and diffuse ST elevation

b. Normalization of the ST segment

c. T-wave inversion with or without ST-segment *depression*

d. Normalization of ECG

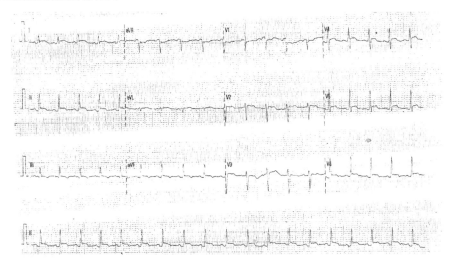

Figure 33.1 Pericarditis: ECG showing widespread ST elevation except in aVR and V1 and PR-segment elevation in aVR.

DOI: 10.1201/9781003027584-33

Table 33.2: Role of ECG in Differentiating the Important Causes of ST Elevation

ECG Feature	Acute Pericarditis	Early Repolarization	Acute Infarction
ST elevation	Concave up	Concave up	Convex up
ST elevation height/T wave height in V6	>0.25	<0.25	Variable
ST depression in reciprocal leads	None except in aVR	None	Present
ST-segment localization	Diffuse	Usually, inferolateral	Localized to coronary territories
PR elevation aVR	Present	None	None
Evolution of T-wave inversion	After ST normalizes	None	T inverts before ST-segment normalization
Q waves	None	None	Present

Pericardial effusion: Two-thirds may show a pericardial effusion on echocardiogram, but the chest X-ray may be normal until >300 mL of pericardial fluid collection takes place.

Additional findings:

a. *Elevated inflammatory markers*: ESR, CRP

b. Pericardial effusion by an imaging technique, e.g., CT scan/MRI

3. What are the causes of acute pericarditis?

The common causes of pericarditis in most parts of the world.

a. Idiopathic (80%) – Viral (Coxsackie, herpes, parvo, influenza and hepatitis, corona)

b. Tubercular

c. Neoplastic

d. Autoimmune

e. Purulent

4. What are the markers of poor prognosis/non-idiopathic causes?

The presence of any of the following factors warrants looking beyond the idiopathic variety

Major

■ Fever >38°C

■ Subacute onset

■ Large pericardial effusion (>20 mm)

■ Cardiac tamponade

■ Lack of response to aspirin or NSAID after 1 week of therapy

Minor

■ Associated myocarditis

■ Immunosuppression

■ Trauma

■ Anticoagulation

5. What is the empiric therapy for acute pericarditis?

The cornerstone of treatment for acute pericarditis is rest and aspirin/NSAID + colchicine. The commonly used dosages are given in Table 33.3.

Table 33.3: Therapy for Acute Pericarditis

Drug	Dose	Duration	Regimen
Aspirin	750 mg thrice daily	1–2 weeks	Taper to 600 mg TDS then 300 mg TDS then stop
Ibuprofen	400 mg TDS	1–2 weeks	Can stop after 2 weeks
Colchicine	0.5 mg once (<70 kg) or 0.5 mg twice daily (>70 kg)	3 months	• *<70 kg*: 0.5 mg alternate days × 1 week – stop • *>70 kg*: 0.5 mg OD × 1 week – stop

6. What is the role of steroids?

Use of corticosteroids is avoided except in the case of aspirin/NSAID allergy or already on steroids for connective tissue disease or in pregnancy with pericarditis. Low doses (prednisolone 0.2–0.5 mg/kg/day or equivalent) should be used for 4 weeks and then tapered gradually.

If during steroid taper when the dose reaches below 15 mg/day and there is recurrence, add aspirin + colchicine to control symptoms without increasing the steroid dose.

7. What are the clinical features of cardiac tamponade?

Tamponade is a clinical- and echocardiography-based diagnosis in critical care. The pathophysiology of tamponade is a stiff, fluid-filled pericardium that restricts right atrial (RA) and right ventricle (RV) filling in diastole and equalizes the diastolic intrapericardial, RA and RV pressures at a higher level, at about 20 mmHg, especially during inspiration. The end result is a reduction of chamber volume and preload resulting in decreased stroke volume.

Clinical features of tamponade—Pulse: Tachycardia and pulsus paradoxus. Systolic blood pressure (SBP) decreases of >10 mmHg during inspiration (pulse may be absent during inspiration). Pulsus paradoxus may also occur in constrictive pericarditis (CP), pulmonary embolism and rarely in chronic obstructive pulmonary disease (COPD). Pulsus paradoxus may not occur even in the presence of tamponade in cases of left ventricular dysfunction (LV) dysfunction, severe aortic regurgitation (AR), aortic dissection with AR and atrial septal defect (ASD). Hypotension indicates tachycardia is not sufficient to compensate for loss of stroke volume.

The jugular venous pressure (JVP) is usually raised, but there may be an inspiratory decline of JVP (Kussmaul sign absent) with absent y descent. Lack of decline of JVP may suggest effusive and constrictive pathology.

Heart sounds: Muffled in advanced cases.

Beck triad: Hypotension, raised JVP and muffled heart sounds suggest advanced tamponade.

Ewart sign: Dullness to percussion in the left paraspinal region due to lung collapse due to a large pericardial effusion.

Low-pressure tamponade: When there is decreased blood volume in the setting of pericardial effusion that otherwise is unlikely to cause compromise of cardiac output. In the presence of volume loss, modest effusion can cause lowering of stroke volume. Examples: Haemodialysis, blood loss, diuretics in the presence of effusion.

Subacute tamponade can have normotension or even hypertension.

Chest X-ray (CXR): Flask-like enlarged heart shadow. Fat pad sign in the lateral CXR view is a linear lucency that exists between the posterior wall of the sternum and the anterior wall of the heart. It is due to separation of the fat pad on the epicardium from the parietal pericardium.

ECG: Tachycardia with low-voltage complexes. Occasionally QRS alternans with alternate large and small QRS complexes may be present. This is due to an anteroposterior swinging motion of the heart in large pericardial effusion.

Echocardiography features: 2D finding: Large effusion (echo estimation of effusion small effusion <10 mm, moderate effusion 10–20 mm, large effusion >20 mm, posterior echo-free space in diastole, **Figure 33.2**).

M-mode and ECG-timed 2D findings

Late diastolic RA collapse – sensitive sign

Early diastolic RV collapse – specific sign

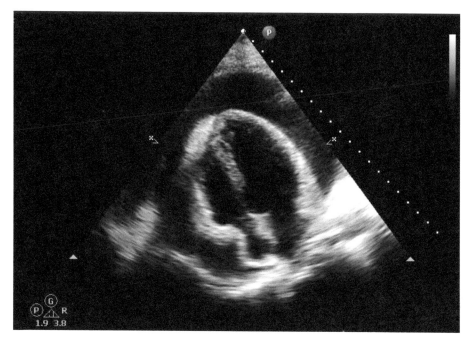

Figure 33.2 Echocardiogram of cardiac tamponade showing a large effusion with RA collapse.

Doppler finding: Reciprocal relation of right ventricular outflow tract (RVOT) flow (velocity time integral [VTI]) vs left ventricular outflow tract (LVOT) flow (VTI), e.g., during inspiration RVOT flow increases but LVOT flow decreases

8. What are the echocardiographic signs of cardiac tamponade and pericardial constriction?

The difference between tamponade and pure constriction is more an echocardiographic exercise as the clinical presentations are usually different (Table 33.4).

Table 33.4: Distinguishing Tamponade from Effusion + Constriction

Parameter	Tamponade	Constriction
Pericardium	Effusion predominant	Thickening predominant
2D/M-mode	• Late diastolic RA collapse – sensitive sign • Early diastolic RV collapse –specific sign	a. Exaggerated leftward septal shift with inspiration b. Septal bounce c. Flattened posterior wall on diastole
IVC dilated	Yes	Yes
PW Doppler	Reciprocal relation of RVOT flow (VTI) vs LVOT flow (VTI), e.g., during inspiration RVOT flow increases but LVOT decreases	Exaggerated respiratory variation of tricuspid and mitral inflow velocity, e.g., during expiration there is >25% increase in mitral inflow velocity
Diastolic pattern	–	Restrictive (E/A >>2)
Tissue Doppler	–	Annulus paradoxus (medial E' > lateral E')
Hepatic vein	–	Expiratory flow reversal

9. What is the clinical presentation of Chronic Constrictive Pericarditis (CCP)?

CCP is the end result of subacute and chronic inflammation of the pericardium with subsequent haemodynamic effects due to restriction of cardiac filling. The pathophysiology hinges on two factors: (a) The dissociation of intrapleural and intracardiac pressures due to the thick shell of pericardium – during inspiration, decreased intrapleural pressure is not transmitted to the left atrium (LA), and the pulmonary vein–LA flow gradient is reduced, leading to decreased filling of the LV and shift of the ventricular septum to left. (b) Enhanced ventricular interdependence – because the cardiac volume is fixed, increased diastolic filling of the LV in expiration leads to a reduction in flow into the RV.

Aetiology: Tuberculosis (TB) is the most common cause of CCP in developing countries (about 50%). Other important causes include radiation, post-cardiac surgery, connective tissue disease, malignancy, trauma, sarcoidosis, drug induced and uraemia.

Presentation: Fatigue and symptoms of right-sided heart failure (dyspnoea, oedema) dominate the clinical picture. On examination, the JVP is raised with a steep y descent, and it increases with inspiration (Kussmaul sign), as the inspiratory fall of intrathoracic pressure is not transmitted to the heart. Pulsus paradoxus may be present. Oedema is universal, and ascites may be present. On auscultation there is a pericardial knock (just before the timing of S3) in early diastole because of a sudden cessation of ventricular filling. On auscultation, features of pleural effusion are present.

Diagnosis: Since the ECG may only show nonspecific ST-T changes, occasionally low voltage and rarely atrial fibrillation (**Figure 33.3**), other imaging tests are more important.

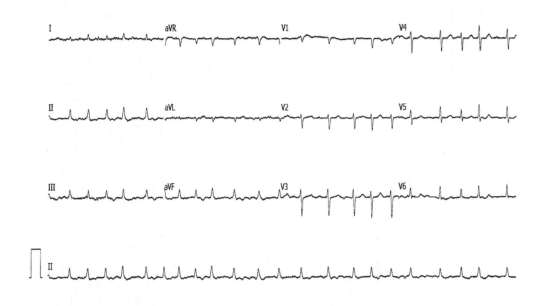

Figure 33.3 ECG of a patient with effusive constrictive pericarditis: AF and low QRS voltage.

CXR: The presence of pericardial calcification in the appropriate setting suggests the diagnosis. It is present in one-third of cases of CCP.

Echocardiography is the principal modality of bedside diagnosis in the cardiac care unit (CCU) and the findings are given in the table earlier (**Figure 33.4**).

CT Scan: Pericardial thickening (>4 mm), calcification, deformation of cardiac contour and inferior vena cava (IVC) congestion.

MRI with contrast: Apart from pericardial thickness, other information includes:

Tagging sequences: Pericardial – myocardial adherence

Real-time cine: Ventricular septal shift on respiration

Contrast: Pericardial enhancement suggestive of inflammation

Cardiac catheterization may be done during the coronary angiogram (CAG) prior to surgery referral and shows diastolic pressure equalization of all chambers and discordance of right- and left-sided ventricular pressure in systole (during inspiration RVSP increases and LVSP falls).

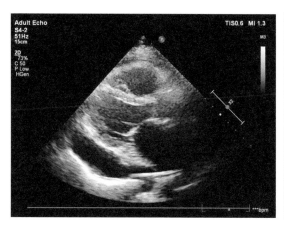 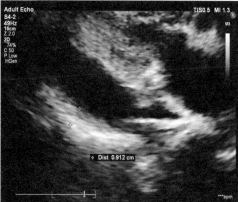

Figure 33.4 2D echocardiogram of the same patient showing pericardial effusion and thickened pericardium.

Treatment: Few cases of effusive CP respond to medical therapy: (a) Those showing inflammation by MRI or PET-CT may respond to colchicine or oral steroids (2–3 months) or (b) those related to the early phase of tubercular constriction, which responds to ATT (6 months). In the vast majority of cases of CCP, including idiopathic CCP, pericardiectomy is the treatment of choice with a perioperative mortality of 6%. Idiopathic CCP has the best prognosis post-surgery (80% survival in 5–7 years), while radiation-induced CCP has the worst outcome (30% in 7 years).

10. How do you differentiate CP vs restrictive cardiomyopathy (RCMP)?

Table 33.5: Differentiating Constrictive from Restrictive Cardiomyopathy

Parameter	CP	RCMP
Atrium	Normal	Dilated
Pericardium	Thick, bright	Normal
Septal motion	Bounce/Paradoxical, left shift with inspiration	Normal
Restrictive mitral Inflow	Present	Present
Annular velocity on TDI (annulus paradoxus)	Medial E′ > lateral E′	Medial E′ < lateral E′
Respiratory variation of mitral E velocity (Figure 33.5)	>25% expiratory increase	<25%
Pulmonary hypertension	Rare	Frequent
Hepatic veins	Systolic antegrade flow increased in inspiration Diastolic reversal of forward flow in expiration – specific for CCP	Diastolic flow > systolic flow in inspiration
Regurgitation in AV valves	Nil	Common (TR > MR)

11. What are the characteristics of tuberculous pericarditis (TBP)?

Epidemiology: TBP is the most important cause of pericardial effusion in the immunocompromised (especially HIV infected), where in some series this aetiology accounts for 90% of cases. TB is responsible for approximately 70% of cases of large pericardial effusion and most cases of constrictive pericarditis in developing countries, as compared to 4% in developed economies.

Pathogenesis and pathology: The tubercular bacilli commonly spread retrogradely by lymphatics from paratracheal, peribronchial and mediastinal lymph nodes and rarely by contiguous spread from the lungs, pleura and diaphragm. If a septic foci discharges in the pericardial space, the development is dramatic. Protein antigens of the bacillus induce delayed hypersensitivity responses,

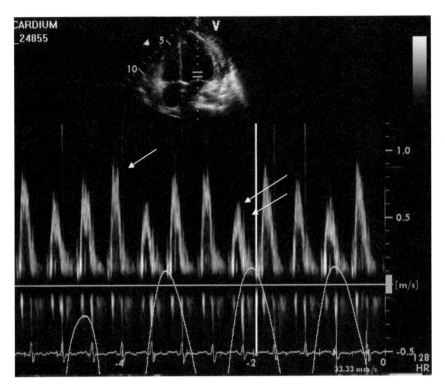

Figure 33.5 Constrictive pericarditis: Respiratory variation of mitral inflow with inspiratory decline (Exp Velocity – Insp velocity/Exp Velocity > 25%).

stimulating lymphocytes (TH 1) to release lymphokines that activate macrophages and induce granuloma formation. Cytolysis mediated by antimyolemmal antibodies may contribute to the development of exudative TBP. There are four stages of TBP:

a. *Fibrinous exudation*: Abundant mycobacteria and leucocytes, early granuloma

b. *Serosanguineous effusion*: Lymphocytes and monocytes predominate

c. Organization with caseous granuloma formation and pericardial thickening

d. *Constrictive scarring*: Fibrosis and calcification of the parietal and visceral pericardium leading to constrictive pericarditis in 30% of cases.

In HIV infection due to depletion of T cells, granulomas are few and CCP is less likely.

Presentation: The entity usually presents with cough (94%), dyspnoea (88%), chest pain, fever (70%), orthopnoea, night sweats and weight loss.

Outcomes: Immunocompromised patients have worse outcomes, including increased mortality, compared to immunocompetent patients. TBP has a mortality rate of 17%–40% at 6 months after diagnosis. Constriction generally develops within 6 months of presentation with effusive pericarditis. The mortality rate from pericarditis at 10 years was 6.5% with ATT, with all deaths occurring within the first 12 months.

Diagnosis: A "definite" diagnosis of TBP is based on the presence of tubercle bacilli in the pericardial fluid or on histological section of the pericardium – caseous granuloma, by culture or by polymerase chain reaction (PCR) (Xpert MTB/RIF) testing.

A "probable" diagnosis is made when there is TB elsewhere in a patient with unexplained pericarditis, a lymphocytic pericardial exudate with elevated adenosine deaminase (ADA) and/or an appropriate response to antituberculosis chemotherapy in endemic areas.

Imaging: Chest X-ray shows evidence of pulmonary Koch disease in one-third of cases and pleural effusion in two-thirds. Echocardiography shows fibrinous strands suggestive of exudative effusion. CT scan of the chest with contrast shows pericardial effusion and thickening (>3 mm) and typical mediastinal and tracheobronchial lymphadenopathy (>10 mm, *hypodense centres*, matting), with *sparing of hilar lymph nodes*.

Pericardial fluid: Pericardiocentesis is recommended in all patients in whom TB is suspected. Cardiac tamponade (present in only 10% in some series) is an absolute indication for pericardiocentesis. The pericardial fluid is bloodstained in more than 80% of cases of TBP. Tuberculous pericardial effusion is typically exudative by Light criteria and characterized by a high protein content and increased leukocyte count, with a predominance of lymphocytes and monocytes. Direct visualization of tubercle bacilli in pericardial fluid is highly variable and ranges from 0% to 40%, while culture positivity is about 50%. Direct inoculation into double-strength liquid Kirchner culture medium at the bedside improves the yield to 75%. The diagnostic sensitivity of pericardial biopsy for TB (demonstrating caseous granuloma) ranges from 10% to 64% and is reportedly less than culture of the fluid. The effusive stage gives the highest yield in either of these methods. Among biochemical tests of the pericardial fluid, ADA >40 U/L has a sensitivity of 87% and specificity of 84% and is useful also for T-cell-depleted HIV patients. Interferon gamma >50 pg/L and lysozyme >6.5 mcg/dL have even more sensitivity and specificity.

Ancillary tests: Culture of sputum, gastric aspirate and/or urine for *Mycobacterium tuberculosis* should be considered in all patients. Lymph node biopsy (e.g., scalene) is a useful way of obtaining a diagnosis if lymphadenopathy is present.

The tuberculin test is not useful in adults.

Treatment: In a young patient with a large pericardial effusion living in TB-endemic area with (1) HIV infection or (2) exudative effusion, the presumptive diagnosis is a tuberculous aetiology. However, in elderly patients or in non-endemic zones, further tests are required.

Antituberculosis chemotherapy (ATT) increases survival dramatically in TBP. It reduces mortality from 80% to 90% in the pre-antibiotic era to 17% to 40% currently.

Regimen: Rifampicin, isoniazid, pyrazinamide and ethambutol (RHZE) for at least 2 months followed by isoniazid and rifampicin (RH) for 4 months (total of 6 months of therapy) has been shown to be highly effective. Extending for 9 months or longer does not give better results.

Role of corticosteroids: There is a trend, but there is no statistically significant reduction of mortality, constriction or tamponade due to the use of steroids in different studies, if corticosteroids are used along with ATT. Since rifampicin is an enzyme inducer, the dosage of prednisolone used (1 mg/kg) in most studies may have been inadequate. On the other hand, steroid side effects in immunocompromised patients with HIV infection are a cause of worry. Hence, the role of systemic steroids is yet to be defined.

Routine pericardiotomy and fluid drainage at the initial stage does not prevent constriction and so is not indicated.

Treatment of TBP: CP occurs in approximately 18% to 46% of patients with tuberculous pericardial effusion despite treatment with ATT and corticosteroids. Subclinical effusive-constrictive disease is the most frequently identified predicting factor for subsequent constrictive evolution. In the patients who are diagnosed as having TBP de novo, ATT for 6 months is the treatment of choice. If there is no improvement or if there is calcific CP on the initial presentation, surgery is the treatment. Some physicians would wait for 6–8 weeks on ATT and refer to surgery if there is no improvement of the symptoms of constriction.

12. Can ATT be started empirically if the option of pericardiocentesis is not available?

In *endemic areas* a diagnostic score can be used. Independently predictive were fever (1), night sweats (1), weight loss (2), globulin level >40 g/L (3) and peripheral leucocyte count <10 × 10^9/L (3). A total score of ≥6 indicates TBP in a patient with a large pericardial effusion, with a sensitivity of 86% and a specificity of 85%.

FURTHER READING
1. Syed F F, Mayosi B M. A Modern Approach to Tuberculous Pericarditis. Progress in Cardiovascular Diseases. (November/December 2007), 50(3): pp 218–236.
2. Adler Y, Charron P, Imazio M, et al. 2015 ESC Guidelines for the Diagnosis and Management of Pericardial Diseases. European Heart Journal (2015), 36: 2921–2964.

34 Acute Limb Ischaemia

Sunandan Sikdar and Saujatya Chakraborty

1. What is acute limb ischaemia (ALI)?

ALI occurs due to abrupt interruption of arterial flow to an extremity, which may lead to loss of the limb and even life.

2. How do you classify ALI?

The classification is given in **Table 34.1**.

Table 34.1: Acute Limb Ischaemia SVS Categories

Category	Status	Description	Sensory Loss	Motor Loss	Arterial Doppler	Venous Doppler
I	Viable	Not immediate threat	None	None	Audible	Audible
IIa	Marginally threatened	Salvageable if prompt Rx	Minimal	None	Inaudible	Audible
IIb	Immediately threatened	Salvageable if immediate Rx	Partial	Mild-Mod	Inaudible	Audible
III	Irreversible	Non-viable	Anaesthetic	Profound	Inaudible	Inaudible

3. What is the prognosis for untreated and treated ALI?

After 12 hr, in untreated cases, limb loss is about 20% and mortality 30% (**Table 34.2**).

In treated cases, the prognosis is definitely improved. The data for catheter-directed thrombolysis (CDT) appears better than surgery, maybe because it is utilized at an earlier time point and has less morbidity.

Table 34.2: Prognosis in ALI

Technique	Mortality	Limb Salvage
Surgery	25%	65%–80%
CDT	4%–8%	80%–90%

4. What are the causes of ALI?

The most common cause is progression of peripheral arterial disease (**Table 34.3**). Embolization (usually from a cardiac cause, frequently atrial fibrillation) accounts for 15% of cases. Embolization from aortic dissection, popliteal aneurysm, intraaortic balloon pump and catheter/devices are rarer causes. An important cause is graft thrombosis.

Table 34.3: Common Causes of ALI

Embolic	Thrombotic
Atrial fibrillation	Progression of PAD
LV apical thrombus	Trauma
IABP/ECMO/Catheterization	Graft thrombosis
Aortic aneurysm/Dissection	Arteritis
Endocarditis	Compression by surrounding structure

5. How do you differentiate embolic from thrombotic causes of occlusion?

Suggestive features to recognize embolic from thrombotic occlusion are given in **Table 34.4**.

DOI: 10.1201/9781003027584-34

Table 34.4: Differentiating Embolic from Thrombotic ALI

Feature	Embolic	Thrombotic
Onset	Sudden	Progressive
Cardiac history	Yes	No
History of claudication	No	Yes
History of surgery/PTA	No	Yes
AF	Common	Less common
Ischaemia severity	Severe ischaemia, cold extremity	Less severe
Contralateral limb	Normal	Affected

6. How do you recognize a viable versus nonviable limb?

Revascularization of a nonviable limb is catastrophic (**Table 34.5**). Hence, great care should be taken to sort out viable limbs before intervention. Signs of ischaemia are usually most pronounced in one joint distal to the level of occlusion. Pallor is often due to vasospasm and does not imply nonviability, while blanching is a sign of reversibility. Paraesthesia occurs in the order of the diameter of the nerve fibres. It begins with light touch, vibration and proprioception and then much later deep pain and pressure sense. Paralysis is a sign of near irreversibility.

Table 34.5: Acute Limb Ischaemia – Time Is Limb (*Revascularization of a Nonviable Limb Is Catastrophic*)

Presentation	Mortality	Limb Salvage
<12 hr	19%	93%
> 12 hr	31%	78%

- Signs of ischaemia are usually most pronounced in one joint distal to the level of occlusion.
- Pallor is due to vasospasm.
- Blanching is a sign of reversibility.
- Paresthesia occurs in the order of the diameter of the nerve fibres, beginning with light touch, vibration and proprioception and then much later deep pain and pressure sense.
- Paralysis is sign of near irreversibility and reperfusion injury.

7. What is the best option?

The three options available for treating ALI should be used as per the situation: Viability of the limb, duration of ischaemia and general condition of the patient:

- Thromboembolectomy
- CDT/Pharmacomechanical thrombolysis (AngioJet)
- Amputation

For deciding which procedure to use in a viable limb, there are two rules of thumb, though these rules can be changed depending on the individual case:

Rule 1: ALI early presentation, CDT preferred over surgery

Rule 2: ALI infrainguinal location of occlusion, CDT preferred over surgery

In any case, except for a nonviable limb, we must proceed for a peripheral angiogram as early as possible.

8. What are the merits and demerits of thrombolectomy?

The procedure is useful in an IIB situation where without immediate patency, limb loss will occur. Demerits of the procedure are:

- Comorbidity, frailty
- Leaves residual thrombus (35%–85%)

- Cannot clear branch vessel occlusion
- Causes endothelial injury – thrombogenic and vasospastic
- Inferior result if extensive thrombus >30 cm

9. What are the salient points of CDT?

- Give a loading dose of aspirin, clopidogrel and atorvastatin.
- Guidewire traversal test (**Figure 34.1**) – In this case, a wire is used to cross the lesion, and passage of the wire usually implies a good prognosis.

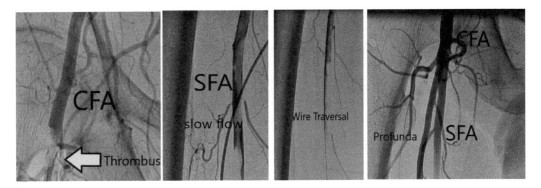

Figure 34.1 Thromboembolism to common femoral artery and treatment by catheter-directed thrombolysis. *Abbreviations*: CFA: Common Femoral Artery, SFA: Superficial Femoral Artery.

- Route of administration of thrombolysis is via a catheter with an end hole and side holes, which is embedded in the thrombus. The catheter is introduced from the contralateral limb (e.g. left femoral artery for right common femoral artery thrombus).
- Newer thrombolytics are usually used: Tenecteplase 1–5 mg then infusion 0.125–0.25 mg/hr, reteplase bolus 2–5 U then infusion 0.25 U/hr or alteplase 2–5 mg loading dose and then 0.5 mg/hr.
- At the end of 12 hr of infusion, a check angiogram may be done. A further 12-hr infusion may be given if the angiogram shows persistence of the clot/haziness.
- The longer the duration of the infusion, the greater the risk of bleeding. Hence, as soon as patency and good distal runoff are achieved, the infusion needs to be stopped.

10. What are the CDT-specific complications?

Though CDT-related complications are rare, they still occur:

1. *Bleeding complication (including intracranial haemorrhage [ICH])*: 5%–20%
2. *Distal embolization*: 5%–15%
3. *Pericatheter thrombosis*: 2%–4%
4. *Dissection*: 2%

11. How do you treat the limb post-revascularization?

- Restart anticoagulation.
- Aspirin may be continued.
- Look out for compartment syndrome.
- Follow-up angiography is necessary to identify any residual significant disease requiring revascularization.

12. How do you recognize compartment syndrome?

This is a catastrophic complication of reperfusion therapy of ALI. The limb is painful and swollen. There is hypoesthesia of the limb. Creatinine phosphokinase rises to very high levels. Commonly the anterior compartment containing the peroneal nerve is involved and signs of nerve involvement are evident. Treatment of choice is urgent fasciotomy.

FURTHER READING

1. Kinlay S. Intervention for Lower Extremity Arterial Disease, in Bhatt D L (Ed) Cardiovascular Intervention: A Companion to Braunwald's Heart Disease, (2016) Elsevier, pp 291–310.
2. Morrison H L. Catheter Directed Thrombolysis. Semin Intervent Radiol 2006;23:258–269.

35 Use of Sedation, Analgesia and Anaesthesia in CCU

Sunandan Sikdar, Swarup Paul, and Jitendra Ladhania

Chapter 35 may be accessed online at: www.routledge.com/9780367462215

DOI: 10.1201/9781003027584-35

36A Preoperative Assessment of Patients with Ischaemic Heart Disease

Anuradha Patel, Sunandan Sikdar, and Rakesh Garg

1. What is the relevant history in patients with ischaemic heart disease (IHD)?

Patients require a thorough assessment, including elicitation of an appropriate history for preoperative workup. A history suggestive of angina pectoris, recent myocardial infarction (MI), unstable angina and cerebrovascular disease is significant for preoperative workup. History of other comorbidities and risk factors (hypertension, diabetes mellitus, chronic kidney disease, stroke, peripheral arterial disease) and symptoms (syncope, palpitation and dyspnoea) should be evaluated and documented. Evaluation of functional capacity is quantitively done by estimating metabolic equivalents (METs) (1 MET is the oxygen requirement while sitting at rest and is equal to 3.5 mL/kg/min). The drug history also needs to be elicited, especially for drugs like antiplatelets and antihypertensives. If the patient has undergone coronary revascularization, then the time of stenting or coronary artery bypass grafting (CABG) is important, in addition to ongoing pharmacological treatment.

The estimated METs and the relevant activities are enumerated here:

- *1 MET*: Walking indoors
- *4 METs*: Climbing one flight of stairs
- *10 METs*: Playing tennis

2. What are the relevant examination findings?

The patient needs to be examined for blood pressure (blood pressure charting, in case of higher readings to rule out white coat hypertension), auscultation of the heart (murmur) and lung (rhonchi, crepitation), abdominal palpation (ascites, distended liver), palpating the abdomen (excluding aneurysm) and the examination of extremities for oedema and vascular integrity (peripheral vascular disease, PVD). The examination findings have subtle implications for perioperative care (**Table 36.1**).

Table 36.1: Examination and Findings of Concern in Patients with IHD

Findings	Implications
Hypertension	• Whether it is controlled or uncontrolled • Uncontrolled blood pressure might need further cardiologist referral
Auscultation of lung fields: Crepitus, distended jugular vein	• Identify the signs for congestive heart failure (CHF) • The presence of incipient CHF increases perioperative morbidity and mortality and requires cautious use of fluid management and modifying anaesthesia and surgical technique accordingly • Optimal analgesia is also required to prevent overt CHF
Auscultation of heart: Murmur	Might indicate valvular heart disease
Abdominal palpation: Ascites, distended liver	Suggestive of CHF
Examination of extremities for oedema	Pedal oedema may indicate renal insufficiency
Increased respiratory rate, METs <4	Decreased functional capacity indicates poor cardiorespiratory reserves and in the absence of any respiratory dysfunction, it is suggestive of poor cardiac reserve
Peripheral vascular disease (PVD), diabetes mellitus (DM), cerebrovascular accident (CVA)	Associated comorbidities

3. When do you require a cardiology consultation in patients with IHD?

A cardiologist's opinion is required in patients scheduled for surgery if the patient is having any active cardiac disease or remains unoptimized for any previous therapy or new symptoms arise in a patient with known cardiac disease. This referral allows assessment, optimization and risk

DOI: 10.1201/9781003027584-36

stratification from the cardiovascular status of the patient. This is especially true if a patient has signs and symptoms suggestive of persistent ischaemia, is in heart failure, has left ventricular dysfunction or has moderate to severe valvular heart disease. Patients with aortic aneurysms also require specialist evaluation. Patients who have undergone coronary interventions in the last 5 years and remain asymptomatic may be scheduled for surgery with low perioperative risk, and no further cardiac evaluation or testing is required. However, patients who have recently undergone revascularization (<1 yr) require specialist evaluation.

4. What are the surgical risk categories for perioperative major adverse cardiovascular events (MACEs) for non-cardiac surgery?

Based on the risk of major cardiac events (cardiac death or acute MI), patients are typically stratified as high- (>5%), intermediate- (1%–5%), or low- (<1%) risk cases (**Table 36.2**).

Low-risk procedure: The combined surgical and patient characteristics predict the risk of a MACE of death or MI of <1%, e.g., cataract and plastic surgery.

Elevated-risk procedure: MACE >1%

Table 36.2: Surgical Interventions and Cardiac Risk

Low Cardiac Risk (<1%)	Intermediate Cardiac Risk (1%–5%)	High Risk (>5%)
Lumpectomy	Transurethral resection of bladder cancer (TURBT)	Laparoscopic total colectomy with ileostomy
Arthroscopic rotator cuff repair	Laparoscopic prostatectomy	Breast reconstruction with free flap
Simple mastectomy	Total hip arthroplasty	Open cholecystectomy
Laparoscopic appendicectomy	Open appendicectomy	Whipple surgery
Laparoscopic cholecystectomy	Laparoscopic radical hysterectomy with bilateral salpingo-oophorectomy	Open ventral hernia repair
Breast surgery	Carotid endarterectomy	Emergency surgery
Cataract surgery	Head and neck surgery	Aortic or other major vascular surgical interventions
Superficial procedure	Intraperitoneal/Intrathoracic surgery	Peripheral artery surgery
Endoscopic procedure	Orthopaedic surgery	
Ambulatory surgery	Prostate surgery	

5. What are the principles of preoperative medication management?

Patients with IHD are initiated with medical management to optimize the cardiac status. The perioperative medications in patients with cardiac diseases usually considered are:

1. *Beta-blockers*: Beta-blockers are one of the treatment strategies for patients with IHD. It has been observed that cardiac function, exercise capacity and long-term survival in patients with heart failure due to MI, hypertrophic cardiomyopathy or idiopathic dilated cardiomyopathy are improved with the administration of beta-blockers. It is also initiated in patients with diastolic dysfunction and secondary to hypertension. The drug dosages are titrated to achieve a target heart rate of 60–80 beats/min without significant hypotension. This control of heart rate improves diastolic filling and myocardial perfusion. The drugs should be continued with regular doses in the perioperative period. This prevents rebound tachycardia and the risk of myocardial ischaemia. Sudden stoppage of the beta-blockers may precipitate acute MI or exacerbation of symptoms in patients with a history of unstable angina. However, acute administration of beta-blockers in the immediate preoperative period should be avoided unless recommended by a consulting cardiologist.

2. *Statins*: Patients taking statins should continue this therapy throughout the perioperative period. A consultant cardiologist may recommend initiation of statin therapy in previously untreated patients.

3. *Calcium channel blockers, digoxin and diuretics*: These need to be continued in the perioperative period. However, these drugs may affect electrolyte levels and need to be monitored.

4. *Antihypertensives*: The antihypertensive drugs should be continued in the perioperative period except for angiotensin-converting enzyme (ACE) inhibitors or angiotensin-receptor blockers (ARB), which are stopped on the morning of surgery in case of haemodynamic instability, hypovolemia, increased creatinine and in patients where large perioperative fluid shifts are anticipated. Clonidine is continued in the perioperative period, as there is a risk of rebound hypertension with abrupt withdrawal. Beta-blockers should also be continued if the patient is already taking them.

5. *Anticoagulants*: Certain patients with cardiac diseases may be receiving anticoagulant therapy or antiplatelet therapies. The minor procedures without significant risk of bleeding like cataract or minor soft tissue surgeries may be done even with these drugs, including warfarin. In surgeries with a high risk of bleeding, longer-acting anticoagulants need to be converted to shorter-acting agents like low-molecular-weight heparin (LMWH) as bridge therapy, and this needs to be stopped 12 hr before surgery.

6. *Herbal medicines (ginseng, garlic and gingko)*: Certain herbal food items like garlic have an impact on coagulation, and these have been even used as extracts for herbal medicines. So, assessment should elicit the use of these herbal ingredients, as these may increase the risk of bleeding in the perioperative period. In case, the patient is taking these, they need to be stopped at least 2 weeks before surgery, though the optimal time effect of these ingredients is not well known.

7. *Aspirin*: Dual antiplatelet therapy (DAPT), including aspirin, is the standard regimen in patients receiving a drug-eluting stent. This is primarily to prevent stent thrombosis after the coronary angioplasty intervention. Its stoppage may lead to stent thrombosis and acute MI, and on the other hand continuation of antiplatelet therapy increases the risk of perioperative bleeding. Low-dose aspirin (75 mg/day) is safer with regard to the risk of bleeding and should be continued in the perioperative period in such patients.

The American College of Cardiology/American Heart Association (ACC/AHA) has recommended postponing the planned routine surgeries by at least 6 weeks when bare metal stents have been used for coronary intervention, for IHD guidelines recommend a delay of at least 6 weeks between insertion of the bare metal stent and non-cardiac surgery and for 6 months (preferably one year) in cases where drug-eluting stents have been used (**Figure 36A.1**).

6. How do you do perioperative bridging of antiplatelet therapy?

Certain patients remain at high risk for thrombosis and their DAPT needs to be continued. In cases where the planned surgery cannot be postponed and surgery with DAPT carries a risk of bleeding, anticoagulant bridging therapy may be considered. Conventionally heparin infusion and LMWH are used for bridging therapy. Other pharmacological agents like tirofiban, eptifibatide and cangrelor can also be used for bridging therapy. Usually, the antiplatelet drugs are stopped 5–7 days before planned surgical interventions and bridging therapy is started, which may be stopped preoperatively. The last dose of these drugs depends on the drug used and usually remains to be 4–12 hr. The drugs need to be restarted postoperatively once surgical haemostasis is ensured. However, in most instances, starting GP IIb/IIIa is not necessary, except in cases where the thrombotic risk is very high. Nowadays, most stents have thin struts, and stent thrombosis is uncommon in the case of well-deployed stents. A detailed discussion is available in the chapter on antiplatelets and anticoagulants.

7. What are the relevant laboratory investigations in IHD patients?

The various investigative strategies in patients with IHD for surgical interventions include:

■ Metabolic panel (serum electrolytes including sodium, potassium, chloride; carbon dioxide, glucose, blood urea nitrogen, creatinine) in patients receiving diuretic therapy chronically and in patients with renal insufficiency.

■ A preoperative baseline resting 12-lead electrocardiogram (ECG) is obtained for all patients with symptoms of MI and asymptomatic patients at high risk for myocardial injury after non-cardiac surgery (MINS). ECG remains a useful screening modality for identifying various cardiac conditions like myocardial ischaemia, MI, conduction abnormalities, hypertensive changes and electrolyte imbalance.

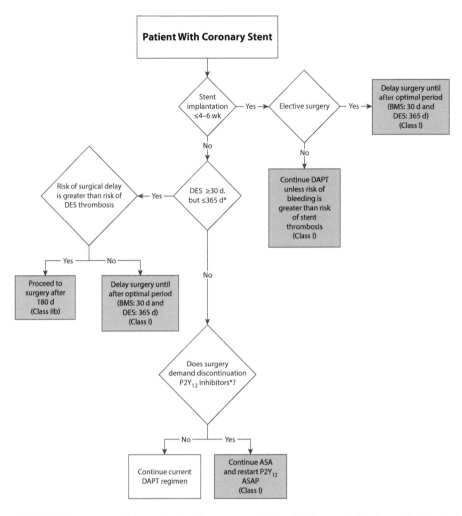

Figure 36A.1 Management of the patient with coronary stents. (With permission from Fleisher L A et al. Perioperative cardiovascular evaluation and management. JACC 2014;64:e77–137.)

- Resting echocardiography
  - Stress testing
  - With exercise
- Pharmacologic stress testing with cardiac imaging
- The stress testing, including ECG and echocardiography, mimics the perioperative stress response and also the sympathetic response during interventions like laryngoscopy and tracheal intubation. Any changes in ECG or echocardiography indicate compromised cardiac function and thus need further assessment, optimization and risk stratification. The exercise ECG simulates stimulation of the sympathetic nervous system and effects that may accompany perioperative events such as laryngoscopy and surgical simulation. Also, the use of pharmacological agents for cardiac stress like dobutamine remains useful in patients who cannot perform the exercise for such cardiac testing. The imaging modalities include dipyridamole, thallium myocardium imaging and dobutamine stress echocardiography.

- *Other investigations*: Complete blood counts, renal function test, chest X-ray.

- *Brain natriuretic peptide (BNP)*: Used in a patient who is considered for possible stress testing where a low value would help downgrade the estimated risk. It is also useful to diagnose incipient heart failure.

8. What are the indications for ECG preoperatively?

A 12-lead ECG is usually done in all patients preoperatively; however, it is especially useful in:

- Known cardiovascular disease
- Significant arrhythmia
- Significant structural heart disease
- High-risk surgery
- Symptoms of acute coronary syndrome

9. What are the ECG findings you can get in a patient with IHD?

The ECG changes are described in detail in the chapter on ECG in critical care. The specific changes in the ECG provide a useful clue for a particular condition of the cardiac status (**Table 36A.3**). Some of the changes are the presence of a (1) Q wave, (2) ST-segment elevation/depression, (3) QTc prolongation and (4) arrhythmia.

Table 36A.3: ECG Findings and Their Significance

Finding	Interpretation	Significance
LBBB	Conduction problem/Dilated LV	Increased mortality
Q wave	Old infarct	Mortality
Deep T inversion	Ischaemia	Perioperative MI
Bradycardia	AV block/Sick sinus	The requirement of temporary pacer
Atrial fibrillation	Scarred atrium	Stroke/HF

10. What are the indications for echocardiography?

Echocardiography is indicated in the following situations as part of the preoperative assessment:

- Dyspnoea of unknown origin
- Worsening dyspnoea/change in clinical status
- Clinically stable, no echocardiography in the last year
- To evaluate valve function in a patient with a murmur
- To evaluate left ventricular systolic function in a patient with heart failure

11. What is the role of biomarkers?

Among the rare scenarios where biomarker levels may impact therapies are occult heart failure or those with the possibility of an acute coronary syndrome. A positive result may mean elevated risk. However, they have been demonstrated to predict risk even if they do not change the line of management.

Elevated troponin level predicts increased mortality, which is not necessarily cardiac. Thus, it may be a measure of "sickness." In the VISION study by Devereaux et al., mortality was 16.9% with a troponin T level of 0.3 ng/mL or higher, but 1% in the group with a normal troponin level.

Preoperative BNP elevation was associated with approximately a 20-fold increase in MACEs, a 9-fold increase in all-cause mortality and a 24-fold increase in cardiac death. Elevated postoperative BNP increases the rate of death and MI by 3.7-fold.

12. What are the principles of regional anaesthesia in IHD patients?

Regional anaesthesia and analgesia techniques are one of the important techniques for perioperative care of the patient for surgical intervention. It has many advantages like the provision of good analgesia and reduction of intravenous polypharmacy but has certain limitations as well, especially in patients with cardiac dysfunction. Patients with IHD may be receiving medications that have anticoagulant/antiplatelet effects. Neuraxial needles or catheters are avoided in patients currently receiving anticoagulant drugs or antiplatelet therapy (other than aspirin alone) because of increased risk for spinal/epidural haematoma. The epidural catheter may be placed using LMWH as bridging therapy for other longer-acting anticoagulants like warfarin or clopidogrel. The LMWH needs to stop 12 hr before administration of a regional central neuraxial block. It should be resumed at the earliest point in the postoperative period. However, if the catheter has been used for neuraxial block, then timing of its removal should be done as per the usage of the anticoagulant.

13. What is the algorithm for perioperative cardiac assessment for coronary artery disease (CAD)?

See **Figure 36A.2**.

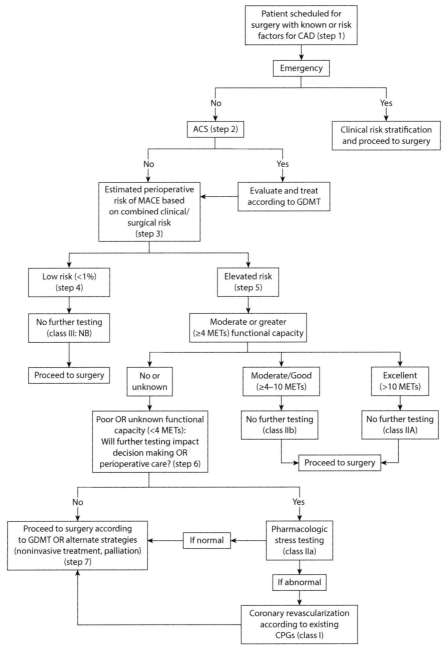

Figure 36A.2 The algorithm for perioperative cardiac assessment for CAD. (Modified with permission from Fleisher L A et al. Perioperative cardiovascular evaluation and management JACC 2014;64:e77–137.)

14. How do you stratify cardiac risk for non-cardiac surgical patients?

It is essential to risk-stratify the patient with IHD based on multiple risk parameters for prognostication and, more importantly, planning of perioperative care. Risk stratification is based on the following parameters:

1. History and physical examination

2. Investigations

3. Functional capacity expressed in METs

4. Type of surgery

5. Risk prediction models

6. Clinical risk factors

15. How do you assess for functional capacity?

1. MET (1 MET is equivalent to resting oxygen uptake of 3.5 mL/kg/min)

2. *Duke Activity Status Index (DASI)*: Score ranges from 0 to 58.2

3. *Cardiopulmonary exercise test (CPET)*: Deficiencies in CPET-derived variables: Ventilatory anaerobic threshold (AT), peak oxygen consumption (VO_2 peak) and ventilatory efficiency for carbon dioxide (VE/VCO_2) are associated with poor postoperative outcomes. A nine-point plot is useful.

METs: METs should be more than 4.

■ 1 MET = self-care, eating, dressing

■ 4 METs = 1 flight of stairs/hill

■ 4–10 METs = 2 flights of stairs, scrubbing the floor or moving heavy furniture

■ >10 METs = swimming, skiing, playing basketball or football

DASI: DASI is a set of standardized 11 questions. A higher score implies a higher functional capacity. A DASI score less than 34 implies an increased risk of perioperative complications.

CPET: CPET is a non-invasive method to assess cardiopulmonary function. A VO_2 max of more than 20 mL/kg/min implies good functional status. A VO_2 max less than 10 ml/kg/min implies high-risk patients.

16. What are the clinical risk factors for adverse cardiac events?

Patients with cardiac disease may manifest various adverse events in the perioperative period. The clinical risk factors which are of importance include:

■ CAD

■ Heart failure

■ Cardiomyopathy

■ Valvular heart disease

■ Arrhythmias and conduction disorders

17. What are the clinical predictors of increased perioperative cardiovascular risk?

Patients with cardiac diseases may be categorized based on various clinical predictors (**Table 36A.4**).

Table 36A.4: Cardiac Risk and Clinical Predictors

Level of Risk	Clinical Predictors
Major (cardiac risk >5%)	• Unstable coronary syndromes
	• Decompensated CHF
	• Significant arrhythmias
	• Severe valvular disease

(Continued)

Table 36A.4 (*Continued*): Cardiac Risk and Clinical Predictors

Level of Risk	Clinical Predictors
Intermediate (cardiac risk <5 %)	• Mild angina pectoris • Prior MI • Compensated or prior HF • DM • Renal insufficiency
Minor (cardiac risk <1%)	• Advanced age • Abnormal ECG • Rhythm other than sinus • Low functional capacity • History of stroke • Uncontrolled systemic hypertension

18. What are the risk prediction models?

There are multiple models with risk prediction for patients with cardiac diseases:

■ Revised Cardiac Risk Index (RCRI)

■ American College of Surgeons National Surgical Quality Improvement Program (NSQIP) risk score: riskcalculator.facs.org

■ Gupta's Myocardial Infarction and Cardiac Arrest score (MICA) calculator

■ AUB-POCES index (American University of Beirut-Preoperative CVS evaluation study)

■ Vascular Study Group of New England (VSGNE) risk index

■ Vascular Quality Initiative (VQI) cardiac risk index

19. What are the components of the RCRI?

RCRI is one of the important risk prediction models in patients with cardiac diseases. It has the following components:

■ A high-risk type of surgery (examples include vascular surgery and any open intraperitoneal or intrathoracic procedure)

■ History of IHD (history of MI or a positive exercise test, current complaint of chest pain considered to be secondary to myocardial ischaemia, use of nitrate therapy or ECG with pathological Q waves; do not count prior coronary revascularization procedure sunless one of the other criteria for IHD is present)

■ History of congestive heart failure

■ History of cerebrovascular disease

■ Diabetes mellitus requiring treatment with insulin

■ Preoperative serum creatinine >2.0 mg/dL (177 micromol/L)

20. What are the implications for RCRI?

Rate of cardiac death, nonfatal MI and nonfatal cardiac arrest according to the number of predictors:

■ No risk factors – 0.4% (95% confidence interval [CI]: 0.1–0.8)

■ One risk factor – 1.0% (95% CI: 0.5–1.4)

■ Two risk factors – 2.4% (95% CI: 1.3–3.5)

■ Three or more risk factors – 5.4% (95% CI: 2.8–7.9)

21. The MICA score is based on which parameters?

The MICA score is based on the following:

- Increasing age
- Type of surgery
- American Society of Anesthesiologists (ASA) physical status
- Abnormal creatinine
- Functional status

22. What are the perioperative complications in IHD patients undergoing non-cardiac surgery?

Patients with IHD can manifest various perioperative complications when undergoing non-cardiac surgeries. The perioperative complications include myocardial ischaemia, MI, cardiac failure, arrhythmia and cardiac arrest. The occurrence of these complications primarily depends on the severity of the underlying cardiac disease, its optimization and the extent of surgical intervention.

23. What are the recommendations for perioperative coronary angiography (CAG)?

CAG may be considered preoperatively in a selected group of patients. The class 1 recommendations for preoperative CAG apply only to patients with:

- Evidence for high risk of adverse outcome based on non-invasive test results
- Angina pectoris unresponsive to medical therapy
- Unstable angina, particularly when facing intermediate- or high-risk non-cardiac surgery
- Equivocal non-invasive tests result in patients with high clinical risk undergoing high-risk surgery

24. What are the indications for preoperative coronary artery revascularization?

Indications for preoperative coronary artery revascularization are as follows:

- Acceptable coronary revascularization risk and a large amount of viable myocardium with left main coronary artery stenosis
- Three-vessel CAD with left ventricular dysfunction
- Left main equivalent (high-grade block in the left anterior descending artery and circumflex artery)
- Intractable coronary ischaemia despite maximal medical therapy

25. How will you premedicate IHD patients?

Anxiolytics such as short-acting benzodiazepines like midazolam can be prescribed to these patients, as anxiety can cause tachycardia and hypertension and remains deleterious in patients with IHD. Also, the patient's routine medications like antihypertensive and antianginal drugs should be continued preoperatively and need to be resumed at the earliest point in the postoperative period.

26. What are the special precautions in compromised left ventricular systolic function?

The left ventricular function assessment remains an important aspect in the patient evaluation. The appropriate assessment modalities include a medical history for the presence of angina or MI, presence of symptoms suggestive of left ventricular failure like dyspnoea at rest or exercise and nocturnal orthopnoea and imaging findings on echocardiography and/or angiography.

27. What type of anaesthesia is preferred for patients with IHD requiring surgical intervention?

A balanced anaesthetic technique is preferred for patients with IHD undergoing non-cardiac surgery. The choice of anaesthetic agents remains debatable, and the choice needs to be individualized as per patient assessment. The technique for anaesthesia depends on various factors like proposed surgical procedures, their extent and duration, patient baseline cardiac status and optimization of the patient's cardiac condition. Patients should be sedated using appropriate agents like benzodiazepines (midazolam 1–2 mg) once monitors have been attached. The use of benzodiazepine has been found to delay recovery and increase the risk of postoperative delirium, especially in elderly patients. So routine use of benzodiazepine-based premedication is not advisable. The combined approach of regional and general anaesthesia is usually preferred for major surgeries. The induction of anaesthesia remains opioid-based, and fentanyl is the preferred opioid. Etomidate 0.2 mg per kg may be administered for induction and remains the drug of choice for patients with cardiac compromise. However, this is associated with adrenal suppression. The induction technique and airway management elicit a strong sympathetic response leading to haemodynamic perturbations, and hence smooth induction and careful airway management to prevent hypotension, hypertension and tachycardia need to be planned. In the case of patients with preserved left ventricular function, inhalational vs propofol-based anaesthetic regimens remain safe. Both inhalations, intravenous and combined agents, have been reported for their use in patients with IHD. But in patients with poor left ventricular function, potent inhalation agents such as isoflurane, sevoflurane and desflurane are avoided during induction and maintenance of anaesthesia or are cautiously used, as these can lead to haemodynamic compromise. A combination of fentanyl and isoflurane (or propofol) is a popular choice in such patients. The depth of anaesthesia should be monitored, and adequate depth should be maintained intraoperatively. The various neuromuscular blocking agents are safe in patients with IHD undergoing non-cardiac surgeries. So, any of the available agents may be used in these patients. Early extubation is desirable in these patients; hence shorter-acting agents remain preferred.

28. What are postsurgical challenges?

The patient should be monitored postoperatively for any ischaemic changes, as the perioperative phase remains a procoagulant phase, and there is increased oxygen demand. Early identification and management remain key for an optimal outcome. The more common modality of monitoring remains the ECG ST-T segment changes and measurement of cardiac markers in cases of ECG changes. The use of transthoracic and transoesophageal echocardiography has also emerged as bedside tools for cardiac function monitoring.

29. Extubating challenge in IHD: How and when?

Early extubation is desirable in patients with IHD. In case early extubation is not feasible for surgical reasons or haemodynamically instability, patients should be sedated appropriately to prevent the stress response. The shorter-acting agents like atracurium and cisatracurium are used, and residual neuromuscular blockade may be reversed with intravenous neostigmine and glycopyrrolate. Smooth extubation is desirable, and optimal pain relief needs to be ensured at the time of extubation as well.

30. Which patients will require intensive care?

Patients on beta-blockers have an obtunded compensatory response and respond poorly to hypovolemia, inhalational agents, induction agents like propofol and surgical intervention leading to hypotension. In the absence of a specific antagonist to beta-blockers, hypotension needs to be managed with correction of the reversible causes or the agent causing hypotension like the reduction of the doses of inhalational agents. The other drugs like atropine for symptomatic bradycardia, epinephrine, isoproterenol, glucagon and calcium may also be used as per the individualized case.

31. What is the transfusion trigger in a patient with IHD?

Caution is the key. There is no consensus regarding the transfusion trigger. Intuitively we restrict transfusion in left ventricular dysfunction patients and those patients who have established critical coronary disease on angiography where there is a presumed risk of thrombosis due to the rise of haematocrit. These risks versus the risk of tissue hypoxia have yet to be settled. However, the greater the degree of anaemia, the higher the benefit of transfusion is an accepted fact.

CASE STUDY 36A.1: REAL-WORLD CASE

Personal experience: Stent thrombosis during cholecystectomy, management and implications
    A 64-year-old, non-diabetic, non-hypertensive woman had a 3 mm × 23 mm sirolimus-eluting stent (Cypher®) for a 90% mid–left anterior descending (LAD) coronary artery eccentric lesion implanted 5 years back. She was on a regular dual antiplatelet. She came for

---

cardiac clearance for laparoscopic cholecystectomy a week before surgery, with a history of typical chest pain. A CAG was done which revealed only minor plaque in the mid-LAD proximal to the stented portion. Other coronary arteries were normal. Clearance was granted. She was taken off dual antiplatelet 5 days before surgery with the concurrence of the cardiologist as per usual practice. At the time she was taken to the operating theatre (OT) her ECG and echocardiogram were normal. Half an hour into surgery she developed hypotension (BP 80/60 mmHg), ST elevation in lead I in intraoperative ECG monitor leads and falling oxygen saturation. A 12-lead ECG showed anteroseptal STEMI. Echocardiography suggested that the LAD territory was hypokinetic with a left ventricular ejection fraction (LVEF) of 40%. CAG revealed stent thrombosis with a filling defect visible inside the stent with the sluggish distal flow (**Figure 36A.3**). An XB 3.5 guiding catheter (Johnson & Johnson Medical) was used to engage the left system and the LAD was wired. A thrombosuction run was done and a white clot aspirated. There was the resolution of the ST-segment elevation post-thrombosuction, and the patient made an uneventful recovery.

This case highlights several important points. Firstly, a pre-procedure normal CAG *does not guarantee* a smooth surgery. Second, any patient with a first-generation stent runs a risk of stent thrombosis once DAPT is taken off even as late as 5 years. Third, the on-site catheterization lab may be lifesaving.

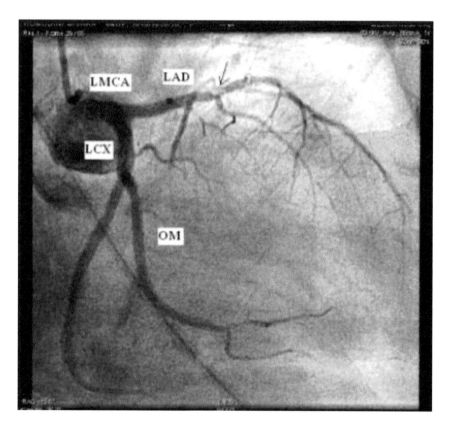

Figure 36A.3 CAG showing the eccentric intrastent filling defect in the LAD artery suggesting a freshly evolving thrombus (*arrow*).

FURTHER READING

1. Eagle KA, Berger PB, Calkins H. ACC/AHA guideline update for perioperative cardiovascular evaluation for noncardiac surgery executive summary. A report of the American College of Cardiology/American Heart Association Task Force on Practice Guidelines (Committee to update the 1996 Guidelines on Perioperative Cardiovascular Evaluation for Non Cardiac Surgery) Anesth Analg 2002;94:1052.

2. Hedge J, Balajibabu PR and Sivaraman T. The patient with ischaemic heart disease undergoing non cardiac surgery. Indian J Anaesth 2017;61:705–711.

3. Lee TH, Marcantonio ER, Mangione CM, et al. Derivation and prospective validation of a simple index for prediction of cardiac risk of major noncardiac surgery. Circulation 1999;100:1043–1049

4. Devereaux PJ, Chan MT, Alonso-Coello P, et al. Association between postoperative troponinn levels and 30-day mortality among patients undergoing noncardiac surgery. Vascular Events in Noncardiac Surgery Patients Cohort Evaluation Study I. JAMA 2012;307:2295–2304.

5. Sikdar S, Kumar D, Basu S, Mohanty V, Naik J, Banerjee S. Perioperative very late thrombosis treated with thrombosuction. Med J Malaysia 2012;67:129–130.

36B Perioperative Assessment and Management of Patients with Valvular Heart Disease for Non-Cardiac Surgery

Neha Pangasa and Dalim Kumar Baidya

36B.1 MITRAL STENOSIS (MS)

1. How would you grade the functional status in MS?

We assess functional status according to metabolic equivalents of task (METs): If a patient is able to climb one flight of stairs or climb uphill, the METs are >4.

2. How will you decide whether a patient can be taken for non-cardiac surgery or needs further evaluation?

This decision has to be made on a case-by-case basis depending on the urgency of surgery and the patient's functional status.

If it's an emergency surgery, then irrespective of functional status, perform clinical risk stratification and proceed for surgery.

If it's an elective surgery, assess the risk of major adverse cardiac events (MACEs). If there is an elevated risk for Major Adverse Cardiac Events (MACEs) but METs >4, proceed for surgery. However, if there is an elevated risk for MACEs and METs <4, then further testing like pharmacological stress testing is warranted.

3. How will you assess the risk for MACEs?

The risk for MACEs is estimated by the Revised Cardiac Risk Index (RCRI), which is described in terms of six predictors based on American College of Cardiology/American Heart Association (ACC/AHA) guidelines:

1. History of ischaemic heart disease (IHD)

2. History of congestive heart failure (CHF)

3. History of cerebrovascular disease (stroke/transient ischaemic attack)

4. History of diabetes mellitus requiring perioperative insulin use

5. Chronic kidney disease (serum creatinine >2 mg/dL)

6. *High-risk surgery*: Intrathoracic, intraperitoneal and suprainguinal, vascular

   - *0–1 predictors*: Low risk of MACE (<1%)

   - *≥2 predictors*: Elevated risk of MACE (>1%)

MACEs: Acute coronary syndrome (ACS), myocardial infarction (MI), heart failure (HF), unstable arrhythmia, death

4. What investigations would you order for patients with MS posted for non-cardiac surgery?

The following investigations should be done:

1. *Blood investigations*: Complete haemogram, liver and renal function tests with serum electrolytes (patients on digoxin, diuretics), coagulation profile (patients with atrial fibrillation [AF] and left atrial [LA] clot are likely to be on anticoagulants).

2. *Chest X-ray*: To look for:

   i. LA enlargement

   ii. Straightening of left heart border

   iii. Elevated left main bronchus

   iv. Pulmonary vascular congestion

   v. Kerley B lines

   vi. Double contour of right heart border

DOI: 10.1201/9781003027584-37

3. *ECG*: To look for:

   i. Atrial fibrillation: With ventricular rate

   ii. Left atrial hypertrophy: P mitrale

4. *2D echocardiography*: In patients with known MS and no 2D echocardiogram in the last year, or those with worsening dyspnoea, 2D echocardiogram should be done to look for:

   i. Gradient across the mitral valve

   ii. LA dilatation, LA clot, LA pressure

   iii. Pulmonary artery pressure

   iv. Right ventricular (RV) and left ventricular (LV) dysfunction

5. Why is the treatment history of these patients important?

Patients with AF are usually on beta-blockers, calcium channel blockers and/or digoxin for heart rate control, and those with AF or LA clots are on anticoagulants. Many patients are on diuretics for pulmonary congestion or HF. Angiotensin-converting enzyme (ACE) inhibitors are often prescribed for LV remodelling in patients with heart failure.

It is reasonable to continue beta-blockers until the day of surgery (ACC/AHA guidelines). Calcium channel blockers can also be continued. Serum electrolytes must be obtained preoperatively for patients on diuretics or digoxin. It is also reasonable to continue ACE inhibitors until the day of surgery (ACC/AHA guidelines). But ACE inhibitors and diuretics can be discontinued 1 day prior if excessive blood loss or fluid shifts are expected during the surgery.

Anticoagulants must be stopped according to American Society of Regional Anesthesia (ASRA) guidelines if neuraxial analgesia is planned.

6. What preoperative orders are given?

   i. Nil per oral for 6 hours after a light meal; 2 hours (clear fluids).

   ii. *Anxiolysis*: Sedation and anxiolysis should be given in order to avoid tachycardia, which would decrease the diastolic time and hence increase the gradient across the mitral valve. But at the same time, oversedation should be avoided to prevent hypoxemia and increase in pulmonary artery (PA) pressures. Alprazolam 0.25 mg on the day before and on the morning of surgery is usually given.

   iii. Anticoagulants (if neuraxial procedure is planned and a major surgery is planned). Warfarin is stopped 5 days prior and bridge with unfractionated heparin/low-molecular-weight heparin (UFH/LMWH) (target international normalized ratio [INR] <1.5). LMWH is withheld 12–24 hours prior depending on the prophylactic or therapeutic dose. UFH is stopped 4 hours prior (activated partial thromboplastin time [aPTT] must be done) (ASRA guidelines).

7. What are the haemodynamic goals in a patient with MS?

The goals are given in **Table 36B.1**.

Table 36B.1: Haemodynamic Goals in Mitral Stenosis

S. No.	Parameters	Goals
1.	Heart rate and rhythm	*Avoid tachycardia*: Maintain sinus rhythm
2.	Contractility	• Maintain • Avoid cardiodepressant drugs
3.	Preload	• Maintain • *Increased*: Pulmonary oedema • *Decreased*: Decreases already compromised LV filling
4.	Afterload	• Maintain • *Increased*: Decrease CO and functional MR • *Decreased*: Reflex tachycardia
5.	Pulmonary arterial pressure	• Maintain/Decrease • Avoid hypoxia, hypercarbia, acidosis, N_2O

8. What monitoring will you do if the patient is planned for a major surgery?

We use the following:

1. Five-lead electrocardiography (ECG), non-invasive blood pressure (NIBP) and pulse oximetry monitors and temperature probe.

2. Triple-lumen central line in the internal jugular vein inserted by ultrasound guidance prior to induction to monitor central venous pressure and give vasopressors if required intraoperatively.

3. Radial artery cannula inserted pre-induction for invasive blood pressure monitoring and arterial blood gas analysis in the perioperative period.

4. Pulse contour-derived cardiac output (CO) monitoring can be done if available.

9. How will you plan induction in this patient?

We use a generous amount of fentanyl (2–5 μcg/kg) to avoid tachycardia during intubation. We often use etomidate as an induction agent (0.2–0.6 mg/kg) due to its haemodynamic stability and vecuronium (0.1 mg/kg) or rocuronium (0.6 mg/kg) as muscle relaxants. Pancuronium is avoided due to its vagolytic effect, and atracurium can lead to hypotension due to histamine release.

10. How will you maintain anaesthesia in this case?

Volatile agents (isoflurane, sevoflurane, desflurane) can be used along with intermittent boluses of fentanyl or morphine and a muscle relaxant. N_2O is avoided in patients with pulmonary hypertension.

Good analgesia must be planned either with regional technique or IV opioids with supplemental NSAIDs/paracetamol, as sympathetic stimulation might increase the pressure gradient across the stenotic mitral valve.

Fluids must be judiciously administered to avoid overloading the LA and hence causing pulmonary oedema.

The heart rate must be controlled and sinus rhythm maintained. In the case of precipitation of AF, short-acting beta-blockers: Metoprolol (5 mg intermittent boluses), esmolol (500 mcg/kg) or calcium channel blockers like diltiazem can be given.

A controlled mode of ventilation should be used, and hypercarbia, hypoxia and acidosis must be avoided in the intraoperative period, as they lead to increased PA pressures. To maintain BP, titrated doses of vasopressors like phenylephrine can be used or an infusion of noradrenaline if required.

11. How will you plan to extubate this patient?

If it is not a major surgery or massive blood loss or fluid shifts have not occurred, the patient can be extubated in the operating room (OR). The haemodynamic response to extubation must be blunted with either IV lignocaine 1.5 mg/kg, 90 sec prior to extubation or esmolol 0.5–1 mg/kg.

12. Is neuraxial anaesthesia safe in a patient with MS?

In mild and moderate MS neuraxial anaesthesia can be considered with careful planning and monitoring. A low-dose spinal and graded epidural can be planned to prevent a precipitous fall in systemic vascular resistance (SVR) and reflex tachycardia, which might occur after a high dose of a local anaesthetic agent given intrathecally or epidurally. Intra-arterial BP must be continuously monitored. *Neuraxial blockade should be avoided in cases of severe MS.* ASRA guidelines must be followed in patients on anticoagulants if neuraxial block is planned.

36B.2 MITRAL REGURGITATION (MR)

13. What investigations would you order for patients with moderate MR posted for non-cardiac surgery?

The following investigations should be done:

1. *Blood investigations*: Complete haemogram, liver and renal function tests with serum electrolytes (patients on digoxin, diuretics), coagulation profile (patients with AF and LA clot are likely to be on anticoagulants)

2. *Chest X-ray*: To look for:

   i. Enlarged LA and LV (LA hypertrophy [LAH] and LV hypertrophy [LVH])

  ii. Enlarged RV (RV hypertrophy [RVH])

  iii. Signs of pulmonary congestion

3. *ECG*: To look for:

  i.   *LAH*: P mitrale

  ii. LVH

  iii. RVH

  iv. *AF*: With ventricular rate

4. *2D echocardiography*: In patients with known MR and no 2D echocardiography in the last year, or those with worsening dyspnoea (ACC/AHA guidelines), to look for:

  i.   Mitral valve/leaflet pathology

  ii. *Doppler*: Quantitative assessment of regurgitant volume, fraction and orifice area

  iii. LA, LV and RV dilatation and hypertrophy

  iv. RV and LV dysfunction

  v.   Pulmonary artery pressure

14. What medications is a patient with MR likely to be taking and how important is this?

Patients with MR could be taking:

1. *Digoxin and diuretics for CHF*: We have to check serum electrolytes before surgery; both can be continued up to the day of surgery, but diuretics may be omitted in the case of major surgery with anticipated massive blood loss or fluid shifts.

2. Beta-blockers, calcium channel blockers and digoxin for AF: Can be continued up to the day of surgery.

3. *Vasodilators (nitrates, ACE inhibitors) to decrease the regurgitant fraction and promote forward flow*: It is reasonable to continue ACE inhibitors up to the day of surgery (ACC/AHA guidelines), but they may be omitted in cases with anticipated massive blood loss or fluid shifts.

4. *Anticoagulants for AF/LA thrombus*: Follow ASRA guidelines if neuraxial analgesia is planned.

15. What preoperative orders will you give for this patient with moderate MR posted for non-cardiac surgery?

Nil per oral, anxiolysis and withhold anticoagulants (similar to MS):

  i.   Nil per oral for six hours after a light meal; two hours (clear fluids)

  ii. *Anxiolysis*: As in MS

  iii. *Anticoagulants*: As in MS

16. What are the haemodynamic goals in this patient?

These are given in **Table 36B.2**.

Table 36B.2: Haemodynamic Goals in Mitral Regurgitation

S. No.	Parameters	Goals
1.	Heart rate and rhythm	• *Maintain/Increased*: To maintain forward flow • Avoid bradycardia • Maintain sinus rhythm
2.	Contractility	• *Maintain/Increased*: To allow forward flow • Avoid cardiodepressant drugs
3.	Preload	• Maintain/Slightly increase • *Decreased*: Can increase regurgitant fraction
4.	Afterload	• Maintain/Decrease • *Increased*: Increased regurgitant fraction and cause pulmonary oedema
5.	Pulmonary arterial pressure	• Maintain/Decrease • Avoid hypoxia, hypercarbia, acidosis, N_2O

17. What monitoring will you do if a patient is planned for a major surgery?

As in MS.

18. Can you use any advanced monitoring in addition to what was noted earlier, and what are the recommendations for use?

A pulmonary artery catheter (PAC) can be used to measure RA pressure, RV pressure, pulmonary artery pressure (PAP) and pulmonary artery occlusion pressure (PAOP). In cases of severe MR, right heart output often overestimates the true CO. Routine use of PAC is not recommended but may be used if significant haemodynamic instability is present (ACC/AHA guidelines; class IIb recommendation).

Transoesophageal echocardiography (TEE) gives the advantage of monitoring left and right ventricular function as well as PAP in the intraoperative period. ACC/AHA guidelines suggest that it is reasonable to use TEE in the perioperative period in patients with haemodynamic instability if expertise is available.

19. Do you prefer neuraxial anaesthesia in a patient with moderate MR?

Neuraxial blockade is very safe in these patients, as a fall in SVR will promote forward flow and reduce the regurgitant fraction. Reflex tachycardia, which might occur in response to hypotension, will also promote a forward flow.

20. How do you plan induction of general anaesthesia in this patient?

Most of the induction agents can be safely used in patients with MR, as they cause a fall in SVR, which is beneficial in these cases. So, we will use fentanyl (2 mcg/kg) with propofol (2 mg/kg) in this case.

However, in patients where MR is secondary to IHD, a precipitous fall in SVR and reflex tachycardia would lead to an imbalance between myocardial oxygen supply and demand and impair myocardial perfusion. So, in such cases, induction agents which lead to haemodynamic stability like etomidate should be preferred. Any muscle relaxant can be used. But vecuronium along with fentanyl has been shown to cause bradycardia, which should be avoided.

21. How will you maintain anaesthesia in this patient?

Inhalational agents with intravenous opioids and muscle relaxants are quite safe in MR. Nitrous oxide is best avoided in patients with pulmonary arterial hypertension (PAH).

The depth of anaesthesia and analgesia must be adequate to prevent any sympathetic response and hypertension in the perioperative period, which would reduce the forward flow. Fluid administration must be judicious, as these patients are at risk of pulmonary oedema. Controlled ventilation, avoiding hypoxia, hypercarbia and acidosis, is preferred to prevent worsening of PAH.

In patients with MR secondary to IHD, a precipitous fall in SVR and reflex tachycardia are deleterious and can be managed with boluses of ephedrine (alpha- and beta-agonist) rather than phenylephrine (only an alpha-agonist).

Any RV dysfunction can be managed with inodilators like milrinone.

22. How will you plan extubation in this patient?

Avoid the sympathetic response and hypertension during extubation, as it can increase the regurgitant fraction. In cases of ischaemic MR, tachycardia should also be prevented by giving IV lignocaine 1.5 mg/kg, 90 sec prior to extubation or esmolol 1 mg/kg.

23. What is the plan for the postoperative period for this patient?

We will closely monitor the patient in the high-dependency unit/intensive care unit (HDU/ICU) in the postoperative period, as patients with moderate to severe MR are at risk of developing pulmonary oedema in the postoperative, period especially after a major surgery with massive fluid shifts.

36B.3 AORTIC STENOSIS (AS)

24. Can a non-cardiac surgery be done in a patient with severe AS?

A symptomatic patient with severe AS must undergo aortic valve replacement (AVR) before planning for an elective non-cardiac surgery. However, if such a patient has to undergo an emergency surgery, clinical risk stratification should be done and then proceed for surgery.

25. How will you investigate a patient with mild-moderate AS posted for non-cardiac surgery?

The following investigations should be done:

1. *Blood investigations*: Complete haemogram, liver and renal function tests with serum electrolytes (patients on digoxin, diuretics), coagulation profile.

2. *Chest X-ray*: To look for:

   i. Enlarged LA and LV (LAH and LVH)

   ii. Signs of pulmonary congestion

   iii. Enlarged RV (RVH)

   iv. Post-stenotic dilatation of the ascending aorta

3. *ECG*: To look for:

   i. *Signs of myocardial ischaemia (MI)*: Frequently co-exists with AS

   ii. LVH

   iii. *LAH*: P mitrale

   iv. RVH

   v. *AF*: With ventricular rate

4. *2D echocardiography*: To look for:

   i. Aortic valve pathology

   ii. Severity of AS (AV area, mean transvalvular gradient [TVG], peak aortic velocity)

   iii. LA, LV and RV dilatation and hypertrophy

   iv. RV and LV dysfunction

   v. PAP

26. What preoperative orders will you give for a patient with moderate AS posted for non-cardiac surgery?

Apart from standard NPO orders, we will advise sedation and anxiolysis with caution. Oversedation may lead to hypoxia (worsening PAH) or hypotension. Undersedation leads to tachycardia and thus compromised myocardial perfusion.

27. What are the haemodynamic goals in this patient?

These are given in **Table 36B.3**.

Table 36B.3: Haemodynamic Goals in Aortic Stenosis

S. No.	Parameters	Goals
1.	Heart rate	• *Avoid tachycardia*: Decreases diastolic filling time and hence cardiac output (CO); precipitates MI • *Avoid bradycardia*: Decreases CO due to low fixed flow across AV
2.	Rhythm	• Maintain sinus rhythm • Arrhythmias are poorly tolerated (apply defibrillation pads pre-induction) • Atrial kick for maintaining CO must be preserved in the setting of LV diastolic dysfunction
3.	Contractility	• *Maintain*: Avoid cardio-depressant drugs
4.	Preload	• *Maintain/Increase*: These patients are preload dependant • *Decreased preload*: Decreases already compromised LV filling
5.	Afterload	• *Maintain/Increased*: To maintain coronary perfusion • *Decreased afterload*: Reflex tachycardia
6.	Pulmonary artery pressure	• Maintain/Decrease • Avoid hypoxia, hypercarbia, acidosis, N_2O

28. What monitoring will you do if the patient is planned for a major surgery?

ECG, triple-lumen central line and radial artery monitoring are as usual. A defibrillator must be prepared, as these patients do not tolerate any arrhythmias (arrhythmias result in loss of atrial kick and reduced LV preload). If the surgical site is close to the heart, defibrillator pads should be attached prior to induction of anaesthesia. PAC may be used if significant haemodynamic instability is present (ACC/AHA guidelines; class IIb recommendation). However, pulmonary capillary wedge pressure (PCWP) is a poor predictor of preload in AS. TEE gives the advantage of continuously monitoring contractility, regional wall motion abnormalities and preload in the intraoperative period.

29. Do you prefer neuraxial anaesthesia in patients with moderate AS?

Neuraxial anaesthesia should be avoided in patients with moderate AS, as the slightest fall in SVR will not be tolerated by these patients with low, fixed CO. However, if planned, graded epidural blockade is preferred over combined spinal-epidural or spinal anaesthesia, with beat-to-beat monitoring of arterial BP and vasopressor infusion if needed. These patients are preload dependent and might need some fluid preloading before neuraxial blockade. Any fall in BP must be promptly treated with vasopressors, preferentially an alpha-agonist like phenylephrine to increase SVR and improve coronary perfusion pressure without causing tachycardia.

30. How will you induce general anaesthesia in this patient?

Induction agents which maintain haemodynamic stability should be preferred. Hence etomidate with opioids is the preferred choice for induction. Propofol and thiopentone are best avoided, as they decrease contractility and cause hypotension. Ketamine is also avoided as it causes tachycardia. Vecuronium and rocuronium are safe muscle relaxants. Pancuronium should be avoided due to its vagolytic effect, and atracurium can lead to hypotension due to histamine release.

The sympathetic response to laryngoscopy and intubation must be blunted to prevent tachycardia by giving lidocaine or esmolol intravenously before intubation.

31. How will you maintain anaesthesia in this patient?

Anaesthesia will be maintained with a combination of opioids and inhalational agents (sevoflurane), maintaining the contractility and SVR at all times and thus ensuring an adequate CO.

The depth of anaesthesia and analgesia must be adequate to prevent tachycardia in the perioperative period, as it will lead to decreased diastolic filling time in an already failing LV. Fluid administration should be targeted towards maintaining a good preload. Hypotension shall be promptly managed with vasopressors. Alpha-agonists like phenylephrine are preferred as they case vasoconstriction without causing tachycardia.

32. How will you plan extubation in this patient?

We will extubate the patient after administering IV lidocaine or esmolol to blunt the sympathetic response to extubation. The patient will be monitored in an HDU/ICU post-extubation, as these patients are at high risk of developing pulmonary oedema in the immediate postoperative period, especially after a major surgery.

36B.4 AORTIC REGURGITATION (AR)

33. What are the haemodynamic goals in a patient with AR?

These are given in **Table 36B.4**.

Table 36B.4: Haemodynamic Goals in Mitral Regurgitation

S. No.	Parameters	Goals
1.	Heart rate and rhythm	• *Maintain/Increased*: To maintain forward flow and decreased diastolic time and decrease regurgitant fraction • Avoid bradycardia • Maintain sinus rhythm
2.	Contractility	• *Maintain/Increased*: To allow forward flow • Avoid cardiodepressant drugs

(Continued)

Table 36B.4 (*Continued*): Haemodynamic Goals in Mitral Regurgitation

S. No.	Parameters	Goals
3.	Preload	• Maintain/Slightly increase • *Decreased*: Can increase regurgitant fraction
4.	Afterload	• Maintain/Decrease • *Increased*: Increased regurgitant fraction can cause pulmonary oedema
5.	Pulmonary arterial pressure	• Maintain/Decrease • Avoid hypoxia, hypercarbia, acidosis, N_2O

34. What investigations would you order and what preoperative advice will you give for a patient with moderate AR posted for non-cardiac surgery?

The investigations and preoperative orders will be essentially the same as in patients with moderate MR (discussed earlier).

35. What monitoring will you do if the patient is planned for a major surgery?

Same as MR.

36. Will you prefer neuraxial anaesthesia in a patient with moderate AR?

Neuraxial anaesthesia can be safely given in these patients, as a fall in SVR promotes forward flow.

37. How will you induce general anaesthesia in this patient?

Most of the induction agents can be safely used in patients with AR, as they cause a fall in SVR, which is beneficial in these cases. We use fentanyl (2 mcg/kg) with propofol (2 mg/kg) in this case.

Any muscle relaxant can be used. But vecuronium along with fentanyl has been shown to cause bradycardia, which should be avoided.

38. How will you maintain anaesthesia in this patient?

The principles are same as in MR. Depth of anaesthesia and analgesia must be adequate to prevent any sympathetic response and hypertension in the perioperative period, which would reduce the forward flow. Fluid administration must be judicious, as these patients are at risk of pulmonary oedema.

Controlled ventilation avoiding hypoxia, hypercarbia and acidosis is preferred to prevent worsening of PAH. Any RV dysfunction can be managed with inodilators like milrinone.

39. How will you plan extubation in this patient?

Avoid a hypertensive response during extubation, as it can increase the regurgitant fraction, with IV lignocaine 1.5 mg/kg, 90 sec prior to extubation.

40. What is the plan for the postoperative period for this patient?

We will closely monitor the patient in the HDU/ICU in the postoperative period, as patients with moderate to severe AR are at risk of developing pulmonary oedema in the postoperative period, especially after a major surgery with massive fluid shifts.

FURTHER READING

1. Otto MC, Nishimura RA, Bonow RO, et al. 2020 ACC/AHA guideline for management of patients with valvular heart disease. Circulation 2020;143(5):e72–e227.

37 Mechanical Ventilation

Basics for CCU Clinicians

Swarup Paul and Sunandan Sikdar

Chapter 37 may be accessed online at: www.routledge.com/9780367462215

DOI: 10.1201/9781003027584-38

38 Basics of Non-Invasive Ventilation

Abhradip Das and Sunandan Sikdar

1. What is non-invasive ventilation (NIV)?

NIV is defined as augmentation of ventilation without a conduit access to the airway.

2. What are the types of NIV?

1. *Pressure-targeted*: The operator sets the *inspiratory* pressure. The volume of air the patient receives is a function of the impedance to inflation of the lungs and chest wall and the inspiratory time (Ti). Ti should be of sufficient length to achieve an adequate volume and at a frequency that allows the patient time to fully exhale.

2. *Volume-targeted*: The operator sets the tidal volume to be delivered and the duration of inspiration (Ti). The ventilator generates the necessary pressure required to deliver this volume within this time.

3. What are the types of pressured-targeted ventilation?

- *Negative pressure ventilation*: Iron lung (used in the early days in cases of polio)

- *Positive pressure ventilation*: Continuous positive airway pressure (CPAP) and bilevel positive airway pressure (BIPAP)

4. What are the advantages of pressure (positive) targeted NIV?

1. *Pressure* delivered to the patient is *constant*, and this avoids the sudden and uncomfortable pressure increase that occurs with volume control.

2. It *compensates for an air leak*, which is an inevitable consequence of the interfaces used for NIV.

3. Positive pressure throughout expiration (EPAP) *flushes exhaled CO_2* from the mask and distal ventilator tubing and aids triggering and counteracts the tendency for upper airway collapse during expiration.

5. What is CPAP?

It is a continuous positive pressure provided to the airway throughout the respiratory cycle. CPAP actually does not provide a volume change, nor does it support minute ventilation. *It recruits lung units and improves V/Q matching.* It increases the functional residual capacity (FRC) and decreases the rate and work of breathing. It reduces airway resistance. It improves haemodynamics in pulmonary oedema by decreasing venous return, afterload and rate and increasing the cardiac index. CPAP is used most commonly in obstructive sleep apnoea (OSA) and pulmonary oedema.

6. What is BIPAP?

It is a bilevel support comprising inspiratory positive airway pressure **(IPAP) and EPAP.** IPAP is the pressure support that the device provides to help in the patient's own inspiration. EPAP is essentially positive end-expiratory pressure (PEEP), which helps to prevent alveolar collapse after the lung empties (**Figure 38.1**).

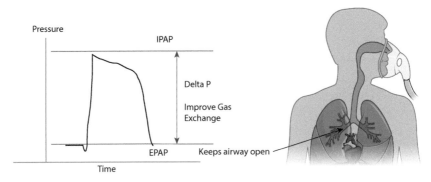

Figure 38.1 Principle of NIV.

DOI: 10.1201/9781003027584-39

7. What are the advantages of NIV?

1. Preservation of the airway defence mechanism
2. *Early support*: No need to wait for intubation
3. Intermittent ventilation possible
4. *Patient friendly*: Patient can eat/drink/communicate
5. Easy application and removal
6. Patient can cooperate with chest physiotherapy
7. Reduced requirement for sedation
8. Outside hospital use possible
9. Avoidance of complications of intubation and ventilator-associated events
10. Reduced infection rate

8. What are the goals of NIV use?

I. Acute care setting

- To augment ventilation and gas exchange (decrease CO_2 and improve oxygenation)
- To reduce work of breathing
- To avoid intubation
- To improve the patient's comfort
- To reduce the hospital stay

II. Chronic care setting

- To relieve or improve symptoms
- To improve quality of life
- To reduce hospital admission

9. What are the indications for the use of NIV in the acute care setting?

Level A

- Acute hypercapnic respiratory failure → Acute exacerbation of chronic obstructive pulmonary disease (COPD), obesity hypoventilation syndrome, neuromuscular disorder
- Weaning (in case of COPD)
- Cardiogenic pulmonary oedema
- Immunocompromised patient

Level B

- Acute respiratory failure in OSA
- Mild acute respiratory distress syndrome (ARDS)
- Postoperative respiratory failure
- Pre-intubation oxygenation (with 100% O_2)

Level C

- Asthma exacerbation
- In selected cases of ARDS
- Do not intubate state
- Pneumonia
- Cystic fibrosis

10. What are the contraindications to NIV?

- Non-availability of trained medical personnel
- Inability to fix the interface
  - Facial abnormality/anomaly
  - Facial burn, trauma
- Inability to protect the airway
  - Comatose patient
  - Stroke or neurological disease with bulbar involvement (poor gag reflex)
  - Confused and agitated
  - Fixed upper airway obstruction
- Haemodynamic instability
  - Uncontrolled arrhythmia
  - On high dose of inotropes
  - Recent/acute myocardial infarction (AMI)
- Severe gastrointestinal (GI) symptoms
  - Vomiting
  - Bowel obstruction
  - Recent GI surgery
  - Upper GI bleeding
- Life-threatening hypoxemia
- Copious secretions

11. What are the protocols for initiation of NIV in acute care settings?

- Explanation to the patient regarding the procedure in detail and giving assurance
- Set up the NIV machine at the bed side
- Propped-up position
- Choose the correct interface
- Hold the mask over the patient's face until the patient becomes comfortable with it. Strap on the face mask and *minimize air leak* without discomfort.
- *Monitor the patient*: Whether NIV is being tolerated and dyssynchrony is not occurring.
- Provide information to the patient and/or relatives regarding the risk of NIV failure and the requirement for invasive ventilation.

12. What are the parameters to be monitored during NIV support?

- *Sensorium*: If drowsy, discontinue NIV
- Mask comfort
- Tolerance for ventilator settings
- *Respiratory rate*: Usually respiratory rate reduces with adequate NIV setting
- Accessory muscle use, abdominal paradox indicates improper setting
- Ventilator parameters
- Air leaking

- Adequacy of pressure support
- Adequacy of PEEP
- Tidal volume (5–7 mL/kg)
- Patient-ventilator synchrony
- Continuous oximetry (until stable)
- Arterial blood gas (ABG) baseline and 1–2 hr after initiation of NIV support, then as clinically indicated

13. What are the interface and circuit in NIV?

Interface: There are three types of interfaces:

- Oro-facial mask/full-face mask
- Nasal mask/nasal pillow
- Helmet for NIV

Advantages of the oro-facial mask/full-face mask

- Better for more severe illness
- Effective in mouth breathing, pursed-lip breathing
- Delivers effective ventilation, so more effective in acute cases

Disadvantages of facial mask

- More claustrophobic
- Hinders cough, clearance of respiratory secretions and more risk of aspiration

Advantages of nasal mask

- Best suited for a cooperative patient
- Better with lesser severity of disease
- Not claustrophobic

Disadvantages of nasal mask

- More leak possible (in mouth breather)
- Less effective with patients with nasal deformities

A full-face mask should usually be the first type of interface used. A range of masks and sizes is required, and staff involved in delivering NIV need training in and experience with using them.

Circuit: The NIV circuit must allow adequate clearance of exhaled air through an exhalation valve or an integral exhalation port on the mask. It may be single limbed (for conventional bilevel NIV) or dual limbed (for critical care ventilators) (**Figure 38.2**).

14. How do you start modes and settings in NIV?

Mode

- *S*: *Spontaneous (also known as assist mode)*: Ventilator delivers assisted breaths in response to patient inspiratory effort. If the patient fails to make an adequate inspiratory effort, no ventilator support is delivered.

- *T*: *Timed mode (also known as control mode)*: Ventilator delivers breaths at a rate set by the operator regardless of patient inspiratory effort. The operator sets the inspiratory pressure, the length of inspiration and the inspiratory rate.

- *S/T*: *Spontaneous/Timed (assist-control)*: A backup rate is set by the operator. If the patient's respiratory rate is slower than the backup rate, machine-determined breaths will be delivered (i.e., controlled ventilation). If the patient breathes faster than the backup rate, no machine-determined breaths will be delivered and all triggered breaths will be assisted. The proportion of controlled and assisted breaths often varies, depending on the patient's state of alertness and respiratory drive.

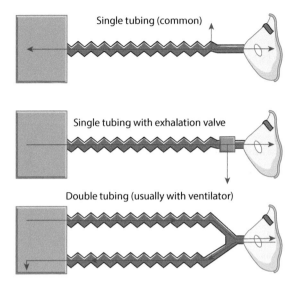

Figure 38.2 Single vs double tubing in NIV.

IPAP (**Figure 38.1**)

- It improves ventilation and increases tidal volume.
- IPAP required in COPD/OSA is around 15 cmH$_2$O to start with. Higher IPAP (>20 cmH$_2$O) is required if pH <7.25. If required IPAP is more than 30, it indicates demand for invasive mechanical ventilation.

EPAP (**Figure 38.1**)

- It improves oxygenation, opens up the upper airway and neutralizes auto-PEEP.
- To start, 3 or 4 cmH$_2$O of pressure is used (higher EPAP is required in OSA) and can be increased to 8 cmH$_2$O safely.

Pressure support (PS/ΔP) (**Figure 38.1**)

- ΔP = IPAP − EPAP
- Difference between IPAP and EPAP should be 4 cm H$_2$O at least to augment ventilation.

Rise time (**Figure 38.3**)

- Rise time is the time required to increase pressure from EPAP to IPAP.
- It should be kept at a minimum in the obstructive airway disease patient (rise time: 100–300 msec [<150 msec]) in fulfilment of their high respiratory demand. On the other hand, a wider rise time is beneficial for the restrictive physiology patient (rise time: 300–600 msec).

Trigger (**Figure 38.3**)

- The trigger (inspiratory) is an input required by the device to initiate a pressure increase from EPAP to IPAP. It may be a flow, pressure or time trigger. Usually, a flow trigger is preferred over pressure triggering in assisted modes (S, S/T), as it provides better patient-ventilator synchrony. Especially in COPD patients, flow triggering has been found to benefit auto-PEEP.
- Spontaneous triggering by the patient should always be encouraged in NIV.
- *Failure to trigger*: Causes are intrinsic PEEP in COPD or upper airway obstruction. Increasing EPAP/PEEP almost always solves the problem. If it persists, trigger sensitivity can be increased.
- *Auto-triggering*: Causes are the trigger is too sensitive, recoiling of the tube and a leak (at the interface or tubing) by mimicking inspiratory flow by dragging the EPAP below the trigger threshold. Reduced trigger sensitivity can overcome this problem

Cycle

- Cycle is when inspiration ends, and expiration begins. It may be **flow cycled or timed cycled**.

- *When flow drops to 25%, expiration begins*. However, in COPD, a drop of flow up to 40% is required to prevent dynamic hyperinflation and air trapping. It is recommended to keep higher (flow) cycle sensitivity in COPD patients to promote early cycling and lower sensitivity in restrictive patients. A high leak hampers the flow cycle and causes asynchrony. Time-cycled breaths have been shown to provide better synchrony in the presence of large leaks.

Ramp

- Usually EPAP and IPAP start low and gradually increase to the prescribed levels during the set time (ramp). Usually, up-titration is done over 10–30 min to achieve adequate augmentation of chest/abdominal movement and slow down the respiratory rate to meet the patient's demand. A shorter ramp is recommended for COPD.

Respiratory rate

- *Target rate*: Where you want your patient to be ideally breathing as per his or her pathological condition.

- *Backup rate*: Set the backup rate two to three breaths below the patient's spontaneous breath or target rate. This prevents asynchrony and ensures adequate ventilation.

- S-mode does not have a backup rate.

Inspiratory time (Ti) (**Figure 38.3**)

- Ti is very important but often missed. Ti eventually decides the I:E ratio. It is always good to have control over the minimum limit **(Ti Min)** for restrictive lung pathology and the maximum limit **(Ti Max)** for obstructive diseases.

- *Ti Max*: Should be limited in COPD so that there is enough time for exhalation.

- *Ti Min*: Should be higher for restrictive patients, as these patients tend to take very feeble, shallow breaths.

- Ti should be from 25% to 33% (called %Ti) of the respiratory cycle (0.8–1.2 sec) in obstructive cases and 33%–50% of the respiratory cycle (1.2–1.5 sec) in restrictive cases.
  Ti(Second) = {(60/RR) × %Ti}.

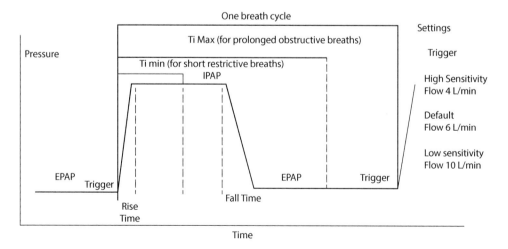

Figure 38.3 NIV nomenclature.

I:E ratio (inspiratory:expiratory ratio)

- I:E should be 1:2.5–1:3 in obstructive cases. In the case of neuromuscular disease (NMD), I:E should be 1:1. It should be titrated according to pH, pCO_2 (**Figure 38.4**).

| Respiratory Frequency (BPM) | Restrictive | | COPD | Normal |
	Ti Max	Ti Min	Ti Max	Ti Max
30	1.0	0.5	0.7	1.0
29	1.0	0.5	0.7	1.0
28	1.1	0.5	0.7	1.1
27	1.1	0.6	0.7	1.1
26	1.2	0.6	0.8	1.2
25	1.2	0.6	0.8	1.2
24	1.3	0.6	0.8	1.3
23	1.3	0.7	0.9	1.3
22	1.4	0.7	0.9	1.4
21	1.4	0.7	0.9	1.4
20	1.5	0.8	1.0	1.5
19	1.6	0.8	1.0	1.6
18	1.7	0.8	1.1	1.7
17	1.8	0.9	1.2	1.8
16	1.9	0.9	1.2	1.9
15	2.0	1.0	1.3	2.0
14	2.1	1.1	1.4	2.1
13	2.3	1.2	1.5	2.3
12	2.5	1.3	1.7	2.5

Figure 38.4 Tentative settings for NIV. (Courtesy Resmed Company.)

15. How do you care for the patient on NIV?

Sedation

- A non-pharmacological approach to calm the patient (reassuring the patient, proper environment) should always be tried before administrating sedatives. The risk of respiratory depression is given as the reason for non-use.

- In patients on NIV, sedation may be used with extremely close monitoring and only in an intensive care unit (ICU) setting with lookout for signs of NIV failure.

- Sedation in patients on NIV, if used appropriately and with the correct precautions, improves patient comfort and reduces chances of NIV failure.

- No preference for any drug can be recommended specifically for use in patients with acute respiratory failure (ARF) on NIV.

- Drugs which have been used in several trials are dexmedetomidine, propofol, remifentanil, and they have been found safe and effective to use.

Inhaled bronchodilator therapy/Aerosol delivery

- Use of an inhaled bronchodilator/aerosol is an integral part of therapy in COPD and asthma. Aerosol delivery is affected by leaks, inspiratory flow rates and position of the expiratory port.

- Brief discontinuation of NIV for the administration of bronchodilators appears to be safe. Bronchodilator therapy is probably better given during breaks in NIV. This may also facilitate coughing and the clearing of respiratory secretions.

- If the patient is **dependent on NIV**, bronchodilator drugs can be given by placing the nebulizer between the mask with or without expiratory port and the respiratory circuit (at least 30 cm distal from the mask in a single-limb circuit). A metered-dose inhaler (MDI) can be given successfully through the designated port in the circuit. A critical care ventilator used for providing NIV support has an integrated aerosol delivery system.

O_2 delivery

- Oxygen enrichment should be adjusted to achieve SaO_2 88%–92% in all causes of acute hypercapnic respiratory failure (AHRF) treated by NIV.

- Oxygen should be entrained as close to the patient as possible (in cases with a low flow rate).

- As gas exchange improves with increased alveolar ventilation, and NIV settings should be optimized before increasing the FiO_2. The flow rate of supplemental oxygen may need to be increased when the ventilatory pressure is increased to maintain the same SaO_2 target.

- Mask leak and delayed triggering may be caused by oxygen flow rates >4 L/min, which risks promoting or exacerbating patient-ventilator asynchrony by resulting a delay in triggering.

- A ventilator with an integral oxygen blender is recommended if the oxygen requirement is >4 L/min to maintain SaO_2 >88%.

Humidification

- Humidification is not routinely required. Heated humidification or heat and moisture exchanger (HME) may be considered if the patient reports mucosal dryness or if respiratory secretions are thick and tenacious. HMEs act by "catching" the heat and moisture of the expired air, filtering the microbes and transferring it to inspired air.

Chest physiotherapy

- This is an integral part of NIV support. It helps to clear respiratory secretions. Sputum retention can be a precipitant for AHRF and can cause NIV to fail. It is a common reason for respiratory distress post-extubation in patients initially managed by intermittent mandatory ventilation (IMV). Excessive sputum production characterizes bronchiectasis and cystic fibrosis and complicates some patients with acute exacerbation of COPD (AECOPD). Promoting sputum clearance can be particularly challenging in those with NMD and in the morbidly obese.

- Techniques such as manually assisted cough and mechanical insufflation-exsufflation (Mi-E) aid sputum clearance in patients with NMD and are beneficial.

16. How do you make a choice of ventilator?

- It can easily trigger into the inspiratory phase in response to the patient's effort (preferably flow based)

- It can be easily cycled to the expiratory phase in synchrony with the patient's breathing

- It should have adequate flow to meet the patient's demand (60–100 L/min)

- *Pressure pre-set*: Pressure support (at least up to 30 cm H_2O)

- It should have a spontaneous timed (S-T) option

- Capable of supporting a breath rate of at least 40/min

- Basic alarms

- Adjustable pressure rise-time, inspiratory/expiratory trigger

- Lightweight/portable/battery backup/user friendly

Both critical care ventilators with leak compensation (dedicated NIV mode) and bilevel ventilators (**Table 38.1**) have been equally effective in decreasing the work of breathing, respiratory rate and $PaCO_2$.

17. What are the precautions to be taken in case of infectious disease?

The following precautions should be taken when using NIV on a patient with infectious disease:

- Minimize leaks in the circuit.

- Non-vented face mask or a helmet with the best fit to the facial contour.

Table 38.1: Comparison of Three Different Types of Ventilator Systems

	Bilevel Ventilators	Critical Care Ventilators	Intermediate Non-Invasive Ventilators
Circuit	Single limb	Dual limb	Single/Dual limb
Exhalation valve	Passive exhalation valve (whisper swivel)	Active exhalation valve	Active exhalation valve
Type of ventilation	• Old models provided only pressure targeted ventilation. • Newer models provide both	Volume- and pressure-targeted ventilation	Volume- and pressure-targeted ventilation
Advantages	• Portable, easy to use • Most home ventilators	Predictable FiO_2 delivery	Predictable FiO_2 delivery
Disadvantages	• Unpredictable FiO_2 delivery, as it lacks a blender • May fail in patients with high O_2 requirement • Risk of rebreathing due to single limb	• Lack of leak compensation, affects the smooth functioning • Newer ICU ventilators have "NIV modes" with leak compensation.	• Some have an incomplete dual-limb circuit, in which the expiratory limb is only a short tube with a PEEP valve • This has negative effects on triggering and cycling

■ Secure the mask prior to turning on the ventilator. Turn off the ventilator before removing the mask.

■ A viral/bacterial filter (to filter particles 0.3 mm in size) at the outlet of the ventilator and also at the expiratory side of the circuit.

■ Complete decontamination of the ventilator before use in other patients.

18. What are the predictors of NIV failure?

Although use of NIV is safe, it needs careful observation to detect failure at the earliest. Various studies have shown the following criteria/risk factors for NIV failure:

■ High severity score of illness (APACHE II, SAPS II, SOFA scores)

■ Older age

■ Failure to improve after 1 hr on NIV

■ Multiorgan involvement

■ Premorbid status (inability to perform self-care)

■ Mean pH <7.25, mean $PaCO_2$ ≥75 mmHg after 2 hr of NIV initiation in patients with hypercapnic failure

■ Difficult to identify the aetiology of ARF

It is very important to know when to discontinue NIV and intubate and ventilate the patient.

■ *NIV failure*: Worsening mental status, deterioration of pH and $PaCO_2$ after 1–3 hr of therapy, refractory hypoxemia – when even a brief discontinuation of NIV leads to significant fall in oxygen saturation

■ Intolerance to NIV

■ Haemodynamic instability

■ Inability to clear secretions

19. How can weaning from NIV be done?

NIV can be discontinued when there has been a normalization of pH and pCO_2 and a general improvement in the patient's condition. When the patient is tolerating periods of NIV breaks, NIV support should be given intermittently during the day with continuous support overnight. In 2–3 days, the patient can be weaned off NIV initial during the day, but later at night also.

20. What are the common problems and troubleshooting in NIV?

Table 38.2: Troubleshooting NIV

Problem	Causes	Solutions
Ventilator cycling independently of patient's effort	• Inspiratory trigger sensitivity is too high • Excessive mask leak	• Adjust trigger • Reduce mask leak
Ventilator not triggering despite visible patient effort	• Excessive mask leak • Inspiratory trigger sensitivity too low	• Reduce mask leak • Adjust trigger • For NMD patients consider switch to PCV
Inadequate chest expansion despite apparent triggering	Inadequate tidal volume	• Increase IPAP. • In NMD or chest wall disease consider longer Ti
Chest/Abdominal paradox	Upper airway obstruction	• Avoid neck flexion • Increase EPAP
Premature expiratory effort by patient	Excessive Ti or IPAP	Adjust as necessary

21. What are the complications of NIV, and how can we minimize or rectify those complications?

1. It is extremely important for the air seal to be tight. Ulceration and pressure necrosis related to local skin effects commonly occur at the bridge of the nose.

   • Protective synthetic coverings may help prevent skin breakdown and ulceration on the bridge of the nose.

2. Eye irritation and pain or congestion of the nasal sinuses may occur.

   • Put some decongestant nasal drops.

3. Distension of the stomach due to aerophagia and aspiration may occur secondary to vomiting.

   • A nasogastric [NG] tube can be used to relieve the distension while still allowing the mask to seal.

4. Adverse haemodynamic effects from NIV are unusual.

   • Although preload reduction and hypotension may occur. Give intravenous fluids.

5. Previous episodes of ventilator-associated pneumothorax warrant consideration of admission to high-dependency unit (HDU)/ICU and use of NIV at lower-than-normal inspiratory pressures.

6. The development of a pneumothorax usually requires intercostal drainage and review of whether to continue with NIV.

FURTHER READING

1. Eliott M, Nava B, Schonhofer S. Non Invasive Ventilation and Weaning: Principles and Practice. Second Edition (2019). Taylor and Francis.
2. Spoleteni G, Hill N S. Non-invasive positive-pressure ventilation. Webb A, Angus D, Finfer S et al (Ed) Oxford Textbook of Critical Care. Second Edition (2016), pp 411–413.

39 Nutrition in Cardiac Intensive Care

Sunandan Sikdar and Swarup Paul

Chapter 39 may be accessed online at: www.routledge.com/9780367462215

DOI: 10.1201/9781003027584-40

40 Cardiac Aspects of Diabetes

Sunandan Sikdar and Kaushik Sen

1. What are the glycaemia parameters that influence outcomes in intensive care?

Hyperglycaemia, hypoglycaemia and blood glucose variability all influence intensive care outcomes.

2. What is the optimum target in intensive care?

Insulin should be initiated at a threshold of >180 mg/dL (10 mmol/L). Once insulin therapy is started, a target of 140–180 mg/dL should be maintained for the majority of critical care patients. More stringent goals, such as 110–140 mg/dL (6.1–7.8 mmol/L), may be appropriate for selected patients (e.g., critically ill postsurgical patients or patients with cardiac surgery), as long as they can be achieved without significant hypoglycaemia. The guideline-based antihyperglycaemic protocol for oral therapy is given in **Figure 40.1**. This, however is applicable to haemodynamically stable patients, especially those before discharge.

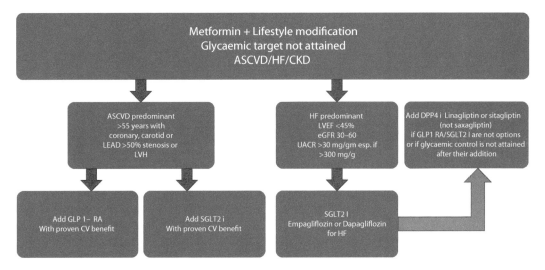

Figure 40.1   Oral antidiabetic drugs: Simplified algorithm for the cardiac care unit (CCU).

3. What are the methods of glucose measurement?

Capillary blood glucose (CBG) is the commonly used in intensive care. But it has inaccuracies, especially if the patient is on vasopressors, if there is reduced perfusion, oedema, anaemia (especially sickle cell anaemia), a hyperosmolar state and several medications commonly used in the hospital (paracetamol, high-dose vitamin C and dopamine). Further, CBG is obtained by "milking" the fingertip – this practice introduces interstitial fluid with a potentially different glucose concentration into the sample. In addition, a lag time between central and peripheral compartments may introduce inaccuracies. CBG at the postprandial state is higher than venous whole blood glucose by 1 mmol/L (1 mmol/L = 18 mg/dL), and the difference is maximum at 1 hour after food. The cut-off for diabetes in venous *plasma* glucose (gold standard) for fasting and the postprandial state is 126 mg/dL and 200 mg/dL, respectively (while in capillary blood, the corresponding values are 117 mg/dL and 185 mg/dL).

   Arterial blood glucose (ABG) by an ABG machine may be an acceptable alternative with lesser limitations than CBG. However, cost and the need for recurrent flushing of the arterial line limit its use. Flushing should never be done with glucose-containing solution.

4. What is the frequency of blood glucose measurement?

When on an insulin infusion protocol, it can vary from 15 min (mostly 30 min) to 2 hours but usually 1 hourly. When on a sliding scale, it is usually 6 hourly.

DOI: 10.1201/9781003027584-41

5. What is an acceptable sliding-dose insulin scale?

First of all, isolated use of sliding-scale insulin (SSI) is strongly discouraged now, especially if insulin is required after the first 1–2 days. The insulin requirement in any given patient can be divided into three parts: (1) basal, (2) prandial and (3) correctional. SSI should correspond to the correctional component only. So, a patient who is taking optimally orally insulin should be given a basal insulin, preferably once-daily injection glargine, or injection of detemir or NPH twice daily and fixed-dose prandial insulin (three times before food if short-acting human insulin or three to four times before food if rapid-acting analogues, e.g. Lispro/Aspart/Glulisine are used). As the glycaemic target is 140–180 mg/dL, if the *preprandial* CBG is beyond 180 mg/dL, one needs to add a correctional dose with SSI. A graded increase of 1–4 units for every 50 mg/dL increase beyond the target is a reasonable option. Initiate with a lower dose in the elderly, frail, patients with renal failure, those with multiple comorbidities or those with limited life expectancy.

A tentative published protocol for hospitalized Indian patients undergoing cardiac surgery is given in Reference 1.

6. Who is administered insulin?

Patients who are able to intake orally and are haemodynamically stable with a normal respiratory pattern can be administered oral antidiabetics. On the other hand, critical patients with hyperglycaemia (CBG >180 mg/dL) not on an oral diet or on enteral/parenteral feed or on vasopressors or on ventilation (invasive/non-invasive) require insulin (**Figure 40.2**). Infusion rates to achieve the same blood glucose concentration may vary widely between patients and in the same patient over time, as insulin sensitivity and resistance can change over time; they are also affected by other treatments.

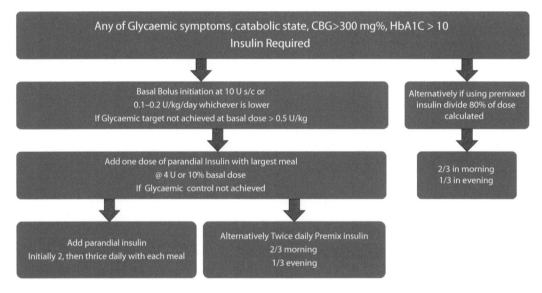

Figure 40.2 Simplified regimen for insulin use.

Hospitalized patients who are not critically ill are best managed with subcutaneous insulin if their blood glucose levels are beyond 180 mg/dL. Insulin infusion should be used in patients who are critically ill. Oral antidiabetic drugs should only be used in entirely stable patients who are taking adequately nutrition orally and are expected to have a short hospital stay.

7. What is the relation between diabetes and heart failure?

Diabetics have twice the prevalence of heart failure compared to non-diabetics. In large heart failure trials, the prevalence of diabetes is between 20% and 40%. The reasons why diabetes predisposes to heart failure can be grouped under the following heads:

a. *Altered myocardial characteristics*: Adverse myocardial energetics (decreased glucose oxidation and increased beta-oxidation), mitochondrial dysfunction, inflammation and fibrosis (so-called diabetic cardiomyopathy).

b. *Macrovascular and atherosclerotic involvement*: Ischaemic heart disease leads to myocardial infarction (MI) and left ventricular (LV) dysfunction. Both heart failure with reduced ejection fraction (HFrEF) and heart failure with preserved ejection fraction (HFpEF) can occur.

c. Endothelial dysfunction and microvascular involvement.

d. Diabetic nephropathy/diabetes-related renovascular disease additionally causes fluid overload, hypertension and HFpEF.

8. What is the treatment for diabetes and heart failure?

The standard treatment for heart failure using an angiotensin-converting enzyme inhibitor (ACEI), angiotensin receptor blocker/angiotensin receptor/neprilysin inhibitor (ARB/ARNI), beta-blocker or aldosterone antagonist holds true in diabetics too. In addition, the EMPA-REG OUTCOME and DAPA-HF trials have established the role of sodium glucose co-transporter-2 inhibitors (SGLT-2Is) empagliflozin and dapagliflozin in reducing heart failure hospitalization (nearly 35% reduction). Empagliflozin has also been shown to improve mortality. The glucagon-like peptide 1 (GLP-1) analogue liraglutide also reduced composite outcomes, which included heart failure. Dipeptidyl peptidase 4 (DPP-4) inhibitors are commonly used antidiabetics, of which saxagliptin (SAVOR-TIMI trial 53) has been reported to significantly increase hospitalization for heart failure and should not be used. Alogliptin (in the EXAMINE trial) reportedly increased heart failure in patients who did not have heart failure at baseline, although it included high-risk patients within 15–90 days of acute coronary syndrome (ACS). So, it should also be used with caution. Fortunately, the more commonly used linagliptin (CAROLINA and CARMELINA trials) and sitagliptin (TECOS trial) are heart failure neutral. There is a lack of randomized data for vildagliptin. Thiazolidinedione (TZD) and pioglitazone are known to cause fluid retention and can precipitate heart failure and should not be used or stopped if already in use. Metformin can be used as a first-line drug if advanced renal disease (estimated glomerular filtration rate [eGFR] <30 mL/min/1.73 m^2) is absent (**Figure 40.1**).

9. What are the salient points about revascularization in diabetes in stable ischaemic heart disease (IHD)?

In stable IHD, the role of routine invasive therapy (percutaneous coronary intervention/coronary artery bypass graft [PCI/CABG]) in reducing death, MI or stroke was negated by the COURAGE and ISCHEMIA trials. In the ISCHEMIA trial at 3.3 years, stable IHD patients, even those with moderate to severe ischaemia on non-invasive testing but with normal LV function, invasive strategy was no better than medical therapy. The benefit of invasive therapy occurs in the following situations: (a) In LV ejection fraction (LVEF) <35% or those in heart failure, (b) significant left main stenosis and (c) highly symptomatic patients. While the choice of therapy in diabetes with critical single-vessel disease or double-vessel disease not involving the proximal left anterior descending artery (LAD) (SYNTAX <23) is usually PCI, in those with two- or three-vessel disease with proximal LAD involvement or SYNTAX >23 or LV dysfunction, a heart team discussion is more appropriate. FREEDOM and other trials have shown that in multivessel disease with diabetes, CABG was superior to PCI in reducing all-cause mortality, MI and stroke at a follow-up of 5 years. This superiority of CABG is not maintained in non-diabetics.

10. What are the principles of management of ACS in diabetics?

The following principles should be followed:

a. All ACS patients must be screened for diabetes (HbA1c >6.5%).

b. Diabetes increases the risk of mortality by two times, and diabetic women have a higher mortality than men.

c. All patients with ST-elevation MI (STEMI), ACS with haemodynamic instability and ACS with dynamic ST changes or those with GRACE score >140 must proceed for early cardiac catheterization. Immediate for STEMI and <24 hours for ACS.

d. The use of drug-eluting stents has significantly improved outcomes in diabetics.

e. For those with non-ACS presentation with multivessel disease + SYNTAX >22 or proximal LAD involvement, CABG is preferred if the surgical risk is acceptable.

f. For STEMI with an occluded major vessel, for non-ACS multivessel disease with SYNTAX <22 without proximal LAD involvement, PCI is the procedure of choice.

g. Ticagrelor or prasugrel should be used as dual antiplatelet therapy (DAPT) during and after intervention. Clopidogrel should be used in those with high bleeding risk or those in whom a non-vitamin K antagonist is to be used concomitantly due to atrial fibrillation.

h. Hyperglycaemia must be managed with a target CBG <180 mg/dL without causing hypoglycaemia.

i. Though some benefit was found in an insulin-glucose-potassium infusion in the IMMEDIATE trial, the role of such therapy in reducing in-hospital mortality is yet to be established in routine practice.

j. Renal function should be monitored 2 days after coronary angiogram (CAG).

11. What is the role of diabetes in lower extremity arterial disease (LEAD)?

Diabetes is strongly associated with LEAD, with an odds ratio between 1.9 and 4. This risk is determined by the duration of diabetes, degree of glycaemic control and insulin requirement. LEAD in diabetics has a strong preponderance for below-knee-only disease (nearly 40%). Chronic limb-threatening ischaemia (CLTI) leads to gangrene, usually starting from the toe and then progressively involving the foot and ankle. The presence of neuropathy adds to delayed recognition due to the absence of pain, increasing the risk of foot infection, non-healing ulcers and increased risk of amputation. Early recognition may be possible by routinely screening for LEAD with the Ankle-Brachial Index (ABI). An ABI <0.9 implies LEAD, while an ABI >1.4 implies calcified arteries, both of which are associated with increased cardiovascular risk. In diabetics ABI has reduced sensitivity because the presence of arterial calcification makes the arteries stiffer and hence falsely elevates the ABI. The Toe-Brachial Index (abnormal <0.7) may more accurate. Due to the very distal nature of the disease and the presence of calcification, CT or MR angiography may be less accurate, and invasive digital subtraction angiography may be preferred.

12. How do you manage LEAD with critical ischaemia?

In the case of diabetics, limb salvage following revascularization has continued to improve. Open surgery with saphenous vein graft to tibial/pedal vessels may give a more durable result than endovascular techniques in many cases. However, medical therapy with antiplatelets (aspirin 75 mg, clopidogrel 75 mg whether to give dual antipaltelets in symptomatic patients should be individualized), atorvastatin 80 mg, cilostazol (100 mg twice daily), antihypertensives (ACEI/ARB) and antidiabetics is also of paramount importance. In advanced disease there is an emerging role of low-dose rivaroxaban (2.5 mg twice daily) in improving limb-related outcomes.

13. How does diabetes relate to atrial fibrillation (AF) and stroke risk?

Apart from being a stroke risk factor in AF scores like CHADVAS, diabetes frequently coexists with AF. The causative role of diabetes in development of AF is not certain. Development of AF leads to heart failure due to loss of late diastolic atrial kick with a stiff ventricle.

FURTHER READING

1. Bansal B, Mithal A. Carvalho P et al. Medanta insulin protocols in patients undergoing cardiac surgery. Indian Journal of Endocrinology and Metabolism 2014. 18: 455–461
2. American Diabetes Association: Diabetes Care in the Hospital: Standards of Medical Care in Diabetes 2020. Diabetes Care Volume 43, Supplement 1 2020: S193–202

41 Cardiac Arrest

Resuscitation and After

Sunandan Sikdar and Kowshik Paul

1. What are the outcomes of cardiac arrest (CA) in the cardiac care unit (CCU)?

The CCU may be the best place to resuscitate a CA. Only a third of CAs outside the hospital are resuscitated to be admitted to the hospital. Although there is no specific survival data about arrest in the CCU, as low as 12% of out-of-hospital cardiac arrest (OHCA) and 24% of in-hospital cardiac arrest (IHCA) cases are discharged.

2. What is the adult chain of survival?

1. Recognize symptoms
2. Early cardiopulmonary resuscitation (CPR)
3. Defibrillate with an automatic external defibrillator (AED)
4. Advanced life support
5. Post-CA care

3. What is post-cardiac arrest syndrome (PCAS)?

PCAS is a pathophysiological complex arising from the after-effects of cessation of circulation during CA and consists of four components:

a. Anoxic brain injury (BI)

b. Systemic ischaemia-reperfusion injury (IRI)

c. Post-arrest myocardial dysfunction (PAMD)

d. Persistent precipitating pathology

PCAS consists of the following phases:

Immediate phase: 0–20 min after return of spontaneous circulation

Early phase: 20 min to 12 hr

Intermediate phase: 12 hr to 3 days

Late phase: 3 days onwards

4. What are the components of CA care?

During arrest before restoration of spontaneous circulation (ROSC):

a. CPR

b. Defibrillation/Electrical management (temporary pacing)

c. Airway management and ventilation

d. *Drug therapy*: Antiarrhythmics and vasopressors

After arrest after ROSC:

a. Cautious fluid repletion

b. Vasopressors for maintaining the mean arterial pressure (MAP) 70 mmHg

c. *If comatose*: Temperature-targeted management (TTM)/hypothermia

d. *Optimize organ perfusion*: Assessing use of dobutamine

e. *Mechanical circulatory support*: Intra-arterial balloon pump (IABP), venoarterial extracorporeal membrane oxygenation (VA-ECMO)

DOI: 10.1201/9781003027584-42

f. *Appropriate diagnostic tests*: ECG, early angiography if ST-elevation myocardial infarction (STEMI) is suspected

g. *Appropriate prognostic tests*: EEG, CT brain for BI evaluation

h. De-escalation of therapy in selected cases

5. What are the principles of CPR?

1. Closed-chest cardiac massage (chest compressions) can produce enough forward blood flow to the brain and organs to decrease the extent of ischaemic injury and to delay metabolic deterioration.

2. Change from airway, breathing, circulation (ABC) to compression, airway, breathing (CAB): Early initiation of chest compression has improved outcomes. Start CPR within 10 sec.

3. High-quality chest compressions (**Figure 41.1**) are defined as a rate between 100 and 120 compressions per minute with a depth of at least 2–2.5 inches in adults, allowing full recoil. Compressions faster than 120 per minute may not allow for cardiac refill and reduce perfusion. Chest compressions should be delivered to children (less than 1 year old) at a depth of one-third of the chest, usually about 1.5–2 inches (4–5 cm). Use the heel of one hand on the lower half of the sternum in the middle of the chest, keeping other hand over the top of the first hand. Do not lean on the chest in between compression, as it prevents recoil.

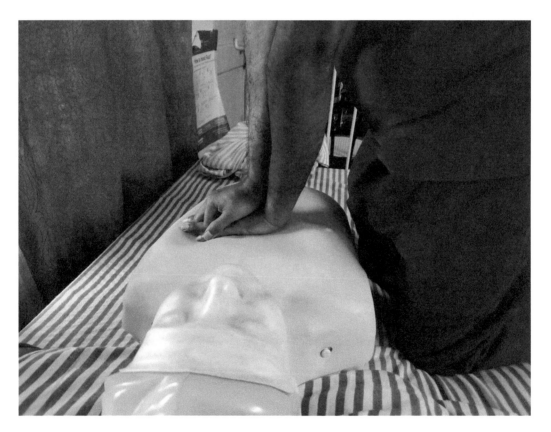

Figure 41.1 Chest compression technique.

4. Interruptions of chest compressions, including pre- and post-AED shocks, should be as short as possible.

5. Compression-to-ventilation ratio remains 30:2 for an individual without an advanced airway in place. For those with an airway, one ventilation every 6 sec.

6. Biphasic defibrillators are more effective in terminating life-threatening rhythms and are preferred to older monophasic defibrillators.

7. Standard-dose epinephrine (1 mg every 3–5 min) is the preferred vasopressor.

8. After 30 compressions, stop compressions and open the airway by tilting the head and lifting the chin with the index and middle fingers to give rescue breaths (except in the case of neck injury). Observe for a rise of the chest.

9. In two-rescuer CPR with bag and mask ventilation, the second rescuer holds the bag-mask with one hand using the thumb and index finger in the shape of a "C" on one side of the mask to form a seal between the mask and the face, while the other fingers open the airway by lifting the person's lower jaw.

10. If the pulse is palpable after initial CPR, one ventilation is given every 6 sec. If the pulse is still not palpable, CPR continues for 2 min and then rhythm is assessed and the cycle continues. If $ETCO_2$ during CPR <10 mmHg, vasopressors should be added.

6. How do you use an AED?

1. The oxygen tubing should not be across the patient's chest while defibrillating.

2. Caregivers must stay away from the patient during shock delivery.

3. Adult/Paediatric pads/paddles should be placed on a bare chest with the jelly provided.

4. One pad on the upper right side beside sternum and the other on the chest a few inches below the left arm near apex.

5. The AED reads the rhythm and then gives for ventricular fibrillation (VF) a defibrillation (unsynchronized) shock (**Figure 41.2**) and for ventricular tachycardia (VT) a (synchronized) shock. For biphasic defibrillators 200 joules and for monophasic one 360 joules are usually recommended.

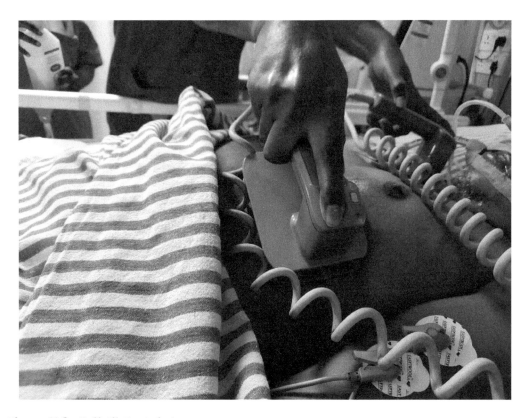

Figure 41.2 Defibrillation technique.

6. If no pulse post-shock, resume CPR immediately.

7. In patients with an electronic device, keep the pads away from the pulse generator.

7. What is the ACLS survey?

1. *Airway*: Advanced airway in a hospital setting.

2. *Breathing*: Give 100% O_2, keep SpO_2 >94%. High-quality CPR should produce a CO_2 between 10 and 20 mmHg. *If the ETCO2 <10 mmHg after 20 min of CPR for an intubated individual, then you may consider stopping resuscitation attempts.*

3. *Circulation*: Use intravenous or intraosseous route to give drugs.

4. *Differential diagnosis*: Rapidly diagnose the cause of CA.

8. What are the drugs used in resuscitation?

- Amiodarone 300 mg (5 mg/kg)
- Lidocaine 100 mg (1.5 mg/kg)
- Epinephrine 1 mg
- Dopamine, noradrenaline, atropine are other drugs that can be used and you can refer to chapter on vasopressors and Reference 3

9. What are the principles of airway management?

Proper bag-mask ventilation in an earlier stage of CA may be more effective than attempting intubation, especially because positive pressure ventilation itself has detrimental effects.

10. What are the types of airways?

Changing from bag-mask ventilation to intubation is done quickly, hampering CPR as little as possible. Two types of routes may be used:

a. Nasopharyngeal airway (NPA) – By nose

b. Oropharyngeal airway (OPA) – By mouth

If gag or cough reflex is present, use NPA.

The main advantage of NPA over OPA is that it can be used in either conscious or unconscious individuals because the device does not stimulate the gag reflex.

Attempts at suctioning should not exceed 10 sec. To avoid hypoxaemia, follow suctioning attempts with a short period of 100% oxygen administration.

11. How do you assess neurologic outcomes?

The first step is proper assessment of neurologic status (Table 41.1). A patient with loss of pain stimuli and brainstem reflexes even after 6 hr after resuscitation has a grim prognosis. An absent pupillary and corneal reflex 72 hr after arrest implies the worst prognosis. A CT scan of the brain suggesting a grey to white matter ratio (GWR) <1.2 is a marker of an adverse neurologic prognosis. CT of the brain may show intracranial haemorrhage unexpectedly, and appropriate corrective action should be taken. EEG is important to rule out continuing status epilepticus or undiagnosed myoclonus. Burst suppression on EEG is a poor prognostic marker in CA.

Table 41.1: Rapid Neurologic Exam

Parameter	Normal Response	Significance
Spontaneous breathing present when in ventilation	Total breathing rate more than set ventilation rate	Intact respiratory centre function
Pupillary reaction to light	Constriction	Intact brainstem
Corneal reflex	Blinking in response to with wisp of cotton	Intact brainstem
Doll's eye	Eyes move in opposite direction to the turning of head	Intact brainstem
Gag reflex	Gag on suction of posterior pharynx	Intact brainstem
Cough reflex	Cough on suction	Intact brainstem
Motor response	Withdrawal of upper and lower limb on pain	Intact pyramidal tract

12. How do you do TTM?

After CA, three waves of neuronal injury occur in the brain: (1) Initial hypotension – hypoxia – low and slow flow; (2) A second wave of ischaemia – reperfusion – injury; and (3) A third wave of injury due to temperature dysregulation and the accompanying cytokine-induced pyrexia. Severe neuronal injury induces death in 24–48 hr after ROSC.

TTM, or controlled hypothermia, by maintaining a temperature of 32–36°C has been shown in some studies to improve neurologic outcomes if started within 6 hr of ROSC.

The contraindications to TTM include refractory shock and bleeding disorders. The relative benefit of 33°C vs 36°C vs normothermia is yet to be determined with certainty. However, for those with unstable haemodynamics, near normothermia is better, while for those judged to have severe neuronal injury, 33°C may be better.

Infusing saline from a refrigerator via a central line or using ice packs or cooling blankets are practical but crude ways of using this technique in situations like the emergency room (ER) where cooling devices with a feedback loop are not available.

Controlling shivering with dexmedetomidine (bradycardia is a side effect) or propofol (*side effect*: hypotension) may improve pyrexia control. Using benzodiazepine may hamper the neurological assessment. Neuromuscular blockers have also been used for this purpose.

13. What are the cardiovascular implications post-CA?

Post-CA, the haemodynamics pass through four phases:

a. *Initial hypertension and tachycardia phase*: Due to vasopressors administered.

b. *Honeymoon period*: Phase of relative haemodynamic stability as the effect of vasopressors wanes.

c. *PAMD phase*: PAMD leads to cardiogenic shock at around 6–8 hr after ROSC.

d. *Phase of vasoplegia*: Between 24 and 48 hr, profound hypotension and shock may be seen – this phase has similarities to septic shock. Vasopressor requirement peaks during this phase.

Shock, persistent acidosis and hypotension (MAP <70 mmHg) are poor prognostic markers after ROSC. Recurrent cardiac arrest occurs in 10%. Post-ROSC, there is a capillary leak syndrome which should be treated with IV fluids. If hypotension does not improve, noradrenaline is the vasopressor of choice. Aggressive fluid resuscitation may lead to pulmonary oedema, especially if there is left ventricular (LV) dysfunction. In the case of PAMD, dobutamine may be helpful in some cases. An $ScvO_2$ <70% indicates requirements for an inotrope.

If arrest is due to a treatable cause, like STEMI/acute coronary syndrome (ACS) or pulmonary embolism, specific treatment is instituted. STEMI/ACS must be subjected to coronary angiogram (CAG) + revascularization after quick stabilization even if the patient is in a coma.

When used in a young patient with a reversible cause, emergent VA-ECMO may of value in two ways: Extracorporeal CPR (ECPR) deployed rapidly during CPR itself and secondly during the post-ROSC phase. Young patients with a reversible cause of CA and shockable rhythms when initiated on ECPR within 20 min from the start of CPR and preferably with $ETCO_2$ >20 mmHg are the optimal candidates for this procedure. However, randomized controlled trials and outcome data are lacking.

Post-ROSC there is myocardial stunning due to the combined effects of oxidative stress from ischaemia-reperfusion injury, cytokine storm and deleterious effects of vasopressors, leading to an LV ejection fraction (LVEF) of 35%–40%. Though it is challenging to differentiate this entity from previously existing structural heart disease, serial echocardiogram will show improvement in ventricular function.

14. What are the respiratory implications for CA?

Respiratory arrest is often a part of cardiac arrest. $ETCO_2$-guided ventilation may be useful. A tidal volume of 6–8 mL/kg body weight and positive end-expiratory pressure (PEEP) of 5–10 mmHg is beneficial in reducing lung injury (**Table 41.2**). Post-ROSC hypoxemia (PaO_2 <60 mmHg) or hyperoxemia (PaO_2 >300 mmHg) both are detrimental and hence should be avoided. PaO_2 80–150 mmHg (SpO_2 94%–99%) is acceptable. The injured brain is still responsive to CO_2. pCO_2 <35 mmHg can trigger cerebral vasoconstriction and hence precipitate injury. Permissive hypercapnia with pCO_2 of 45–50 mmHg is a useful goal in the post-CA situation.

Table 41.2: Respiratory Parameter Settings for Ventilation in Post-Cardiac Arrest Syndrome

1. *Acceptable SpO$_2$*: 94%–97%
2. pO$_2$ 70–100 mmHg
3. PEEP 5–10 cmH$_2$O
4. pCO$_2$ 40–45 mmHg
5. Tidal volume <6 mL/kg if ARDS
6. Tidal volume <8 mL/kg if no ARDS

---

15. What are the neurologic complications of CA?

Two major neurologic complications are cerebral oedema and seizures.

Cerebral oedema is common after hypoxic BI. A CT scan showing a GWR ratio <1.2 is suggestive. Cerebral oedema leading to elevation of intracranial pressure (ICP) is a poor prognostic marker. Elevation of the head of the bed, hyperventilation and osmotherapy with mannitol are unproven therapies in CA patients with this condition. However, maintaining MAP with vasopressors is of great importance to improve brain tissue oxygen levels.

Seizures occur in 25% of patients post-arrest and herald a poorer prognosis. Status epilepticus has a particularly bad prognosis. Similarly, a poor prognosis has been described for status myoclonus, especially if it lasts for >30 min. EEG monitoring and brain imaging are necessary. Levarecitam, valproic acid, phenytoin, phosphenytoin and lacosamide have all been used, with no agent being proved better than the rest.

FURTHER READING

1. Kang Y. Management of post-cardiac arrest syndrome. Acute Crit Care (August 2019);34(3):173–178.
2. Walker Amy C, Johnson Nicholas J. Critical Care of the post-cardiac arrest patient. Cardiol Clin (2018);36:419–428.
3. Disque K. ACLS Advanced Cardiac Life support provider handbook. (2015); Sartori Publishing.

42 Cardiac Assist Devices

Karan Madan, Sourabh Pahuja, and Sunandan Sikdar

1. What are the cardiac assist devices utilized in cardiac critical care?

In a patient with cardiogenic shock (CS) with insufficient response to vasopressors, shifting early to cardiac assist devices before irreversible changes start may be life-saving. The available devices are (**Figure 42.1**):

1. Intra-aortic balloon pump (IABP)

2. Impella device

3. Extracorporeal membrane oxygenation (ECMO)

4. Tandem Heart

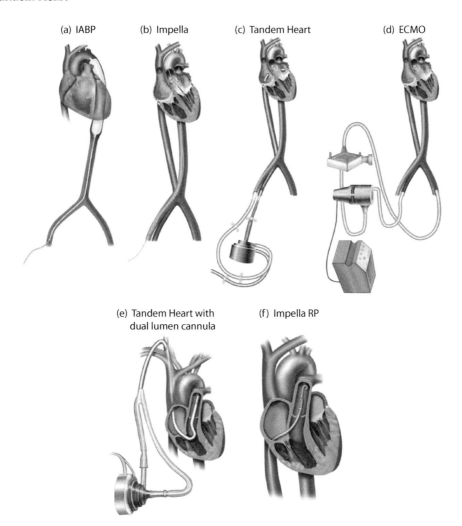

Figure 42.1 Types of mechanical circulatory support. (With permission from Aditya Mandawat, Sunil V. Rao. Percutaneous Mechanical Circulatory Support Devices in Cardiogenic Shock. Circulation: Cardiovascular Intervention. Wolters Kluwer Health, Inc. 2017.)

They are all grouped under the term mechanical circulatory support (MCS). The earliest left ventricular (LV) assist devices (LVADs) used pulsatile flow (devices filled during diastole and ejected

DOI: 10.1201/9781003027584-43

during systole), but these led to cumbersome systems. Nowadays most devices use continuous flow with a smaller number of moving parts. The purpose of using an MCS device can be classified as follows:

1. Acute and temporary support (e.g. in acute myocardial infarction [AMI] with CS – usually IABP/Impella)

2. Bridge to transplant (e.g., advanced heart failure [HF] with CS and long waiting time to transplant)

3. Destination therapy (e.g., advanced HF, CS but not a transplant candidate due to age and comorbidity)

4. Bridge to recovery (e.g., in myocarditis where after a point, recovery is expected)

IABP and ECMO are the more commonly used MCS and hence are discussed in greater detail.

2. What are the indications for IABP?

1. CS after acute coronary syndrome/ST elevation MI (ACS/STEMI) being considered for percutaneous coronary intervention (PCI)

2. CS after ACS/STEMI with ischaemia, ventricular septal defect (VSD), mitral regurgitation (MR)

3. Haemodynamic support awaiting transplant

4. Severe arrhythmia with refractory ischaemia

5. High-risk PCI with LV dysfunction and large territory at risk (left main coronary artery [LMCA]/multivessel PCI)

6. Inability to wean from bypass after cardiac surgery

3. What are the contraindications to IABP?

1. Significant aortic regurgitation (AR)

2. Abdominal aortic aneurysm/dissection

3. Uncontrolled sepsis

4. Bleeding diathesis

5. Bilateral peripheral arterial disease (PAD)/bypass graft

4. What is the principle of IABP?

IABP works on the principle that inflating a balloon in the aorta in diastole will improve coronary perfusion, while abrupt deflation in systole will reduce the LV afterload. The inflation-deflation cycle is generally triggered relative to the R wave of the surface ECG. If ECG triggering is not possible due to arrhythmia, a pressure trigger may be used.

The intra-aortic balloon (IAB) catheter consists of a long cylindrical polyurethane balloon (length roughly 20–30 cm, inflated volume 30–50 mL) mounted on a flexible shaft (**Figure 42.2**). The tip of

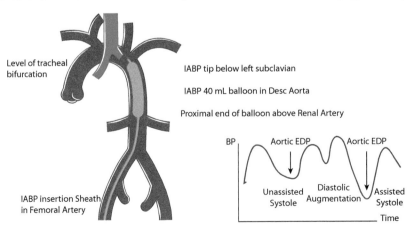

Figure 42.2 IABP and waveforms.

the IAB is ideally positioned in the descending thoracic aorta, 1–2 cm distal to the origin of the left subclavian artery. A 40-mL balloon is used for most patients and 30 mL for those with a smaller body size. Before inserting, we must try to make sure that the balloon is made to its lowest profile by evacuating air (50 cc) by a syringe from the newly opened balloon and flushing with heparinized saline. The inferior (proximal) end of the balloon should be above the level of the renal arteries to avoid occluding them. The catheter is usually dual lumen – one for the guidewire and measuring pressures and the other for quickly shuttling helium gas to and fro. The guidewire lumen is then connected to a pressurized flushing device that delivers a heparin flush 3 mL/hr to maintain lumen patency. However, once in a while care must be taken to avoid inadvertent injection of air bubbles or thrombi through the guidewire lumen, since its tip is only a short distance below the aortic arch. Patients with smaller-size arteries and atherosclerotic arteries can be considered for sheathless insertion, which has a smaller size and causes less trauma.

5. What is the timing for inflation and deflation of the IABP balloon, and how is it adjusted?

Balloon inflation-deflation is fine-tuned in the 1:2 mode. The balloon inflation should coincide with the dicrotic notch and deflation just before ejection begins. First the inflation point is moved rightward (later) until it occurs in late diastole and the dicrotic notch is uncovered. It is then progressively moved left (earlier) until the dicrotic notch on the central aortic tracing just disappears. Again, using the iterative method, the deflation knob is moved left (earlier) and then slowly advanced toward the right (later) until the end-diastolic pressure dips 10–15 mmHg below the patient's unassisted diastolic pressure. Usually, these adjustments are nowadays automated and done by the machine itself.

6. What are the steps for IABP insertion?

1. *Femoral arterial puncture*: 7F sheath inserted.

2. Teflon wire inserted up to the diaphragm.

3. 7F sheath exchanged for IABP sheath and Teflon wire removed. During this process, the groin should be compressed, so that a haematoma does not form.

4. IABP wire inserted up to the left subclavian origin.

5. IABP balloon de-aired, flushed and introduced over the wire, keeping an eye that the distal end of the balloon marker is 2 cm below the left subclavian.

6. The IABP wire is removed, and the lumen is aspirated and flushed.

7. Pressurized saline is then connected.

8. After connection to console, the system is purged with helium.

9. Depending upon the clinical situation, augmentation is set (initially at 1:1).

10. The sheath and balloon shaft are sutured securely and aseptically to the skin, keeping a mark, so that subsequent migration can be detected.

7. How do you anticoagulate in IABP?

If the patient is not on anticoagulation, heparin (5,000 units) should be given intravenously as soon as the balloon is inserted, followed by continuous intravenous heparin titrated to maintain an activated clotting time (ACT) of 1.5–2.0 times the normal

8. What are the complications of IABP?

The complications of IABP include:

1. Sepsis

2. Thrombocytopenia

3. Blood loss

4. Haemolysis

5. Vascular obstruction (i.e. distal leg ischaemia)

6. Thrombus, embolus

7. Vascular dissection

8. Mild to moderate thrombocytopenia may occur owing to platelet destruction, but the platelet count rarely falls below 50,000–1,00,000/mL and should rapidly return to normal following balloon removal

However, major complications related to IABP are about 7%, with amputation, ischaemia and access site bleed each measuring <1% in large registries.

9. What is the monitoring protocol for IABP?

IABP requires intensive medical care.

1. The dorsalis pedis/posterior tibial should be assessed every 8 hours by nursing staff, preferably by handheld Doppler probe for early detection of arterial thrombosis.

2. Regularly checking the platelet count and activated partial thromboplastin time (APTT). APTT should be maintained at 50–70 sec.

3. The IABP monitor should be assessed for proper augmentation. The arterial line should be regularly flushed, especially if arterial blood gas is being drawn from the same source.

10. How do you wean from IABP?

Once the patient has stabilized, the counterpulsation is progressively decreased from 1:1 to 1:2 to 1:3. Then counterpulsation is turned off. Heparin is omitted and ACT monitored; the lines are removed once ACT <160 sec and APTT <50 sec. The site is then firmly compressed by hand or with a mechanical compression device for 30–60 minutes.

11. What is the current role of IABP?

The support provided by IABP with respect to cardiac index is too low to compensate for the reduction of intrinsic stroke volume in CS. The IABP SHOCK II and CRISP AMI trials have shown that IABP does not improve 30-day mortality and reduce infarct size. However, the fact remains that randomized trials up to now have not been able to show that other assist devices (e.g., Impella) fare any better than IABP with respect to 30-day mortality, though their cost is much higher. Hence, IABP continues to be used in many centres worldwide, especially in primary PCI in AMI or during high-risk PCI or cardiac surgeries.

12. What are the relative merits of different types of MCS?

The different MCS and their characteristics are given in **Table 42.1**.

Table 42.1: Characteristics of Different Types of MCS

Parameter	IABP	Impella 2.5	Impella CP	Tandem Heart	ECMO
Mechanism	Pneumatic	Axial	Axial	Centrifugal	Centrifugal
Flow (L/min)	0.5	2.5	2.5–3.5	4–5	Variable
Cardiac Index	Increased	Increased	Increased remarkably	Increased remarkably	Increased remarkably
MAP	Increased	Increased	Increased	Increased	Increased
Coronary perfusion	Increased	Increased	Increased	Increased	May decrease
Femoral access	7–8F	13F	14F	15–19F Venous 21F	15–17F Venous 19–25F
Contraindication	Acute AR Arrhythmia	PAD, AR, LV thrombus	PAD, AR, LV thrombus	PAD, RV failure	PAD

13. What are the indications for ECMO?

The indications for ECMO (**Figure 42.3**) fall broadly into the following categories:

1. CS refractory to multiple vasoactive medications or an existing MCS device, such as an IABP

2. Cardiac arrest unresponsive to conventional cardiopulmonary resuscitation (CPR) (extracorporeal CPR, commonly known as ECPR)

3. Refractory ventricular arrhythmias

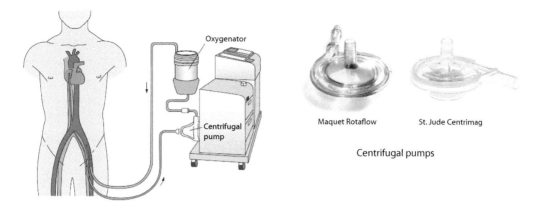

Figure 42.3 VA-ECMO: *Note*: Deoxygenated blood is taken from the right atrium and oxygenated blood is returned via the femoral artery. (With permission from Bermudez C A, Daneshmand M A. The Role of Extracorporeal Membrane Oxygenation in Cardiac Support, Fig 6.3, Fig 6.4, pp 53–70, in Kirklin J K, Rogers J G. Mechanical Circulatory Support: A Companion to Braunwald's Heart Disease, 2nd Edition, Elsevier.)

4. Acute or decompensated right heart failure in the context of pulmonary vascular disease (e.g., pulmonary hypertension or pulmonary embolism)

5. Hypoxemic respiratory failure with a ratio of arterial oxygen tension to fraction of inspired oxygen (PaO_2/FiO_2) of <100 despite optimization of the ventilator settings, including the tidal volume, positive end-expiratory pressure (PEEP) and inspiratory to expiratory (I:E) ratio

6. Hypercapnic respiratory failure with an arterial pH less than 7.20

7. Ventilatory support as a bridge to lung transplantation

Unfortunately, unlike studies on ECMO for respiratory failure, there is an absence of randomized controlled trials examining the efficacy of ECMO for the treatment of CS.

14. What are the contraindications to ECMO?

a. Unsalvageable multiorgan failure or hypoxic brain damage

b. Irreversible cardiac damage where LVAD is not being considered

c. Aortic dissection

d. Aortic regurgitation

e. End-stage malignancy

f. Pre-existing condition that is incompatible with recovery

Relative contraindications:

a. Age >75 years

b. Peripheral vascular disease

c. Coagulopathy/contraindication to anticoagulation

d. Limited vascular access

e. Uncontrollable bleeding and very poor prognosis from the primary condition

15. What are the components of ECMO?

ECMO has the following components (**Figure 42.3**): (1) A pump (centrifugal), (2) membrane oxygenator, (3) cannula and (4) heat exchanger.

The amount of blood flow in the circuit and the fraction of oxygen delivered through the oxygenator are the main determinants of blood oxygenation and circulatory support. The rate of gas flow through the oxygenator, known as the sweep gas flow rate, and the blood flow rate are the major determinants of carbon dioxide removal. As sweep gas flow increases compared to the blood flow, pCO_2 decreases.

First-generation pumps with rotor to motor coupling created a stagnation of flow. These were improved in the second-generation pump (Sorin – Revolution, Maquet – Rotaflow) with open-centre impeller and in third-generation pumps (St Jude Centrimag), where a bearingless magnetically levitated impeller is used to reduce blood trauma.

Developments also took place in oxygenators. Nanoporous hollow fibres with PolyMethyl Pentane (PMP) with reduced pore size (<0.03 µm), high gas permeability and infrequent plasma leakage have revolutionized oxygenator technology, allowing for prolonged support with decreased blood component trauma, decreased platelet activation, lower thromboembolism and decreased device-related bleeding complications.

Modifications of pump and oxygenator technology have contributed to the increasing popularity of ECMO.

16. What are the configurations of ECMO?

- Respiratory support – Venovenous (VV) ECMO

- Circulatory support – Venoarterial (VA) ECMO

For access, the femoral vein and artery are most commonly used. However, in the case of peripheral arterial disease, the subclavian artery may be used rarely. The tip of the arterial cannula is positioned in the distal abdominal aorta or proximal common iliac artery. Peripheral arterial cannulas sized 15–16 Fr are used for smaller patients (<60 kg), and 17–21 Fr cannulae are used for larger patients. For the cannulation of the femoral vein, the cannula tip is positioned in the body of the right atrium. Generally, adequate venous drainage can be achieved with a 22 Fr multi-fenestrated venous cannula in smaller patients (<60 kg) and a 25 Fr multi-fenestrated venous cannula in larger patients; the target ECMO flow rate is 2.0–2.2 LPM/m². Since nearly 30% of ECMO patients have limb ischaemia, placing a distal perfusion catheter (5–10 Fr) in the distal superficial femoral artery is recommended during cannulation.

During VV-ECMO, blood is extracted from the vena cava or right atrium and returned to the right atrium. VV-ECMO provides respiratory support, but the patient is dependent upon his or her own haemodynamics.

During VA-ECMO, blood is extracted from the right atrium and returned to the arterial system, bypassing the heart and lungs. VA-ECMO provides both respiratory and haemodynamic support. The additional benefit of haemodynamic support comes with additional risks, which are discussed later

17. What is north-south syndrome/Harlequin syndrome?

ECMO, unlike IABP, increases LV afterload and LV end-diastolic pressure (LVEDP). This causes pulmonary congestion and central pulmonary shunting, pouring in deoxygenated blood to the LA and LV via pulmonary veins. This deoxygenated blood is ejected in the aortic root and also perfuses head vessels resulting in central hypoxia. On the other hand, oxygenated blood circulates in other parts of body from the outflow of the femoral arterial cannula (**Figure 42.4**).

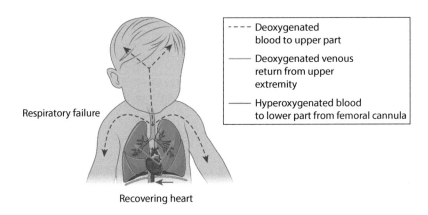

Figure 42.4 Harlequin syndrome.

The solution to this problem is to convert VA to VV ECMO by placing a cannula in the internal jugular vein (IJV). The oxygenated blood now returns back via two routes – the superficial femoral artery (SFA) and IJV. Oxygenated blood in the IJV reduces central hypoxia.

Occasionally a ventricle does not eject while on VA-ECMO, leading to intraventricular, LV outflow tract or sinus of Valsalva thrombus formation, as well as severe LV distention, resulting in coronary ischaemia, arrhythmias or cerebrovascular thromboembolism. This untoward event may be prevented by placing an axial flow pump across the aortic valve (e.g., Impella) or by venting the LV. IABP may also be used.

North-south syndrome does not occur when instead of SFA, central cannulation is done in the aorta, as in cases of CS during cardiothoracic surgery.

18. What level of anticoagulation should be maintained?

Anticoagulation is sustained during ECMO with a continuous infusion of unfractionated heparin, or a direct thrombin inhibitor titrated to an ACT of 180–210 seconds. The ACT target is decreased if bleeding develops. ACT is easily determined at the point of care, but plasma APTT (1.5 times normal) can also be used. Thromboelastography is a useful adjunct. APTT should be between 50 and 70 sec.

Platelets are continuously consumed during ECMO because they are activated by exposure to the foreign surface area. Platelet counts should be maintained greater than 50,000/μL. A significant reduction in count may require platelet transfusion.

19. What are the complications of ECMO?

Apart from the complications of IABP, which can also occur, three other complications are specific to ECMO:

a. *Bleeding*: Bleeding occurs in 30%–50% of patients who receive ECMO and can be life-threatening. It is due to both the continuous anticoagulation and platelet dysfunction. Meticulous surgical technique, maintaining platelet counts greater than 50,000/mm^3 and maintaining the target ACT reduce the likelihood of bleeding.

b. *Thromboembolism*: Systemic thromboembolism due to thrombus formation within the extracorporeal circuit is a complication that can be devastating, with one report suggesting rates of pulmonary embolism as high as 16%; rates of deep venous thrombosis may be higher (up to 70%) and may be associated with cannulation, especially femorofemoral cannulae.

c. *Neurological*: The incidence of neurologic injury in adult respiratory failure patients recorded in the Extracorporeal Life Support Organization (ELSO) registry is 10%.

d. *Cannulation-related*: A variety of complications can occur during cannulation, including vessel perforation with haemorrhage, arterial dissection, distal ischaemia and incorrect location (e.g., venous cannula within the artery). These complications are rare (<5%). A skilled and experienced surgeon is important to avoid or address such complications.

e. *Heparin-induced thrombocytopenia (HIT)*: HIT can occur in patients receiving ECMO. When HIT is proven, the heparin infusion should be replaced by a non-heparin anticoagulant.

VA-ECMO–Specific Complications

a. *Pulmonary haemorrhage*: Pulmonary oedema and haemorrhage can occur in patients who have no LV emptying during VA-ECMO. Oedema occurs when the LA pressure exceeds 25 mmHg. It is treated by venting the LA or LV.

b. *Cardiac thrombosis*: There is retrograde blood flow in the ascending aorta whenever the femoral artery and vein are used for VA-ECMO. Stasis of the blood can occur if LV output is not maintained, which may result in thrombosis.

c. *Coronary or cerebral hypoxia*: During VA-ECMO, fully saturated blood infused into the femoral artery from the ECMO circuit will preferentially perfuse the lower extremities and the abdominal viscera. Blood ejected from the heart will selectively perfuse the heart, brain and upper extremities. As a result, the oxyhaemoglobin saturation of the blood perfusing the lower extremities and abdominal viscera may be substantially higher than that perfusing the heart, brain and upper extremities (see information on Harlequin syndrome earlier).

d. *Neurological injury*: In a report of neurologic injury in cardiac (VA) patients in one institution, approximately 50% suffered neurologic injury which included coma, encephalopathy, anoxic brain injury, stroke, brain death and myoclonus.

e. LV overloading and subsequent north-south syndrome

f. Systemic inflammatory syndrome

20. What are the indications for an Impella?

The Impella 2.5 circulatory support system is intended for providing partial circulatory support using an extracorporeal bypass control unit for periods up to 6 hours. The Impella class of devices has a catheter-mounted (9F catheter) microaxial flow pump with its inlet in the LV cavity and outlet in the aorta, while the device itself straddles the aortic valve. The flow provided by the Impella (graded as per output from P0 to P9) is axial and is in parallel to the pulsatile flow provided by the native ventricle. As the native stroke volume falls, the Impella's flow can be ramped up and vice versa. However, while weaning, the Impella's flow must not be decreased to zero (P0), as in that case the communication from aorta to the ventricle causes a functional aortic regurgitation. Three more common indications for the Impella are:

a. Supporting cardiac output during high-risk PCI, especially in compromised ventricles

b. In CS after AMI/myocarditis/post-cardiotomy/transplant rejection

c. During ablation of refractory ventricular arrhythmias

21. What are the contraindications to the Impella?

Contraindications to the use of Impella include:

a. Mechanical aortic valve

b. Moderate to severe aortic insufficiency

c. LV thrombus

d. Severe peripheral arterial obstructive disease

22. What is the difference in haemodynamics between IABP and Impella?

IABP enhances blood pressure during diastole and reduces systolic ventricular pressure but does not significantly influence ventricular volumes. In contrast, Impella 2.5 markedly reduces ventricular volumes (and preload) and reduces peak ventricular pressure (and afterload) while increasing aortic systolic and diastolic pressures. This reduces the LV work and oxygen consumption, and therefore the infarct size, when Impella is used after MI.

23. What is the arterial pressure trace in LVADs?

Most LVADs (**Figure 42.5**) consist of an extracorporeal, non-pulsatile centrifugal (continuous flow) pump that withdraws blood from the LA (via a 21F trans-septal cannula introduced via the femoral vein) and delivers (3.5–5 L/min) it into one or both femoral arteries through l5F–l6F cannulae. But because it is non-pulsatile, the arterial tracing will be flat, especially if the device flow is far more than the native ventricle (**Figure 42.6**).

24. How do you measure pressure in continuous flow devices?

In continuous flow devices, the pulse may not be palpable because the device ejects continually, provided the native LV is too weak to pump a substantial amount of stroke volume. In this case inflate the cuff and use a Doppler probe. The pressure where the flow reappears is taken as the mean arterial pressure.

25. What are the complications of long-term LVADs?

LVADs are prone to multiple complications, even though they are much better than medical therapy in sick patients:

1. Bleeding (especially GI bleeding due to destruction of Von Willebrand multimers by the pump)

2. Infection (driveline, pocket or device)

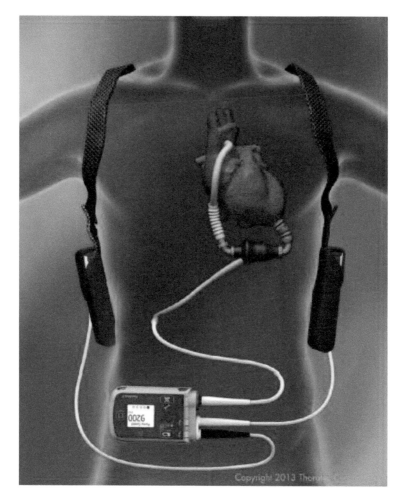

Figure 42.5 Durable LV assist device. (With permission from Gregoric I D, Arabia F A. Current Types of Devices for Durable Mechanical Circulatory Support, Fig 10.2, pp 109–119, in Kirklin J K, Rogers J G. Mechanical Circulatory Support: A Companion to Braunwald's Heart Disease, 2nd Edition.)

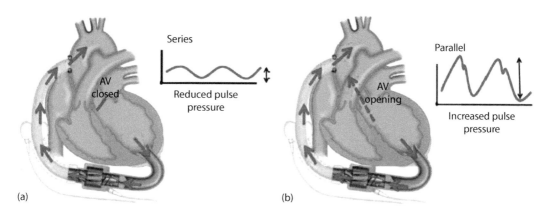

Figure 42.6 Centrifugal pump in (a) series and (b) parallel and the effect on pulse pressure. (With permission from Pagani F. Understanding the Principles of Continuous-Flow Rotary Left Ventricular Assist Devices, Fig 7.8, pp 71–81, in Kirklin J K, Rogers J G. Mechanical Circulatory Support: A Companion to Braunwald's Heart Disease, 2nd Edition.)

3. RV dysfunction (may require RV assist device)

4. Pump thrombosis (may be fatal)

5. Late aortic insufficiency (due to unuse of aortic valve by inactive LV)

6. Stroke

FURTHER READING

1. Arora S, Atreya A R, Birati E Y, et al. Temporary Mechanical Circulatory Support as Bridge to Transplant or Durable LV Assist Device, in Eng M H, Neill B O (Ed) Mechanical Circulatory Support: Interventional Cardiology Clinics. 2021, pp 235–249. Elsevier.
2. Kirklin J, Rogers J G (Ed) Mechanical Circulatory Support: A Companion to Braunwald's Heart Disease. 2nd Ed. 2020. Elsevier.

43 Cardiorenal Syndrome and Heart Kidney Interaction

Sunandan Sikdar and Pinaki Mukhopadhyay

Chapter 43 may be accessed online at: www.routledge.com/9780367462215

DOI: 10.1201/9781003027584-44

44 Cardiac Drugs

Uses and Precautions

Sunandan Sikdar and Rana Rathore Roy

Chapter 44 may be accessed online at: www.routledge.com/9780367462215

DOI: 10.1201/9781003027584-45

Index

Note: Locators in *italics* represent figures and **bold** indicates tables in the text.